Indirect Action

Indirect Action

*Schizophrenia, Epilepsy, AIDS,
and the Course of Health Activism*

Lisa Diedrich

 University of Minnesota Press
Minneapolis • London

An earlier version of chapter 1 was originally published as "Doing Queer Love: Feminism, AIDS, and History," *Theoria* 112, no. 1 (April 2007): 22–50. An earlier version of chapter 2 was originally published as "Que(e)rying the Clinic before AIDS: Practicing Self-Help and Transversality in the 1970s," *Journal of Medical Humanities* 34, no. 2 (June 2013): 122–38; published with kind permission from Springer Science+Business Media. An earlier version of chapter 6 was originally published as "Being the Shadow: Witnessing Schizophrenia," *Journal of Medical Humanities* 31, no. 2 (June 2010): 91–109; published with kind permission from Springer Science+Business Media.

Graphic novel excerpts from *Epileptic* by David B., copyright 2005 by L'Association, Paris, France; reprinted by permission of Pantheon Books, an imprint of the Knopf Doubleday Publishing Group, a division of Penguin Random House LLC. All rights reserved. Any third-party use of this material, outside this publication, is prohibited. Interested parties must apply directly to Penguin Random House LLC for permission.

Published by the University of Minnesota Press
111 Third Avenue South, Suite 290
Minneapolis, MN 55401-2520
http://www.upress.umn.edu

Printed in the United States of America on acid-free paper

The University of Minnesota is an equal-opportunity educator and employer.

23 22 21 20 19 18 17 16   10 9 8 7 6 5 4 3 2 1

Library of Congress Cataloging-in-Publication Data
Diedrich, Lisa, author.
Indirect action : schizophrenia, epilepsy, AIDS, and the course of health activism / Lisa Diedrich.
Minneapolis : University of Minnesota Press, 2016. | Includes bibliographical references and index.
Identifiers: LCCN 2016003048 (print) | ISBN 978-1-5179-0000-7 (hc) | ISBN 978-1-5179-0001-4 (pb)
Subjects: LCSH: Public health—History. | Social medicine. | Social justice. | BISAC: SOCIAL SCIENCE / Disease & Health Issues. | MEDICAL / History.
Classification: LCC RA424 .D48 2016 (print) | DDC 362.19689—dc23
LC record available at https://lccn.loc.gov/2016003048

For Victoria Hesford

Contents

Illness-Thought-Activism

At AIDS/Activism/Art: Looking Backward/Looking Forward, a 2012 event commemorating the twenty-fifth anniversary of the founding of the AIDS Coalition to Unleash Power (ACT UP),[1] writer and activist Sarah Schulman explained that in ACT UP if a particular political strategy or tactic was tried once and did not work, the group did not try it a second time. When asked about the short- and long-term effects of such an instrumental politics, Schulman noted ACT UP was primarily a single-issue reform movement with very specific and immediate goals. ACT UP was not a revolutionary movement, she stated emphatically; people were dying and wanted simply to survive, not foment revolution.[2] Schulman's comments intrigued me at the time and have stuck with me since as I have thought about the relationship between illness, thought, and activism in the period just before and after AIDS arrived. Schulman offered a succinct, if counterintuitive, understanding of the politics of AIDS and especially of ACT UP. I came to realize what was radical in response to AIDS was locatable not in the direct action politics of organized protests at specific targets (the Food and Drug Administration, the National Institutes of Health, the New York City Health Commission, etc.) but in the indirect action of multiple forces operating prior to the emergence of AIDS that made something like ACT UP possible. What Schulman's comments helped me better understand was, then, the simple fact that illness, thought, and activism all operate in multiple temporalities. We do them and they happen to us acutely and chronically, persistently and randomly, directly and indirectly.

The Uses of Indirection

In *Indirect Action* I consider the conceptual and practical uses of indirection. In doing so, I don't mean to suggest ACT UP's direct action response to the AIDS crisis and U.S. government inaction beginning in 1987 was wrongheaded or ineffective. Moreover, although I revisit forms of illness as thought and health activism as practice in the 1960s and 1970s, I am not nostalgic for a revolutionary time associated with that period, a nostalgia Neferti Tadiar has diagnosed as operating in relation to a current desire for a preneoliberal political moment.[3] Rather, the conceptual and practical uses of indirection were first impressed upon me by a decidedly evolutionary not revolutionary theory: Rachel Carson's analysis in *Silent Spring* of the direct and indirect relationships between bodies and environments, illness and chemicals. In the chapter "The Human Price," about pesticides, Carson puts it as follows:

> The new environmental health problems are multiple—created by radiation in all its forms, born of the never-ending stream of chemicals of which pesticides are a part, chemicals now pervading the world in which we live, *acting upon us directly and indirectly, separately and collectively.* Their presence casts a shadow that is no less ominous because it is formless and obscure, no less frightening because it is simply impossible to predict the effects of lifetime exposure to chemical and physical agents that are not part of the biological experience of man.[4] (emphasis added)

I discuss Carson and her work in more detail in chapter 4 but simply want to note here that Carson attempts to provide an ecological method for thinking cause and effect both directly and indirectly.[5] I try to do this too, both in terms of the conjuncture I investigate (illness-thought-activism) and through the overall structure of my investigation. Rather than tell a linear story of the development of specific forms of health activism in response to specific illnesses culminating in a radical transformation of medicine by politics, I assemble, arrange, and examine an illness-thought-activism archive across multiple spaces and temporalities.

This book is about illness, thought, and activism and their interconnectedness in the period just before and just after the emergence of HIV/AIDS in the United States. My intervention is theoretical and methodological as well as political and therapeutic. By expanding the historiographical parameters through which illness and health activism in the United States have tended to be thought, I demonstrate how and why illness figured prominently in the social, political, theoretical, and institutional transformations that took place in the period from around 1960 to when AIDS arrived. I trace the multiple figurations of illness in some key texts of social and critical theory, many of which were later categorized as part of an emergent poststructuralism, as well as in literary, film, medical, and activist texts, many of which are formally innovative and experimental, in order to consider questions about, in the most general terms, being, doing, and becoming in relation to illness experiences and events, therapeutic thought and practices, and clinical and caring institutions and spaces. I engage with the multivalent work of several writer/thinker/health activists— Schulman and Carson figure prominently, but so too do Frantz Fanon and Isaac Julien, Cindy Patton and Gregg Bordowitz, Samuel Delany and Frederick Wiseman, Félix Guattari and David Wojnarowicz, Eve Kosofsky Sedgwick and Gilles Deleuze, Michel Foucault and John Berger. What connects this eclectic group is that each treats the conjuncture illness-thought-politics as a multiplicity in history.

This project began with a simple realization: we cannot apprehend an experience and event of illness—like HIV and AIDS, but not only—through discrete disciplines and categories. This posed a problem of form and method as much as of content and concepts. My methodological solution—or perhaps, more accurate, my methodological work-around—to this problem is to approach illness indirectly as a multiplicity of bodies and minds, concepts and histories, and clinical, critical, and narrative discourses and practices. In attempting to grasp what illness is in different places and times, I look for and deploy various method-images (my term for verbal and visual statements that help articulate through condensation the complexity of an object), in this case, illness as phenomenological experience and epidemiological event, as localized virus and global crisis, and as much more in between. My work attempts to account for the often indirect and unstraightforward relationships between very big things (environments, economies, histories, structures, ideologies) and very small things (genes, cells, viruses, conversations, gestures, and feelings) and between very fast things (a flash, an instant, a glimpse, a glance) and very slow things (the interminable, the evolutionary, the gradual, the glacial). I see my work as participating in an emergent interdisciplinary project, which I call critical medical studies and others have called critical health studies and which, for me, emphasizes the multiplicity of histories of and methods for approaching the conjunction illness-thought-activism in time.

Illness as Thought in Time

Illness is central to the production of thought in the period just before and after the emergence of AIDS.[6] The experience of illness (both mental and physical) figures prominently in the critical thought and activism of the 1960s and 1970s, yet its importance has been largely overlooked in accounts of this period, which have tended to emphasize the figures and practices of sexuality rather than and as mutually exclusive of those of illness. AIDS and poststructuralism both emerge in the 1980s, and while many accounts suggest the influence of poststructuralism in general and queer theory in particular on the political, aesthetic, and conceptual response to AIDS, I want to do something different here. Although a common critical move is to read the 1980s as the apotheosis of a reductive identity politics, which queer and poststructuralist work around 1990 relievedly turned away from, I don't want simply to rehearse this tired narrative in which queer sets us free. By stretching the experience and event of AIDS historically, I hope to upset this critical teleology, which too assuredly positions the theoretical now as more fully realized than a theoretical then.

I argue illness—along with and intimately intertwined with sexuality—is an important underlying condition in the emergence of poststructuralist thought, most persistently in Foucault's work but also in the work of several thinkers writing in the 1960s and 1970s and later associated with poststructuralism, including Deleuze and Guattari, Fanon, and Agamben, and still later in the work of thinkers who contributed to the emergence of queer theory, most notably Eve Kosofsky Sedgwick but also Cindy Patton, Gregg Bordowitz, and other activist/writers/artists. These writers/thinkers/activists do not simply provide theoretical and methodological tools that might help us analyze the experiences and events of illness in this particular historical moment. Rather, I historicize their work as part of the production of thought in relation to illness as a politicized experience and as participating in forms of activism around health—including sexual, mental, and environmental health, all of which became sites of politics and thought in the postwar and postcolonial period from around 1960 to 1980. I consider the relationship of these political, methodological, and conceptual critiques from within and without medicine and ask, how does what illness is—its ontology—change during this time? Or to echo the question Foucault asked in his lectures in 1983, as he was dying of AIDS, what is the present field of possible experiences of illness at the beginning of the 1980s?[7] In grappling with this question, I work transversally across the interconnected domains of politics, aesthetics, theory, and health and medicine that together create illness as multiplicity. In exploring the relation of AIDS activism to what I call its prehistory, Foucault and his work figure prominently. On the one hand, Foucault provides a discourse on and practices of method—both archeological and genealogical—for inquiries into the conditions of possibility—epistemological, clinical, ethical, and practical—that grounded the positivity of the response to AIDS. On the other, his entire oeuvre can be read as part of a prehistory of AIDS, quite literally in the sense that the period in which he was actively thinking, lecturing, and writing—from 1954 to 1984—is the period I explore in relation to the emergence of AIDS and its forms of activism. Read as a history of the present of the 1960s and 1970s, Foucault's work participates in the configuration of the discursive and nondiscursive practices of health and illness at that time, contributing to the extension of politics into domains not previously perceived as domains of political struggle—not just sexual politics but illness politics, too. Although I do not dwell on the biographical fact of Foucault's own death from AIDS in 1984, I argue this loss structures what later becomes a deeventalization of AIDS in particular and illness more generally in queer theory.[8] By taking up Foucault's articulations of illness as thought and politics, I work against this deeventalization of AIDS in contemporary queer theory. The move away from AIDS in queer theory seems to reveal an anxiety of identification with an earlier political desire now perceived as stuck reductively in an identity frame. This deeventalization is most often rendered as a historical cut between feminist critical theories and social movements of the 1970s and queer theory of the 1990s and 2000s.

The deeventalization of AIDS is also an effect of the disaggregation of illness and sexuality in and by queer theory. Yet I contend the intermingling of illness and sexuality forms the theoretical substrate of poststructuralism. By historicizing the turn to "reparative reading" and/or "weak theory" since around 1990,[9] these theoretical shifts can be seen as emerging concurrently with the AIDS crisis, and this emergent strain of theory is not only weak but ill, sick, or debilitated—that is, a historicotheoretical symptom of the AIDS crisis and its deeventalization in queer theory.[10] Despite many recent references to and engagements with Sedgwick's reparative turn,[11] no one seems to have noticed the immediate motivating factor for Sedgwick's supplementing of the paranoid with the reparative is a conversation she had with writer/thinker/AIDS activist Cindy Patton, who argues paranoia, while satisfying on many levels, especially in the face of the hopelessness wrought by AIDS in that moment, is nonetheless not the most productive and immediate strategy for addressing the AIDS crisis. I discuss this conversation at greater length at the end of chapter 2, but for now I simply want to note that the failure to acknowledge or even notice the link between Patton and Sedgwick is one sign of a forgetting of some of the figures who acted as relays between health activism before and after AIDS, a forgetting I work to counter in *Indirect Action*. Even in Robyn Wiegman's brilliant rereading of Sedgwick as practicing antihomophobic and feminist inquiry—rather than, or not yet, queer theory—in an essay that also diagnoses "reparative reading's contemporary allure"[12] as a forgetting of AIDS, Patton and her work and its influence on Sedgwick are not mentioned.

Like Patton and Sedgwick, Schulman acts as a relay between feminism and AIDS activism, and her recent critique of gentrification as a direct effect of AIDS might be read as a howl of protest against this deeventalization and what she sees as two consequences of AIDS in the present moment, both the "suffering and trauma of some, and the vague unknowingness for others."[13] By thinking about the process of transmission in general as well as specific relay figures in particular, I am interested in exploring not only who makes these connections but also how ideas and practices are relayed from one event or movement to another. By returning to AIDS and its prehistory now, I hope to emphasize "a drama of transmission" in which what is transmitted is not, or not only, forms of identity but rather forms of political desire that flow across feminist and queer theories and social movements.[14]

AIDS and Its (Pre)histories

This book is not precisely or only about AIDS or AIDS activism. Yet a feeling about the forgetting of the complexity of the response to AIDS motivates my inquiry throughout, even as the trajectory of my analysis moves away from the experience and event of AIDS and its moment of emergence. Put another way, I began this project as a response to what seemed to me to be a forgetting of the early days—the pre–ACT UP days—of AIDS activism in the United States. In my earlier work *Treatments*, I explored the emergence of a new figure—the politicized patient—and a new genre—the patient's counternarrative to medicine's perception of the experience of illness.[15] I located this emergence around 1980, discussing Susan Sontag's *Illness as Metaphor* (1978) and Audre Lorde's *The Cancer Journals* (1980) as hinge texts between the women's health movement of the 1970s and AIDS activism of the 1980s. I was surprised, however, not to find more historical and critical work on health activism in the period immediately prior to the emergence of AIDS. I was surprised especially because many of the critical theorists whose work was being read and engaged with around this same time were explicitly linking the "critical and clinical"—in Deleuze's apt juxtaposition from 1967[16]—in the period before AIDS. Yet much of the critical work on AIDS activism seemed to suggest health activism itself had emerged ex nihilo with the formation of ACT UP in New York City in 1987.[17] Despite the fact that as early as the mid-1980s Patton was already making the important and already historical point that AIDS activism emerged when the first person got sick from the then unknown virus[18] and despite important recent scholarly work, including Jennifer Brier's excellent history of activist responses to AIDS before the formation of ACT UP and Deborah Gould's powerful sociological analysis of the affective experiences of AIDS activism,[19] I contend the origin story of AIDS activism in particular and health activism more generally in the United States still operates to forget health activism before ACT UP.

This forgetting has taken many forms. In the past few years, popular culture has shown some interest in the early days of AIDS in the United States. This period has been depicted in several feature and documentary films, including Jean-Marc Vallée's *Dallas Buyers Club* (2013), Ryan Murphy's adaptation for HBO of Larry Kramer's 1984 play *The Normal Heart* (2014), and David France's documentary about ACT UP from 1987 to 1996, *How to Survive a Plague* (2012), all of which have been produced and distributed to popular and critical attention and even acclaim, contributing to a feeling that a forgotten history is being recovered. Other events of documentation of the early days of AIDS have included the New York Historical Society's 2013 exhibition *AIDS in New York: The First Five Years* and fairly extensive media coverage in 2012, especially in New York City, of the twenty-fifth anniversary of the founding of ACT UP.[20] Furthermore, in relation to contemporary politics, activists involved in the Occupy Wall Street protests that began in 2011 have cited ACT UP as an inspiration for the direct action tactics of the Occupy movement. Despite this recent attention to the early days of AIDS and ACT UP, these popular accounts often cover over as much as they reveal about the complexity of the response to AIDS in particular and the history of health activism more generally.[21] My project works against this forgetting by drawing links across multiple spaces and temporalities of health activism in the period before and after AIDS crystalized as a substance in history. A direct causal narrative of loss and response simplifies this history by reducing the scale of a historical event that had a more intricate shape and extended duration. This project seeks to begin to map some of the changing contours of that shape across time and space. ACT UP became legendary for confronting the complacency of Reagan-era conservatism with a politics of direct action. My work acknowledges the importance of direct action on the politics and practices of health in the late 1980s but also seeks to discern another politics—what I am calling indirect action—at work not only in how we do health and health activism in the contemporary moment but also in how we do feminist and queer studies of them.

As I was completing this book in the summer of 2015, the first volume of writer/activist Larry Kramer's latest novel, *The American People,* was published at long last.[22] In a 1997 interview Kramer describes the already at that time drawn-out process of writing *The American People.* Kramer tells his fellow AIDS activist Lawrence Mass the novel began as a story about his family, his experience growing up in Washington, D.C., in the symbolic center of American history and politics, and only eventually "lead[s] up to when AIDS came along."[23] In the process of writing his novel, Kramer discovers that in order to tell the story about when AIDS came along, he has to go back in time: "What existed in the '80's was there for a reason, and the reason did not start in 1981."[24] Indeed, he finds he has to keep going back further and further in time—to even before his family or the place of his upbringing existed. Kramer explains his book has "become this enormous thing. It's all over the place. I've got boxes of it over there. It's been an enormous problem technically. How do you keep hold of it all? How do you remember it all?"[25] In Kramer's novel AIDS morphs into a more diffuse, generalized, and generalizing concept, which Kramer names the Underlying Condition, or UC. UC functions in Kramer's massive novel as a kind of literary and historical catachresis, a term Gayatri Chakravorty Spivak defines as a "concept-metaphor without an adequate referent."[26] As Kramer explains to Mass, "UC is traced all the way back to the beginning of time. . . . So it's really a history of the world as reflected through disease, through illness; and that's what gets passed on from generation to generation."[27]

In *Indirect Action* I am interested in the conceptual, methodological, and formal problem of describing the *underlying conditions*—or what Foucault calls the conditions of possibility of present reality—when AIDS arrived in 1981. Kramer's image of an "enormous thing" that is an "enormous problem technically" well captures the methodological complexity of diagnosing what existed in 1981 when people first became aware of AIDS. Indeed, Kramer's image provides another method-image of the conjunction illness-thought-activism that is both useful in its attempt to trace indirect historical trajectories and problematic in its direct association with Kramer's very singular biography. By making Kramer's singular term Underlying Condition plural, I begin the process of moving away from Kramer's singularity. Still, what I think we glimpse in this method-image is an epic struggle to account for the sprawl and mess of historical events and nonevents, as well as the metaevent of historical events becoming nonevents.[28]

I take Kramer's method-image of the forever-unfolding underlying conditions of AIDS to challenge the preeminence of Kramer himself in the origin story that says health activism began with ACT UP. I do so in order to consider something more general: the relationship between direct and indirect forms of action in changing the trajectories of science and medicine, politics and art. I also want to suggest we think illness and activism in other temporal registers—in the register not just of emergency and crisis but also of chronicity and endurance. My many and partial prehistories of AIDS trace back, then, looking for continuities and discontinuities, or "dis/continuities," in Karen Barad's terminology,[29] between AIDS activism in the early 1980s and several earlier transformations of discourses and practices of health and illness during the period immediately prior to the emergence of AIDS.

My choice of 1960 as a starting date for this prehistory is not arbitrary. It was a watershed year in the wars of liberation against colonialism, with seventeen countries in Africa alone gaining independence. I want to suggest links between these decolonizing movements and their practices of health activism before AIDS—as demonstrated, for example, in Fanon's clinical and critical decolonizing work in Algeria during the war of liberation against French colonialism—and those practices of health activism that emerged later. The year 1960 also inaugurated the decade of the rise of new social movements inspired by the steady march of liberation from colonialism around the world, and a common characteristic of these movements was that they had capacious and radical agendas concerned with much more than electoral politics—for example, the Black Panther Party's theories and practices of social health, as described compellingly in Alondra Nelson's historicosociological study of the Black Panther Party's health activism.[30] I am not claiming Fanon's political and therapeutic interventions in Algeria around 1960 led directly to or caused the Black Panther Party's politicotherapeutic interventions around 1970 or led directly to ACT UP's interventions a generation later. Rather, I am interested in pursuing new linkages—indirect ones—between later forms of health activism and the varieties of politicotherapeutic experience in the 1960s and 1970s in the hopes of creating ways around obsolete idioms and petrified social forms that have become sedimented since 1987.[31] Many scholars have considered health activism after AIDS, but I want to explore health activism before AIDS—and AIDS activism not as exemplary but as in relation—in order to find a way around an idiom that has historically linked AIDS and activism and stopped there.[32]

I use "prehistory" not to suggest a fixed period of time or place, nor to suggest a time outside history, but as a methodological incentive to look in advance of the precipitation of a particular substance in history. How does a disease like AIDS become a substance in history? My understanding of the precipitation of AIDS as a substance in history is an echo of Denise Riley's earlier use of the idea of precipitation in relation to the category "woman" in history. In *Am I That Name?* Riley writes that "even the apparently simplest, most innocent ways in which one becomes temporarily a woman *are not* darting returns to a category in a natural and harmless state, but are something else: adoptions of, or precipitations into, a designation there in advance, a characterisation of 'woman.'"[33] Why might it be helpful to think "AIDS" in particular and "illness" more generally as Riley thinks "woman"? For me the concept and practice of prehistory undermines a binary structure in which the natural becomes historical and political, at a specific point in time and once and for all. The process of chemical precipitation is then another method-image that allows us to consider how a category—in this case, the disease category AIDS—is formed in solution and also the ways that it might become unformed through practices of science, medicine, politics, and aesthetics. I want my prehistorical analysis to, in the words of Félix Guattari, "think time against the grain, to imagine that what came 'after' can modify what was 'before' or that changing the past at the root can transform a current state of affairs: what madness! A return to magical thought! It is pure science fiction, and yet ...."[34] Throughout *Indirect Action* I seek to think the time of AIDS against the grain and unfold another narrative alongside medicine's hegemonic heroic narrative of progress and its seemingly relentless push toward ever more specialization. The goal is not to replace the heroic with the magical but to extend the temporal and spatial parameters that shape our encounter with illness and its vicissitudes in the contemporary moment.

In a sense, then, in its attempt to frame an event by what comes before and after, my project is not unlike Kristin Ross's fascinating analysis of May 1968 and its "prehistory," a word she uses but does not gloss, and its "afterlives," or how May 1968 has been remembered—and forgotten—in the years since.[35] Ross's prehistory extends the event of May 1968 both temporally and spatially to include the effects of the Algerian War for liberation against French colonialism and the Vietnam War against U.S. imperialism. Just as my prehistory of AIDS first decenters the gay male activist as the autonomous subject of AIDS activism before tracing back to other figures and forms of health activism, in her account of the events of May 1968 Ross decenters the figure of the student and the dominant story of a rebellious generation (and its developmental narrative arc from radical youth to mature—read: depoliticized—adult).

My approach differs from Ross's in my understanding of the political. Ross is correct to question a frequent interpretation of the shift from the social movements of the 1960s to the neoliberalization beginning in the 1970s as somehow inevitable. But I am less certain about her need to recuperate May 1968 as a rupture rather than as a continuity, or as Ross problematizes the neat and tidy accounts of the afterlives of 1968, "Politics must be excised to allow the great (and inevitable) forward movement of cultural modernization to be celebrated."[36] Yet no singular political event or alternative social form is of a substance different from a set of ideas or an ethos or a representation, as Ross sometimes seems to believe. My aim is not to wistfully look back at the social movements of the 1960s and 1970s in the hopes of returning to the forms of activism associated with that time but to think about the relationship between this period and its forms of therapeutic culture and political activism and the period that immediately followed—and both in relation to the present. I do this not by telling a conventional history of a particular illness or social movement or through a conventional history of medical and political and medicopolitical ideas but by demonstrating the multiplicity illness-thought-politics in history through both the form and the content of *Indirect Action.*

Form Matters

Form matters, and here's how. I first conceived of the overall form of this project diagrammatically as a spatial network of interlinked experiences and events of illness, with shorter chapters, which I call snapshots, as nodes in the network that condense and encapsulate the overall structure. By integrating longer narrative chapters with shorter visual/descriptive snapshots and one final afterimage, I formally convey various ways of see-ing the conjuncture of illness-thought-activism in the period from around 1960 to 1990. Although the concept of the snapshot was part of the struc-ture I diagrammed from the beginning, I wrote the majority of the snap-shots after writing most of the narrative chapters and found they created a space to explore ways of freezing and unfreezing the complexity of illness, thought, and politics in both form and content. What emerged was a kind of "graphic history"[37] or graphic analysis in which multiple and contradic-tory sites of illness, thought, and activism were assembled and juxtaposed.

Indirect Action extends its analysis across fields and historical and so-cial milieus. I begin in the United States in the near contemporary mo-ment with a recent cultural memory of feminism and AIDS activism that forgets the importance of feminism in AIDS activism and feminists as AIDS activists from the earliest days of the epidemic. I queer the origin story of AIDS activism in the United States by recalling its feminist his-tory. In the first chapter, artist/activist Gregg Bordowitz functions as a key relay figure and practitioner of what I call doing queer love, and in the first snapshot I draw on Bordowitz again by combining a reading of his visual image *The Order of Image Production* with his concept "queer structures of feeling," further extending the concept and practice of the relay within the overall structure of the text itself. In form, then, the snapshots operate to both link and separate the chapters, and in content they demonstrate queer couplings—in the first snapshot, as exemplified by Bordowitz's own fantasized sexual, political, and creative link with queer theater impresario Charles Ludlam.

In chapter 2, I continue my work of queering the origin story of health activism by defamiliarizing some of our now taken-for-granted assumptions about the conceptual, institutional, and political milieu into which AIDS emerged. In this chapter I que(e)ry the clinic before AIDS (both asking questions of the clinic and making it queer), circa 1970, through an exploration of clinical discourses, practices, and institutions that emerged in relation to the antipsychiatry movement in France and the women's health movement in the United States. In particular, I look at two practices—self-help and transversality—that demonstrate new therapeutic models that came from outside medicine but influenced the practice of medicine before AIDS. By juxtaposing these two examples of clinical practice in the 1970s, I demonstrate the importance of a comparative method for investigating the transformation of the discourses, institutions, and practices of illness from within and without medicine, especially because the borders between what is inside and outside medicine do not remain fixed. I also consider in the conclusion to this chapter what happens when certain experimental practices like self-help are incorporated into or appropriated by the conventional discourses and institutions of medicine—that is, when they move from outside to inside medicine. Co-optation—or what others have called the "politics of absorption"[38]—is the double bind of health activism, and I return to this problem throughout the book.

A snapshot again interrupts the temporal flow of the chapters in an attempt to challenge the naturalization of a progress narrative in relation to illness, thought, and politics. The second snapshot combines an image of the cover of the catalog for an exhibition of artist/writer/activist David Wojnarowicz's work in 1989 with two quotations: the first, a long quotation from Wojnarowicz himself taken from the catalog foreword written by Guattari, and the second, from Marion Scemama, the woman who brought Wojnarowicz and Guattari together, about their brief collaboration. The snapshot brings together another queer coupling, or ménage à trois—Wojnarowicz, Scemama, and Guattari—connecting AIDS activism of the 1980s with the social movements of the late 1960s and demonstrating the multiple temporalities of creative work and politics and politics as creative work.

I then trace back from around 1970 to investigate the changing spaces of the clinic in the 1960s in order to explore the problem of how, before AIDS, clinical experience in general and the practices of diagnosis and treatment in particular were enacted as categories of historical analysis. I read Foucault's *The Birth of the Clinic* as a history of the present of a shifting clinical experience in the 1960s, and I explore that present, which is now our past, by reading it with and against another exploration of a changing conception of clinical experience, John Berger and Jean Mohr's *A Fortunate Man,* about a rural general practitioner in the United Kingdom in the 1960s.[39]

The third snapshot creates a conceptual and temporal parenthesis at the center of *Indirect Action.* It opens around 1959 with an image of a sketch and a list describing components of the first "happening," Allan Kaprow's *18 Happenings in 6 Parts,* and closes around 1990 with Samuel R. Delany's account of his experience of the event of Kaprow's happening in *The Motion of Light in Water* and Joan W. Scott's two readings of Delany's memoir in her essay "The Evidence of Experience." I extend Scott's readings of Delany by highlighting the way, in *The Motion of Light in Water,* he works to refract his memories of both sexuality and mental illness in order to capture the complicated relationship between his experiences of art, sex, and madness.

My analysis in chapter 4 jumps scale—moving from the clinical to the ecological. Methodologically, this chapter continues my analysis of counterpractices of generalism in science and medicine and, as in chapter 3, links two texts that diagnose the condition of scientific and medical practice at a particular moment—Rachel Carson's *Silent Spring,* published in 1962, and Lewis Thomas's Notes of a Biology Watcher column, published in the *New England Journal of Medicine* from 1971 to 1980.[40] Not unlike Berger and Mohr's text, *Silent Spring* and Thomas's essays were a challenge to an "era of specialists" and were early calls for interdisciplinary and collaborative methods in approaching socioscientific problems. I consider how they problematize the shifting relationship between specialization and generalism by analyzing the way each scientist/writer negotiates the formal aspects and modes of address of writing for both fellow scientists and general readers. Finally, I explore the links between these interdisciplinary and generalist initiatives from within science to what comes after: new social movements around women's health and environmental justice.

The next snapshot draws together the political and therapeutic, exploring several scenes of therapy in a clinic in Algeria during the war of liberation in the late 1950s, the first presented in Frantz Fanon's essay "Colonial War and Mental Disorders" (1961)[41] and the second in Isaac Julien's documentary film *Frantz Fanon: Black Skin, White Mask* (1996). Bringing Fanon's essay together with Julien's later representation of Fanon allows me to draw out some of the continuities and discontinuities between colonial war and mental disorders before AIDS and queer politics and theory after AIDS. This snapshot also introduces the method-image "visualizing critical theory," a phrase Julien takes from a comment Donna Haraway made after seeing *Fanon*, suggesting again both the desire to freeze complexity and the impossibility of doing so.

I then move to two chapters in which I discuss more recent texts that treat the experiences and events of illness in the 1960s and 1970s and the effects of these experiences then and now on individuals, families, and communities. In chapter 5, I offer a graphic analysis of David B.'s graphic narrative of his brother's epilepsy. Through drawing in general and the creation of *Epileptic* in particular, David B. struggles to find a form to answer the question people ask him when they hear about his brother's condition, "So what's it like, a seizure?" David B. draws the experience and event of his brother's epilepsy as it emerges and evolves during the same period in which many writer/thinker/activists, including Foucault and Deleuze and Guattari, are preoccupied with madness. Then, in chapter 6, I look at Foucault's delineation of psychiatric power in relation to two recent treatments—one filmic, the other narrative—by the daughters of Mildred Smiley, an American woman suffering from schizophrenia beginning in the 1960s and continuing to the present.[42] As we look and try to make sense of what we see (and don't see), we too participate in the production of mental illness as a category of analysis.

The snapshot that flashes between the chapters on epilepsy and schizophrenia and the politicization of these illness experiences juxtaposes two attempts to document conditions at Bridgewater State Hospital—one contemporary, Disability Law Center's "Investigation of Bridgewater State Hospital" from 2014, and one historical, Frederick Wiseman's documentary film *Titicut Follies* from 1967. Wiseman's now classic, though not uncontroversial, work of cinéma vérité provides not only an image of the often horrific conditions of state institutions for the mentally ill in the 1960s but also a counterimage to the widespread impression of the institutionalized mentally ill as inarticulate and in need of heroic advocates to speak for them. The snapshot offers ways of thinking about madness through social coordinates other than reductive "familialist coordinates."[43] Wiseman's film shows that many of the inmates diagnosed as mad in the film are not as preoccupied with early childhood experiences—daddy-mommy-me, in

Deleuze and Guattari's intentionally reductive phrase[44]—as are their doctors; rather, they are interested and engaged in the changing social world around them.

My first book, *Treatments*, ended with an ethics of failure, or what I described as the experience of being at a loss yet exploring various routes. I ended this earlier work with failure because I wanted to make a case for the ubiquity and importance of failure in our scientific, political, and artistic practices and to explore how our subjectivities, research methods, and objects of study are constituted by our failures as much as by our successes. *Indirect Action* ends in a different, if related, register with a discussion of what is most often taken as an image of success, ACT UP's phrase and campaign "Drugs into Bodies," a slogan and cause that transformed the experience and event of AIDS and other illnesses in very concrete, material ways. In my afterimage I turn to two recent films—the documentary *How to Survive a Plague* and the feature film *Dallas Buyers Club*—that screen treatment activism in the early days of AIDS in the United States. Rather than serve as a conclusion, however, I want my readings of these films to demonstrate the dual process by which they "screen treatment activism"— how they both make certain practices of activism and particular activists visible and screen others from view. "Drugs into Bodies" is a complex and ambivalent remainder of the radical success of treatment activism. In a moment in which drugs are delivered as the sole therapeutic solution to any and all problems—medical, psychological, and social—the phrase and practice encapsulates a very particular conjuncture of illness-thought-activism in neoliberal times. We are now living the side effects of the success of treatment activism. Could it have been and be otherwise?

1

Doing Queer Love, circa 1985

"Feminists Asleep in AIDS Fight": so asserts the headline of a 2004 editorial in the *Denver Post* by Pius Kamau.[1] The sleeping activist is an evocative figure: what might it mean to sleep through a fight? And how might the image of the sleepless activist suggest a particular—heroic—mode of activism that limits the range of ways of doing health activism?[2] In his opinion piece, written just after the global AIDS conference in Thailand in 2004, Kamau, a thoracic and general surgeon who was born and raised in Kenya and immigrated to the United States in 1971, calls on American feminists, in particular, to address the "feminization of the AIDS crisis in the world."[3] "Who better to lead the charge," Kamau asserts, "than women who have locked horns with the male establishment and won?"[4] Kamau calls for the revival of the "energetic feminist movement of yesterday to help educate children about HIV transmission and the use of condoms, to mobilize female protest in developing countries and to fight monopolistic pharmaceutical companies for inexpensive drug therapy."[5] He says he'll never forget the feminist movement of yesterday, which included, for him, "the bra-burning, the protest marches, and Betty Friedan's *Feminine Mystique*"[6]—his three events already suggesting a feminism out of time or a second-wave feminism condensed to the point of banality. While his reference to bra burning reveals a mainstream media-constructed cultural memory of the movement and his reference to Friedan's *Feminine Mystique*, a sense of the movement as middle class and white and not (yet) radical, nonetheless Kamau has a notably enthusiastic view of the U.S. second-wave feminist movement. Because of this movement, Kamau believes, "American women are today the most free in the world," and he wants to remind them that "women of the world still need you." According to Kamau, then, where AIDS in the developing world is concerned, to paraphrase Gayatri Chakravorty Spivak, white women need to save brown women from brown men.[7]

On the same day Kamau's editorial was published, a message posted on an academic women's studies listserv based in the United States contained a link to Kamau's article, a brief description of his piece, and a request for more information: "Pius Kamau claims feminists have ignored the AIDS crisis in Africa. I know this is absolutely incorrect but I do not have the specific information immediately at hand to counter this claim." The person who posted the message wanted to know if anyone could point her "to research that is women-centered that addresses AIDS in Africa." What followed on the women's studies listserv was strange, at least to me: there seemed a general agreement that Kamau was right that feminists have ignored AIDS, not just in Africa but throughout the world, and a rather defensive need to explain why. One post asserted that feminists shouldn't be expected to do everything, echoing a letter to the *Denver Post* in response to Kamau's column that noted: "There are a lot of bad things happening in the world, and it is not feminists' duty to be working against all of them, even those bad things where half of the victims are women."[8] The message from the women's studies listserv seemed to be, to paraphrase Spivak again, that white women cannot be expected to save brown women in all the situations in which they need to be saved from brown men.

The post that I was most surprised by, which I want to use to introduce the question of what gets brought forward and remembered, or not, when AIDS arrives in the 1980s, presented a peculiar history of AIDS activism and an equally peculiar history of feminism in the United States. It is this peculiar presentation of history I am concerned with in this opening chapter, although one could also, of course, critique the peculiar view of the contemporary efforts to fight AIDS in Africa that suggests feminism—either a feminism originating in the West or a feminism indigenous to Africa, or one that combines elements of the two—is not an influence on these efforts. It is my aim in *Indirect Action* to look back to a past history of illness, thought, and health activism in order to consider how that history might be useful to us now in a different time and in other contexts. Thus, I begin with this near contemporary discussion of that history to demonstrate first how that history gets remembered, and forgotten, today.

According to the post on the women's studies listserv, the history of the relationship between feminism and AIDS goes like this:

HIV/AIDS emerged in the West as a STI [socially transmitted infection] which affected white gay men primarily. But the politics of the prevention movement are often overlooked in the question of why feminists didn't, or don't, join the struggle on this front.

The first 20 years of sexual politics in the Western HIV/AIDS movement have been dominated by sexual libertarianism and sexual liberalism. As such, it is quite hostile to feminist analyses of sex, gender and sexuality. . . .

The shift of HIV infection from white gay men to black, ethnic minority and indigenous women has meant that women have become more of a focus now. 75% of HIV is transmitted through penile-vaginal or anal penetrative sex which makes it impossible for the HIV prevention movement to continue to present the fallacy that sexual behaviour and HIV transmission are unrelated. In the past 5–10 years, there has been an ideological shift away from psychosocial and individualistic explanations of transmission to more structural analyses which open the door for pioneering feminist interventions.

The author of the post also mentions Gabriel Rotello's *Sexual Ecology*[9] as a "good book discussing the ideology of Western HIV prevention" and states that the only woman she heard at the Bangkok conference offering "a feminist analysis of sexuality" was Vicki Tallis, who worked with BRIDGE, an organization working on gender and development issues and affiliated with the Institute for Development Studies at the University of Sussex in the United Kingdom.

I quote at length from the discussion surrounding Kamau's piece to demonstrate the extent of the forgetting that surrounds the history of feminist and AIDS activism in the United States in the early days of the epidemic and, especially, *the forgetting of the intimate and effective relationship between the two*. There are many assumptions in this post, including that feminists were not and are still not AIDS activists, that early AIDS activism in the West was not influenced by feminism, that early AIDS activism did not provide a structural analysis of HIV/AIDS, that contemporary AIDS activism in African countries and the rest of the developing world is not already explicitly feminist or influenced by feminism, that AIDS activists do not make a link between HIV transmission and sexual behavior (or specific sexual practices), and that there are no feminists who espouse a position that might be called "sexual libertarianism" or "sexual liberalism."

In response, sociologist and women's studies scholar Judith Lorber protested the assumptions and forgetting in the listserv discussion by noting, simply, "Feminists have been writing on women, sexuality, gender and AIDS for the last 20 years," and she provided a selected bibliography of some of that work.[10] I want to lodge my own protest by offering a further genealogy of feminist AIDS activism. My goal is not to present a definitive history; rather, in tracing this genealogy I hope to discern some of the historical ties between feminism and U.S. AIDS activism in terms of political tactics, institutions, and the persons involved in order to investigate the politics of illness and health along with and in relation to the politics of history and memory. The historical memory of the early years of AIDS activism in the United States has often been reduced to one figure: the middle-class gay white male involved in the AIDS Coalition to Unleash Power (ACT UP). This figure serves to contain and cover over the complex history of AIDS activism in the United States in the 1980s.[11] Just as AIDS was initially identified as a "gay disease," AIDS activism was initially understood as something that only gay men did. Both of these assumptions about AIDS in the early years of the epidemic have had effects, at that time and into the future, on who was diagnosed; on how the disease was treated, both clinically and politically; and on the historical memory of the response to AIDS in the United States. I believe that by telling a more complex story of illness-thought-activism at a particular moment in time and in a particular place, we will be better prepared to respond more effectively to AIDS and other illnesses in the present.

Listening for Echoes of Health Activism

How and what we remember has a bearing on the politics of the present, which is why Foucault describes his own historical work as an intervention into the history of the present. An important aspect of Foucault's genealogical method is his attempt to discern the discontinuities and surprising continuities of historical events. To locate these discontinuities and continuities, Foucault frequently invokes a method-image that I would characterize as listening for echoes. Foucault's work is frequently criticized for diagnosing a type of power that leaves no space for resistance. Yet all of his work attempts to discern the conditions of possibility for the emergence of new forms of agency. Even in a work like *Discipline and Punish,* where he seeks to describe a new modality of power, the "complex ensemble that constitutes the 'carceral system,'"[12] a modality of power that functions not simply within the institution of the prison but throughout society—even there, amid his description of a power that is all around us, that constitutes us and our relations—Foucault listens for a counternarrative. Thus, in his chapter "Illegalities and Delinquency," Foucault hears a counternarrative in the Fourierists' antipenal polemics published in La Phalange, which take criminal activities not as "monstrosities" but, according to Foucault, "as the fatal return and revolt of what is repressed, the minor illegalities not as the necessary margins of the society, but as a rumbling from the midst of the battle-field."[13] In Foucault's genealogical analysis, the "lessons of La Phalange were not quite wasted"; their echo was heard and, thus, became useful again in the second half of the nineteenth century.[14]

As feminist historian Joan W. Scott has argued, following Foucault, the concept of the echo does "serious analytic work," helping us to understand both the process of writing history and the historicization of identity categories.[15] In her historico-ontological work, Scott utilizes this concept "to demonstrate that feminist identity was an effect of a rhetorical political strategy invoked differently by different feminists at different times."[16] Scott deploys the term "fantasy echo" to suggest repetitions of identities and modes of political struggle that are "not exact"[17] but still resonate across different times and places. Echoes are not, as is often thought, "reproduction[s] of the same."[18] Rather, they "are delayed returns of sound; they are incomplete reproductions, usually giving back only the final fragments of a phrase. An echo spans large gaps of space (sound reverberates between distant points) and time (echoes aren't instantaneous), but it also creates gaps of meaning and intelligibility."[19] An echo is a fold in sound and works by shortening and lengthening intelligibility at the same time. In this chapter I want to follow the methodological and historical interventions of Scott and Foucault by utilizing the concept of the echo to help theorize the historical relationship between health feminism and AIDS activism. It is my hope that by presenting some of the lessons of early feminist AIDS activists in the United States, their lessons will be not quite wasted. Indeed, one of the political purposes of the project of exploring the prehistory of AIDS is an attempt to make some of these lessons useful to us again in the beginning of the twenty-first century. The method-image of the echo, then, but as motivated by the productive power of a fantasy of the future.

One lesson of those early feminist health activists I hope will be not quite wasted is one that I call "doing queer love." This is a historical echo I believe we must try to hear now, not just in order to challenge a particular history of AIDS activism in the United States but also in order to provide a model that can be useful for addressing the continuing problem of AIDS across the globe. I want this opening chapter to echo forward to later chapters, in which clinical spaces, practices, and discourses before AIDS are que(e)ried. Through both its form and content, *Indirect Action* draws links between a multiplicity of micro- and macropractices of care in a variety of therapeutic spaces. In a sense, then, although I begin with queer theory and AIDS activism and trace back from there, I do not intend this structure to secure a progress narrative or a story that is always already inevitable. Rather, I want to think about how we might undo precisely what we take to be most inevitable—politically, conceptually, and clinically. Each component of the concept "doing queer love" is important: the ongoingness, the making strange, and the affective commitments. In this chapter, then, I trace the echoes between health feminism and AIDS activism in order to present a more complex history of both movements and to try to think through the ways that the coming together of these two struggles in a particular place and time—New York City in the 1980s—created particular practices of doing queer love that might be effective in other times and places. This may seem absurd—or even imperialist. After all, queer is a Western identity category, isn't it?

Yet illness itself might be understood as queer, and indeed one of the definitions of *queer,* according to the *OED,* is "not in normal condition; out of sorts; giddy, faint, or ill." Illness queers identity categories, and it queers relationships between individuals, communities, and even nations. If we consider queer not in terms of a particular identity—that is, not as a form of being but as a mode of doing—then we begin to expand the affective and effective possibilities of the concept. So, *doing queer* as opposed to *being queer,* and relatedly, *doing illness* as opposed to *being ill.*[20] What might it mean to do queer rather than be queer, and how might this doing create new forms of not only queer sexuality but also queer love, in this case within the particular domain of the politics of health and illness? By queering love rather than or as well as sexuality, the concept of queer and its multiple lessons and uses expand.

By noting the capaciousness of the term and category "queer," I want to highlight its etymological link to illness and ill feelings. If "queer" is capacious, so too is "illness," perhaps more so or differently from "queer."

It seems to me that this link is useful for extending the analysis of the experiences and events of both illness and queer historically and methodologically.[21] I contend that doing queer love provides a framework through which we might respond both politically and personally to the stigma and shame attached to an illness like AIDS, even in contexts where it is transmitted mainly through heterosexual sex. In making this argument, I consider AIDS activism in terms of a way of life as opposed to an identity, and I return again to Foucault's work to think this ethics in its moment of arising—around 1981.

Queer Ascesis

In his essay "The Subject and Power," Foucault explains that the main objective of his work "has not been to analyze the phenomenon of power" but rather "to create a history of the different modes by which, in our culture, human beings are made subjects."[22] His three-volume *History of Sexuality* might be understood, then, as a history of the modes by which human beings are made and make themselves subjects within the "domain of sexuality"[23] during different historical moments and in different cultures. For Foucault the task of the philosopher is "to investigate not only the metaphysical systems or the foundations of scientific knowledge but a historical event—a recent, even a contemporary event."[24] Foucault marks the beginning of a transformation of the philosopher's task—from investigating metaphysical systems and foundations of knowledge to investigating a historical event—in a fairly obscure text published by Kant in a Berlin newspaper at the end of the eighteenth century entitled "What Is Enlightenment?" According to Foucault's reading of Kant's text, the question for Kant is not, Who am I? as it had been for Descartes, but, "What are we? in a very precise moment of history."[25]

I want to ask the question, What are we? in the very precise moment of the emergence of AIDS activism in the mid- to late 1980s, in the very precise place of New York City. In this opening chapter, I want to ask this question about New York in the 1980s both so that we might know something more or else about that illness event and so that we might know something more or else in anticipation of future illness events in other places. In the chapters that follow, I will trace back from the present reality of the 1980s by exploring the period immediately before AIDS emerged in 1981, specifically in relation to the discourses and practices of health activism, the new objects of clinical and ecological analysis, and the new subjects of care and caring as articulated across a heterotopia of spaces between 1960 and 1980. My goal is not to create a comprehensive or total history of health activism in the period I call the prehistory of AIDS but to explore the complexity of the conjuncture illness-thought-activism in time and space.

In an interview for the French gay magazine *Gai Pied* that appeared in April 1981, Foucault discusses this "problem of the present time, and what we are, in this present moment,"[26] in particular with regard to the event of a specific form of doing social relations and subjectivity that we call "homo-sexuality."[27] Foucault expresses concern for the tendency to "relate the question of homosexuality to the problem of 'Who am I?' and 'What is the secret of my desire?'"[28] Instead, Foucault thinks it "better to ask oneself, 'What relations, through homosexuality, can be established, invented, multiplied, and modulated?'"[29] Such a rethinking of homosexuality not in terms of *the truth of one's identity* but rather in terms of *one's becoming through relations* leads Foucault to speculate on the radical potential of friendship between men. For him the "neat image of homosexuality," which emphasizes the im-mediate pleasure of "two young men meeting in the street, seducing each other with a look, grabbing each other's asses and getting each other off in a quarter of an hour," does not generate unease, despite conservative as-sertions to the contrary.[30] What makes homosexuality more "disturbing," according to Foucault, is its "mode of life, much more than the sexual act itself."[31] Foucault is not interested in defining once and for all a specific mode of life but rather encourages what he calls *ascesis,* which he delineates as "the work that one performs on oneself in order to transform oneself or make the self appear which, happily, one never attains."[32] Foucault wonders if we might create or invent—not discover, which would imply some true identity—a homosexual ascesis or mode of life.

He notes that women have been more able to do something like this in the past because physical contact between women is more tolerated, and he discusses Lillian Faderman's historical account of romantic friendship and love between women as demonstrating the way such a mode of life is invented through intimate gestures.[33] Foucault claims that "man's body has been forbidden to other men in a much more drastic way," insisting that only during war do men have the kind of intimacy that is allowed more generally between women.[34] There are certainly problems with Foucault's schema: on the one hand, although certain personal or private intimacies between women may have been more tolerated historically, I do not at all think that women's social or political movements, for example, which we might understand as expressing a kind of intimacy, have been encouraged or even tolerated, and on the other hand, there are many more domains in which men engage in homosocial, if not explicitly homoerotic, bonding than Foucault acknowledges, including sports, social and business clubs, and, even, many professions that are predominately male.[35] Nevertheless, his interest in the ethics of a particularly gay way of life that is inventive and remains open to new relationships and new social spaces anticipates, for me, what emerges with, or in response to, AIDS in the gay and lesbian community. Foucault might be talking about the history of AIDS and AIDS activism when he notes, "We have to dig deeply to show how things have been historically contingent, for such and such reason intelligible but not necessary. We must make the intelligible appear against a background of emptiness and deny its necessity. We must think that what exists is far from filling all possible spaces."[36] Foucault discussed "friendship as a way of life" just as AIDS was emerging and just as feminism was being transformed in crucial ways by what would come to be known as the "sex wars"—all around 1981.[37] I contend that around that same time, through the experience and event of AIDS in the gay community in the United States, a *queer ascesis* was invented or came into being through the friendship and love not only between gay men but between gay men and lesbians. Illness making queer as much as sexuality.

Beginnings 1: The Origin Story of AIDS Activism in the United States

Although most histories of AIDS in the West begin around 1981, histories of AIDS activism in the United States most often begin with the creation of the AIDS Coalition to Unleash Power (ACT UP) in New York in 1987. Prior to 1987, it is believed, the gay community responded to AIDS through practices of accommodation, not practices of politics. In this prevailing narrative, politics emerges only after the failure of accommodation. Practices of accommodation, on the one hand, as exemplified by many of the policies of Gay Men's Health Crisis (GMHC), founded in New York in 1982, sought to establish a network of services for people with AIDS. This network of services, established initially by and for the gay community, provided resources for caring and strategies for coping with the realities of a terrible new disease that was killing virtually everyone who became ill.

A prime example of this strategy was the AIDS Buddy program to provide practical assistance for people with AIDS in their own homes, a program I would describe as an early form of doing queer love. Practices of political confrontation, on the other hand, came later and sought to challenge the denial of the crisis by the U.S. government and the "general public" and to insist that the government's failure to respond meant that it was abetting, if not outright committing, genocide against the gay community. Or so the story goes.

From the beginning, this origin story of AIDS activism has been challenged. In a collection of her journalism from the 1980s, writer/activist Sarah Schulman notes in her introduction: "Contrary to the recent periodization of the history of AIDS activism, there was resistance and political rebellion before the founding of ACT UP."[38] As discussed in the introduction, Cindy Patton has been working against this origin story since even before the publication of *Inventing AIDS* in 1990. She makes her point again in *Globalizing AIDS,* asserting that while "ACT UP reintroduced agitprop into a rather bland political scene, . . . activism *began* when the first living person was acknowledged to have an unnamed but recognizable syndrome and had to cope with a hostile medical system."[39] More recently, Jennifer Brier has returned to the first two years of the epidemic in the United States to explore the politics, especially as articulated in the radical gay newspaper *Gay Community News (GCN)* in Boston. In particular, she discusses a conversation published in *GCN* between Patton, who was then managing editor, and Bob Andrews, part of the *GCN* collective, in which Patton draws on feminist politics to argue against the conservative call for behavior change emphasizing abstinence as a response to AIDS.[40] Brier's discussion of early AIDS activism in *Infectious Ideas* concurs with my assessment not only that Patton was the first to make this argument but also that she has felt compelled to periodically remake it in the face of narratives that judge the early response as not activism. According to Brier, "Patton was the first to caution against drawing too sharp a distinction between early AIDS activism and early AIDS service work. In *Inventing AIDS,* Patton argues that seeing ACT UP as the first example of radical activism ignores earlier radical roots,"[41] and these radical roots extend back to well before 1981. Furthermore, in interviews for the ACT UP Oral History Project, many interviewees, including Jean Carlomusto and Gregg Bordowitz, are keen to discuss their own AIDS activism before the formation of ACT UP, as I will discuss.

Nonetheless, the narrative that begins with accommodation then moves into confrontation and most often ends with the arrival of the protease inhibitors and successful forms of treatment remains the hegemonic historical narrative of AIDS in gay communities in the United States. This is the case in the recent documentary *How to Survive a Plague,* which I discuss in more detail in this book's concluding afterimage. This is the case even in Deborah Gould's excellent study of ACT UP as social movement, which while acknowledging AIDS activism didn't begin with ACT UP, seems to be emotionally and politically invested in ACT UP's exceptionalism. Toward the end of her introduction, Gould describes attending an exhibit, *Becoming Visible: The Legacy of Stonewall,* at the New York Public Library in 1994 to commemorate the twenty-fifth anniversary of the Stonewall Riots. She is surprised to come "face to face with images, documents, and ephemera from ACT UP, included as part of this history."[42] She feels pride that ACT UP is included in this longer history of LGBTQ activism but also sorrow, because at the time of the exhibit ACT UP was in decline. Thus, for Gould ACT UP's inclusion in the history of activism the exhibit traces is a sign of what she calls, movingly, "the movement of movements into history" and, more specifically, her "belated realization that the movement was indeed coming to an end."[43] Without meaning to diminish Gould's important insight about the affective force of social movements, my approach is interested less in the beginnings and endings of movements and more in the ongoingness of such activism from one moment and movement to the next—how they persist, endure, wax, and wane. Related to this is the question of the multiple temporalities of politics and illness and of illness as politics in direct and indirect ways.

Building on the feminist work of Schulman, Patton, and Brier, in *Indirect Action* I challenge the hegemonic historical narrative of AIDS activism, as well as the temporopolitical modality of crisis that has been used to contain the experience and event of AIDS. When we say AIDS was (and is) a crisis, what do we mean? Or more to the point, what does this particular crisis mode bring into being? The purpose of my challenge is not to revise the understanding of Gay Men's Health Crisis as sometimes accommodationist[44] nor to claim that ACT UP wasn't one of the leading actors in bringing AIDS to the forefront of the American social and political landscape and to the consciousness of the American people and to activists outside the United States. Rather, in this chapter I trace a genealogy of AIDS activism by moving back from 1987 and ACT UP's emergence in order to consider some factors that led to that emergence, before moving in later chapters to illness experiences and events before AIDS. Some of the factors that led to ACT UP are widely known, like Larry Kramer's frustration with and eventual exile from GMHC, but others are less acknowledged, even forgotten, as the discussion on the women's studies listserv indicates, such as the influence of the women's health movement on the forms of activism that emerged with AIDS from the very beginning, not just with ACT UP. In particular, I analyze the link between feminism and AIDS activism, as well as the articulation of a queer ascesis that such a link brings into being, by considering three figures—Sarah Schulman, Ann Cvetkovich, and Gregg Bordowitz—whose work both remembers and continues to perform this link. Schulman, Cvetkovich, and Bordowitz have all sought to document the affective and effective histories of AIDS activism. Their multiple practices—combining art, feminist and poststructuralist theories, and oral history—are modes of doing queer love.

Beginnings 2: "We Like Dykes!"

In *My American History,* Schulman presents what she knows is not a typical account of lesbian and gay history, never mind American history. To explore American history in the Reagan and the first Bush years, Schulman looks back to feminism in the United States in the 1970s, its influence on her own theories and practices, and the way it gets remembered in the 1980s and after. In her introduction she notes that 1970s feminism has been historically revisioned as, paradoxically, "either dominated by dogmatic and prudish lesbians or deeply homophobic."[45] Although she acknowledges some larger feminist organizations "were the site of well-known lesbian purges," she regrets that the dominant account of seventies feminism does not at all capture her own experiences within the diverse and vibrant movement that was "engaged in re-evaluating and re-imagining every aspect of social life."[46] Seventies feminism, as Schulman describes it, exemplifies many of the practices and new forms of relations that Foucault encourages in the interview from 1981. According to Schulman, the practitioners of seventies feminism "opened up new venues for the imagination as they asserted women's lives and lesbian lives as justifiable terrain for autonomous political organizing, challenged male power and hegemony, raised consciousness, and learned to re-conceptualize the social and physical functions and the desire of the female body."[47] Schulman delineates a shift in feminism around 1980 that coincides with the rise of Reaganism and the New Right in the United States, one that we might today describe as the emergence of a neoliberal feminism "focused more on cultural expression and less on direct action."[48] Despite this shift, Schulman, who presents a Foucaultian-style genealogy in her own right, acknowledges echoes of seventies feminism in the emergence of AIDS activism in the 1980s. Indeed, I would argue that many feminists who were driven from, or simply left, the "mainstream" feminist movement for various reasons in the early 1980s continued to work to reconceptualize the interrelationship between gender, race, class, and sexuality through AIDS activism. As Amber Hollibaugh explains in an interview, "AIDS activism as a movement valued my ability to do explicit work around sexuality."[49] Having just experienced the "sex wars" that erupted in the U.S. women's movement at and after the Barnard Conference on Sexuality in 1982, Hollibaugh was ready to participate in a political movement that valued her ability to "talk about sexuality as part of class and race."[50]

Around the same time, both Schulman and Maxine Wolfe found themselves estranged, as lesbians, from the feminist reproductive rights movement in New York, and they, like Hollibaugh, engaged with a movement that needed them and the skills they had learned in the women's liberation movement. Wolfe was one of the early leaders in ACT UP and brought a long activist past to the group. She was one of the few "older" members of ACT UP, becoming involved when she was in her forties and continuing to participate in the group for over ten years. In an appreciation of Larry Kramer entitled "The Mother of Us All," Wolfe acknowledges Kramer's importance to early AIDS activism but also suggests what was unique was the genetic contribution of each of them to the newly born movement:

> Recently, I learned that some ACT UP members would affectionately describe Larry Kramer and myself as the "father" and "mother" of the group, though it wasn't always clear who was who. Though Larry can lay claim to taking part in ACT UP's birth, I cannot. I never even heard of Larry Kramer before my first ACT UP meeting in late June 1987, three months after the group started. Both of us were connected to that elusive entity called "the community," but our worlds were far apart: Yale vs. CUNY; the West

Village vs. Brooklyn; the *New York Native* vs. *Womanews*; gay man with no radical history vs. lesbian with lots of it, especially on the left, in the women's and lesbian feminist movements.[51]

That a social movement might have a father and/or mother is not a particularly radical idea, but the divergent kinship networks Wolfe traces suggest a queer genetic mixing that was, at least initially, an important aspect of ACT UP's character. What was new in early AIDS activism, as Wolfe's statement implies, was not the discourses, tactics, and institutions that the movement brought into being but the social and economic capital that gay men brought to such a movement. Or as Schulman puts it, "The coming together of feminist political perspectives and organizing experience with gay men's high sense of entitlement and huge resources proved to be a historically transforming event."[52]

Schulman's journalism from the period shows that lesbian feminists offered early personal and political support for gay men experiencing AIDS and the hysteria surrounding it. In an article from December 1985 in the *New York Native* entitled "Becoming an Angry Mob in the Best Sense: Lesbians Respond to AIDS Hysteria," Schulman describes the challenges both lesbians and gay men face as a result of "the new homophobia accompanying AIDS hysteria."[53] She acknowledges that relationships between gay men and lesbians, while often individually quite satisfying and emotionally important, have been at the community level more constrained and "historically tenuous."[54] Nonetheless, as she maintains in the opening sentence of her piece, "we're in this together now."[55] What follows this assertion is a feminist analysis into the rather muted response by the gay male community in New York to the closing of the baths and the surprisingly interested (and hardly prudish) response by several well-known lesbian activists. Writer/activist Jewelle Gomez, for example, tells the *Native* that "closing baths and bars is the first sign of political repression. Whether we think bars and baths are wonderful or not, they're not going to stop with the bars. We can't pretend that and still be self-respecting."[56] And Joan Nestle, writer and cofounder of the Lesbian Herstory Archives, worries about being "'lulled into a circle of respectability.'"[57] Nestle links the failure to mount strong protests against the bath closings to a "state of shame" in the gay and lesbian community. "Are we willing to fight for sexual territory that we are being told is death?" she asks. Nestle demonstrates that when trying to counter the paralysis that sometimes accompanies shame, it helps to know one's history: "When I saw the television and I saw policemen standing in front of the bar, it came home to me that this was a fifties image."[58] Schulman explains that "Nestle expressed a belief that a grassroots movement would develop from these events," and her piece ends with a quote from Nestle calling for a reemergence of the activism of her (women's and gay liberation) past: "There's really a chance for street responses like we used to have, by an angry mob. I think we have the potential to be an angry mob and I say that in the best sense of the word."[59] Nestle's connection between history, shame, and the potential of the angry mob anticipates Eve Kosofsky Sedgwick's later theorizing about the importance of the negative affects, in particular shame, for bringing into being a queer politics.[60]

Schulman's later commentary on this piece notes the irony in the fact that "although lesbians are constantly portrayed in the straight and gay media [and, I would add, even at times on women's studies listservs] as prudish and anti-sex, clearly grass-roots lesbian activists were a lot more willing to go on record as opposing the closing of the baths than a good percentage of the gay male leadership."[61] Schulman also contends that while gay men were largely apolitical, lesbians had the critical and practical tools to confront institutional power. Because of their access to greater resources and positions of power, gay men believed that they were included in the "general public" and that their needs would and should be met. Many lesbians, according to Schulman, were "clear on their exclusion from the beginning," and this exclusion gave them a better view of the workings of power.[62] She acknowledges again that some lesbians resented gay men for their sense of entitlement and lack of sociopolitical critique, but she also notes that other lesbians "did not hold grudges, or were willing to work hard to build a more enlightened and effective community."[63] Schulman's notion of an "effective community" denaturalizes a romantic notion of community[64] and captures, I think, the way that, in early AIDS activism, lesbian and feminist activists became useful to gay men in ways that neither group had imagined before. The lessons many lesbians had learned in the 1970s echoed into the 1980s in the domain of AIDS activism. I don't mean to imply that lesbian and feminist activists were used by gay men in a sort of mercenary fashion, although on some levels this may be true, at least unconsciously. I want to consider here how relations, between the "general public" and gays and lesbians, as well as among and between gays and lesbians, are enacted through an event like AIDS and to suggest that usefulness can be a means through which we create not only effective but also affective communities, or, in Patton's terminology, "networks of allegiances."[65] It can be a means through which we begin to do queer love. Usefulness is a multilayered concept in relation to politics and, even more so, in relation to the event of neoliberalization, which is happening concurrently to the event of AIDS. Although I want *Indirect Action* to work against a teleology that arrives at AIDS activism and neoliberalism, part of the point of returning to the prehistory of AIDS is to try to disentangle the response to AIDS after 1981 from an increasingly neoliberalized health care and activism in order to suggest other possible trajectories in the present.

In *People in Trouble,* her novel depicting the early years of AIDS in New York, Schulman portrays the emergence of just such a queer sort of love. Kate, one of the narrators, describes the makeup of the ACT UP–like organization Justice:

No straight men showed up at all.

"Straight men don't know how to take care of other people," Daisy explained. "And they don't work well in groups."

There was a band of veterans from the now defunct women's liberation movement who were the only ones who had been consistently politically active for the last decade, and so knew better than anyone else how to make flyers, how to do phone trees, the quickest way to wheat-paste, and who weren't afraid of getting arrested.

"Being a woman in Justice means being in leadership," Daisy once said. "As soon as you walk in the room all the guys turn around and say, 'Now what?'"

"We like dykes," the guys would chant every once in awhile when the women did something really great.[66]

Working across multiple genres, Schulman reveals that lesbians and feminists were important players in the early AIDS movement and that the AIDS movement brought gay men and lesbians together in remarkable ways, creating new forms of relationships, new kinds of love. Because of their activism in the past, lesbians became the progenitors of the "now what?" of AIDS activism.

Echoes 1: Seizing Our Bodies and the FDA

As the main interviewer for the ACT UP Oral History Project, Schulman continues to do queer love by documenting both the historical links between AIDS activism and other political movements and forms of activism and the affective experiences that come with political activism, especially political activism haunted by loss. Queer love, as practiced by Schulman, becomes a historical methodology, which is itself a form of politics—a "then what?" to link to the "now what?" Although in many of the interviews AIDS activism is understood within a long history of struggles by minority groups for civil rights and self-determination, I want to continue to focus here on what I am arguing is an explicit connection between AIDS activism and the health feminism of the 1970s. I will continue this discussion in the next chapter when I que(e)ry the feminist clinic and its practices of self-help in the 1970s. Schulman herself embodies this connection—and I will argue that she, like Félix Guattari at La Borde, is a figure who acts as a relay between political movements and gestures, and through these relay figures, echoes are transmitted linking movements.

In response to Schulman's question about "ACT UP's greatest achievement and biggest disappointment," Gregg Bordowitz says, "The biggest achievement was the idea that people with AIDS should be in control of the decisions that govern our treatment and cure. It's the one thing I return to, that principle that the people with the disease should be at the center of a discussion about the disease. No more of this notion of patients being taken care of, that patients play an active role in their care. All of that self-care stuff was really important, I think that was the lasting contribution."[67] Bordowitz is certainly right that ACT UP emphasized these things, and he acknowledges elsewhere in his interview the influence of other political fights on ACT UP's theories and practices. What rarely gets recognized explicitly is the continuity between ACT UP's theoretical critique and its political tactics and those of the women's health movement. I will discuss the discourses, practices, and institutions of feminist health activism in more detail in the next chapter, but for now I want to take Claudia Dreifus's 1977 edited volume *Seizing Our Bodies* as an exemplary statement of health feminism and as showing the links—direct and indirect—between movements.[68]

As the title of Dreifus's volume suggests, one of the main goals of the women's health movement was to provide women with the tactics and tools to seize control of their bodies from institutions, such as medicine and the law, as a means to liberation. Health feminism was concerned with women's often negative experience of medicine and, in particular, gynecology. The "radical, anarchic" movement distrusted organized medicine and offered an early critique of the medicalization of supposedly "natural" experiences, which resulted in, for example, the transformation of childbirth into an increasingly technological experience in the hands of usually male obstetricians.[69] The women's health movement established both consciousness-raising groups, in which "expert" medical knowledge could be shared beyond the small coterie of medical professionals, and self-help clinics. As Dreifus explains, these clinics, which would become the Feminist Women's Health Centers, "uniformly have women, often nonprofessionals, doing the bulk of the medical service; their emphasis, always, is on patient involvement in diagnosis and treatment, on deprofessionalization of services."[70]

Just as important and, also, as a means to raise consciousness about the politics of women's bodies, the women's health movement used direct-action tactics to disrupt the specific institutions that affected women's experiences of their bodies. For example, a group of health feminists disrupted the Senate hearings on the safety of oral contraceptives in 1970.[71] As Judith Coburn explained at the time, "We went to the hearings to protest the alliance of drug companies, population control experts, and the government, an alliance we believe has given the Pill a clean bill of health at women's expense."[72] Although AIDS activists would demand something different from the drug companies and the government than was demanded by those women who disrupted the Senate hearings, the notion that one might challenge specific government institutions making health policy, like the Food and Drug Administration, was part of the politics of feminist health activism at this time. Before further exploring drugs and their effects by problematizing a politics narrowed to the specific aim of facilitating drugs into bodies, I want to first draw a link between feminists disrupting Senate hearings on the pill and AIDS activists disrupting business and government as usual at the FDA to point to continuities between these health activisms as well as discontinuities and lost possibilities.

When Schulman asks Gregg Bordowitz to describe some of the big actions that he worked on for ACT UP, he says that the most important one was the nonviolent takeover of the FDA. According to Bordowitz, David

Barr and Mickey Wheatley came to him to propose this action on the floor of an ACT UP meeting, and their rationale for the action won Bordowitz's support. Bordowitz explains to Schulman that Barr and Wheatley told him, "Look, we have this idea for a strategy that would be very different than things that have been tried before in activism. Millions of groups, not millions that's an exaggeration, but many groups have gone to Washington and protested in front of the White House. Many groups have protested in front of Congress. For our movement, we need to go to the Food and Drug Administration. This is very specific. This is an institution that is very specific to the issues that we're facing."[73] The demand of this action, according to Bordowitz, was both to "cut through the bureaucratic red tape of the Food and Drug Administration" and to emphasize "that people with AIDS should be involved in every level of decision-making concerning research for a treatment and a cure for our disease."[74]

In an echo of Dreifus's *Seizing Our Bodies*, Bordowitz goes on to explain that he came up with the slogan for the action—"Seize Control of the FDA"—which, he says, "was frightening to many people, this notion of seizing control. But," he continues:

I was very insistent: "This is what has to be. It has to be that we are just going to take over the agency. The agency is not being run in our interests. People with AIDS are going to take over the agency and run it in our own interests." This is very much the idea, which I think was the lasting historical contribution of ACT UP, that people with AIDS be in control of all decisions concerning our health. It was very significant and it's very consistent within the history of civil rights movements. Primarily, the core principle is self-determination. So this is self-determination for people with a disease. But it's also the heart of the union movement: self-determination for workers to run their work life; the civil rights movement, self-determination of people of color; feminism; gay and lesbian liberation. It's consistent, and you can see actually our demand, as activists, as people with AIDS, or supporters of people with AIDS in the AIDS activist movement is completely consistent with the history of civil rights.[75]

At the same time as Bordowitz is asserting the originality of ACT UP's strategies and tactics, he acknowledges that it is continuous with and echoes a long history of other movements for self-determination. This is what is forgotten in both the hegemonic narrative of AIDS activism that posits such activism emerged with ACT UP and the feminist narrative that sees no direct or indirect connection between the two movements theoretically, strategically, and in terms of participants. Feminists and gay men were able to create an "effective community" precisely through political struggle that, while concerned with AIDS in the present, also remembered and made connections to struggles for self-determination in the past, through the participation of lesbians in particular as transversal figures linking one movement to another across times and places. Listening for these historical echoes in the present helps us to imagine into being new forms of health activism for the future.

Echoes 2: Doing Queer Love through Oral History

Schulman's journalism and fiction from the period and her contemporary oral history work all attempt to counter the loss of this continuity, the silencing of these historical echoes, and, in so doing, attempt to recover, or reinvent, an effective community among lesbians and gay men. According to Schulman, she and filmmaker Jim Hubbard began their video oral history project because she "had long been disheartened by the false AIDS stories told in the few mainstream representations of the crisis."[76] In these false AIDS stories, AIDS activism and the love among gay men and between gay men and lesbians never existed; instead, only once the "general public" "came around" was AIDS finally addressed, in the United States at least. It should be noted that, in many respects, these false AIDS stories are perpetuated not just by the mainstream media but also in some feminist and gay and lesbian histories. What Schulman wants to communicate through this project is "what really took place": "Thousands of people, over many years, dedicated their lives to achieving cultural and scientific transformations."[77]

If anything, Schulman's urgency is more profound now than when she began the project, so much so that, for her, the ACT UP Oral History Project has become a reaction formation against what she describes as the "gentrification of the mind," a phrase that suggests the forgetting of the experiences and events of AIDS in the 1980s, or their disremembering, creating what we might call gentrified memories, a process I return to in the concluding afterimage. She writes of her work on the project with Hubbard: "Jim and I now have more cumulative information about ACT UP than anyone. After each interview we reconceptualize the project, we try to articulate a trajectory, we put together the pieces of what made the organization work and the consequences and impact of its actions on AIDS and on the world. We get ACT UP. And the more I understand what ACT UP was, the more I see what is missing from the contemporary discourse."[78] The "getting" ACT UP is ongoing for Schulman; the more cumulative information intensifies rather than calms the urgency. Like the story of Kramer's long unfinished and ever-lengthening novel that I discuss in the introduction, Schulman's (and Hubbard's) oral history project can never be finished. The gathering of evidence, the reconceptualizing of the project, the trying to articulate a trajectory, this work reveals what is missing in the present. Looking back at the history of AIDS activism is an to attempt to recover the evidence—of cultural and scientific transformations and of the creation of heterogeneous affective and effective communities.

Historian John Howard has noted that oral history has been a particularly "vital methodology" for gay and lesbian and queer history. According to Howard,

> Gay persons who have gone through the stereotypical trajectory—from country to city, from "closetedness" to "awareness"—those who are strongly self-identified as gay and highly politicized make *excellent* oral history narrators. They understand the need for such studies. They feel compelled to participate and often do so via urban-centered, community-based oral history projects, some of the earliest of which were undertaken in Boston, Buffalo, San Francisco, and Toronto.[79]

In his own work, however, Howard wants to supplement these studies that focus on this "stereotypical trajectory" with a study that offers a different trajectory or that recognizes this is not always or the only trajectory for queer people. As a method for documenting both the hegemonic and the nonhegemonic stories, oral history also seems to be a particularly vital methodology for the history of AIDS activism; it is a method well suited to capturing both the effective and the affective dimensions of this history. Doing oral history might itself be a way of doing queer love.

Like the ACT UP Oral History Project, Ann Cvetkovich's own ACT UP oral history project discussed in her *An Archive of Feelings* seeks to counter a mainstream memory of the movement, which as it purportedly remembers that movement paradoxically forgets its complexity. Cvetkovich is interested, therefore, in documenting, in particular, lesbian involvement in ACT UP because, she fears, "with the passage of time, ACT UP is in danger of being remembered as a group of privileged gay white men without a strong political sensibility, and sometimes critiqued on those grounds."[80] Again, the figure of the middle-class gay male as AIDS activist ends up screening our memory of the movement and its complexity. It is perhaps not surprising, considering the devastation in the gay community wrought by AIDS, that two lesbian writer/scholar/activists should take responsibility to witness to the early years of AIDS in the United States through oral history projects. Indeed, as both Schulman and Cvetkovich understand, part of the reason lesbians play a significant role as witnesses to the AIDS crisis is that most of those lesbians who participated in AIDS activism have survived to witness the event, while so many of their gay companions in AIDS activism did not. This phenomenon itself—gay men dying and lesbians surviving and becoming witnesses—becomes part of the event of AIDS that must itself be witnessed.

Like the ACT UP Oral History Project, Cvetkovich's oral history of ACT UP's lesbians is an attempt to present a broader history of AIDS activism that emphasizes both the effective and the affective components of activism. Schulman and Cvetkovich as oral historians are part of the genealogy of feminist AIDS activism that I trace in order to remember past methods of doing queer love, before queer and before AIDS, and in order to bring others into being. Although perhaps inspired and influenced by each other, the preoccupations that Schulman and Cvetkovich bring to their interviews are somewhat different.[81] I want to point briefly to these differences in order to highlight once again the fact that there is not one, singular story of AIDS activism and to note much work is still to be done to document the multiplicity of AIDS activism in particular and forms of doing queer love more generally.

Schulman discusses the personal relationships that formed as a result of ACT UP, and she is clearly interested in and gets many of her interviewees to talk about the fact that several gay men had sexual relationships with both straight women and lesbians in ACT UP. Indeed, Schulman and several of her interviewees discuss Bordowitz, in particular, as the "lesbian boyfriend." Schulman certainly understands that the possibility of a more fluid understanding of sexuality was part of what made ACT UP potentially radical, but at the same time, I maintain she is preoccupied more with the drama of direct action than with the less direct effects of bodies and pleasures in relation to activism. Schulman tries hardest to get her interviewees to speak about ACT UP's countless protests and the myriad organizational details that brought these protests to fruition; she seems more concerned with gathering evidence of ACT UP as an effective community than as an affective community. She shows how each interviewee came to be an activist and what particular organizational, artistic, or performative talents they brought to ACT UP or how they discovered these talents through ACT UP. There is no doubt she herself knows a much longer history of struggles for self-determination, as Bordowitz would have it, but she wants to get at whether her interviewees located themselves within this longer struggle before they came to ACT UP, either actively through past activism or intellectually through knowledge of the history of such struggles. Through her oral history work and her own knowledge of and participation in late twentieth-century social movements, Schulman acts as a relay between feminist and civil rights activism of the 1960s and 1970s and AIDS activism of the 1980s and 1990s. The ACT UP Oral History Project itself also becomes a relay between the activism of ACT UP and activism after ACT UP.

At the same time, Schulman seems determined to be an arbiter of what is political and what isn't, as is made clear in her most recent work on gentrification as a direct effect of the AIDS crisis. Schulman begins *The Gentrification of the Mind* with a recollection from 2001 while in Los Angeles trying to get writing work in film and TV. She hears a report on National Public Radio about the twentieth anniversary of AIDS. "'This is the first time I've heard AIDS being historicized," she explains, and she is horrified by the sanitized—"gentrified"—history that gets told of an America that was initially troubled by people with AIDS but eventually "came around."[82] It is then that Schulman begins to document a different, less sanitized history of AIDS in America. Although my sympathy is with Schulman and her fellow activists, who transformed the response to AIDS—political and medical and politicomedical—in profound ways, I also want to pause to ask whether, as Schulman seems to believe, the political itself has disappeared along with the disappearance of ACT UP and so many of its members.

Cvetkovich, however, is preoccupied with presenting an affective history of ACT UP as a central case in her larger body of work on public feelings.[83] Although her work, like Schulman's, presents the transformation of politics and science brought about by ACT UP, she is equally, if not more, curious about the transformation of desire and the experience of loss that took place within ACT UP. For Cvetkovich, oral history has the radical potential to document not only the political achievements of ACT UP but also its failures and less direct effects: most acutely, the failure to save the lives of so many who died in the early years of the epidemic, in spite of AIDS activism, as well as the forms of love illness-thought-activism brought into being. Cvetkovich explains that oral history documents "lost histories and histories of loss," and she says her goal is "to use interviews to create political history as affective history, a history that captures activism's felt and even traumatic dimensions."[84] Cvetkovich is surprised to discover a gap between "ACT UP's professed reputation as a model for queer intimacies, and the actual practice, which involves a lot of secrecy."[85] She explains that in her interview with Zoe Leonard, one of Bordowitz's lesbian girlfriends, Leonard distinguishes between "oral history as witnessing and oral history as confessional, suggesting that the narrative of one's sexual life in ACT UP might be an important story of personal growth, but not necessarily one of public or collective significance."[86] Although I think Leonard is right that what matters is not the individual sexual relationships between gay men and lesbians that ACT UP spawned but the "larger picture of AIDS," I also think that we might understand doing queer love as a model of witnessing that combines the preoccupations of both Schulman and Cvetkovich and, indeed, that is preoccupied: preoccupied with doing politics and history and with the effective and affective dimensions of both.[87] By doing queer love through oral history, Schulman and Cvetkovich are digging deeply and listening attentively but also showing that things are historically contingent, as Foucault would describe his own method. Neither Schulman nor Cvetkovich offers a definitive history. Rather, both seek to counter the forgetting of the political and emotional complexity of the early years of AIDS activism in the United States and to remind us of the many ways the political relates to the emotional. Their work is meant to inspire further work to trace direct and indirect connections: between lesbians and gay men, between past and future struggles for self determination, between political protest and sexual desire, between being at a loss and doing queer love.

Echoes 3: From New York City 1989 to Durban, South Africa 2000

I conclude this chapter with a final echo and sign that doing queer love might be a model that can travel to other contexts. When we consider the ways that doing queer love as an affective and effective strategy for confronting AIDS might travel and be translated, we need to recall Scott's point that because echoes span gaps in space and time, they also create "gaps in meaning and intelligibility."[88] As Scott contends, these gaps are necessarily transformative, and as such they potentially produce new discourses, practices, and institutions. I want to listen again to Bordowitz, not this time as one of Schulman's interviewees in the ACT UP Oral History Project discussing the way ACT UP took up and transformed the strategies of other movements nor as the "lesbian boyfriend" also discussed in Cvetkovich's archive of the feelings of political activism but as an artist and activist involved with Testing the Limits, a collective of video artists formed in the spring of 1987 "to document emerging forms of activism developed in response to government inaction about the global AIDS epidemic."[89] In "Picture a Coalition," an early statement about the importance of this video work, Bordowitz writes: "People must be able to see themselves making history. People living with AIDS must be able to see themselves not as victims, but as self-empowered activists."[90] Bordowitz's 1988 essay ends with the repetition of the phrase "picture a coalition," which is a performative gesture that suggests how and why we must do queer love: "The most significant challenge to the movement is coalition building, because the AIDS epidemic has engendered a community of people who cannot afford *not* to recognize themselves as a community and to act as one."[91] The sense that people with AIDS must recognize themselves as a community and act as one was necessary in New York City in 1988, and it is still necessary today, in New York and beyond.

Bordowitz's later videos and writings continue to attempt to picture a coalition, in particular between New York in the 1980s and South Africa in the first decade of the twenty-first century. In the essay "More Operative Instructions," he describes the structure of his video *Habit* (2001), which is organized in three sections that "explore the themes of habit, foreignness, and intimacy."[92] Bordowitz first wants to show the distance between him, a relatively privileged person with AIDS (PWA) in the United States, and many PWAs in South Africa, who do not have access to the treatments that

Bordowitz has had access to but whom Bordowitz nonetheless refuses to represent as "victims."[93] One of the questions Bordowitz works through in *Habit* is, "How can people who exist across great divides of geography and resources have meaningful relationships? How can we join our efforts to address structural inequities implicit to global capitalism?"[94] Bordowitz demonstrates the concept of the echo and also does queer love as he attempts to bring into being just such a meaningful relationship across gaps of geography and materiality. This kind of relay work is what I want my project to do, too.

In his essay Bordowitz recalls being in South Africa at the Thirteenth International AIDS Conference in Durban in 2000 and feeling "nostalgia for the eighties activism of ACT UP."[95] Bordowitz describes his sense that he was reliving a moment from his past:

> In Durban there were 5,000 people wearing t-shirts with the words "HIV positive" boldly printed on their chests. I felt the urge to say, "Wow, this is 1989. This is just like 1989 was for us." Of course, that is enormously arrogant and not correct. I had to think that through and I realized that the African situation is singular. It has its own integrity, its own logic. Undeniably, there is a shared history of activism around the world, and at the same time there are unassimilable differences between situations of crisis. In South Africa the well-informed core leadership of TAC [The Treatment Action Campaign] has read Douglas Crimp's work. It has followed ACT UP's history. It has borrowed articulations and signage from all over the globe. Similarities were the first points of entry for me, but they do not yield the deepest understanding.[96]

New York City 1989 echoes forward in time to Durban 2000, but Durban 2000 is not a reproduction of the same, of that earlier time and place. Similarities might be points of entry, but differences are routes to some place new. The leaders of TAC read Crimp and know the history of ACT UP, but they transform that history and theory in a different time and place. How is it that "here" might speak to "there" across gaps of time and space? In *Habit* Bordowitz proposes that "the reconciliation of habit and foreignness is intimacy" and that the "substance of intimacy is love."[97] For Bordowitz, "we can overcome great divisions through chosen affiliations."[98] In his presentation of the relationship between habit, foreignness, and intimacy in *Habit* and in "More Operative Instructions," Bordowitz demonstrates what I describe here as doing queer love. Doing queer love is a method that asks, to paraphrase Foucault, "What relations, through illness and health activism, can be established, invented, multiplied, and modulated?" Doing queer love provides a model for overcoming divisions through chosen affiliations, between lesbians and gay men, between AIDS activists in New York and South Africa, between the very precise moment of 1989 and the very precise moment of 2000.

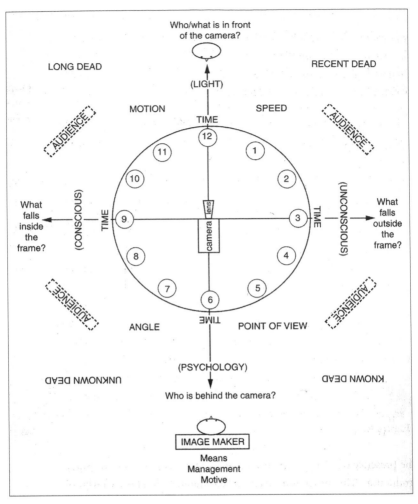

Figure 1. I am drawn to the image's diagrammatic form, the complexity and multiplicity of its components, and Bordowitz's declared hope for what it might do, as I make my own attempt to enumerate some of the forces in play among the dynamic set of relations between illness, thought, and activism in time and place. Gregg Bordowitz, The Order of Image Production, 2003. Reprinted by permission of the artist.

Gregg Bordowitz's *The Order of Image Production* (2003) and "Queer Structures of Feeling" (1993)

As noted in chapter 1, Gregg Bordowitz is one of several key relay figures I take as objects of my analysis in *Indirect Action*. As with the concept of the echo, the concept of the relay works to both link and separate forms of thought and activism across different spaces and times. Bordowitz is one example of such a figure because all of his work explores the complex relations between the experiences and events of illness and new forms of thought, art, and activism. The image/word assemblage that serves as my first snapshot combines a diagram designed by Bordowitz, *The Order of Image Production* (Figure 1), with an analysis of a concept and practice Bordowitz calls "queer structures of feeling." Although they both appear in the same collection of his writing, *The AIDS Crisis Is Ridiculous,* a text I take up in chapter 1, Bordowitz doesn't relate the diagram and concept directly to each other. I do so here by literally and figuratively connecting them via a brief discussion of Bordowitz's fantasy of lineage, a desire for a connection with Ridiculous Theater playwright, actor, and impresario Charles Ludlam. By assembling these materials, I want this opening snapshot, on the one hand, to provide a microcosm of the method and materials of the larger project and, on the other, to demonstrate how the snapshots themselves function as relays in my overall project of historicizing illness, thought, and activism in the period before and after the emergence of AIDS.

Bordowitz himself uses the term "snapshot" to describe the image he has composed to capture *The Order of Image Production.* He says it is "a snapshot of a constantly moving phenomenon. A useful picture, it enumerates the forces in play among a dynamic set of relations."[1] I am drawn to the image's diagrammatic form, the complexity and multiplicity of its components (light, motion, time, speed, angle, point of view, image maker, psychology, audience, the long and recent, known and unknown dead, etc.), and Bordowitz's declared hope for what it might do as I make my own attempt to enumerate some of the forces in play among the dynamic set of relations between illness, thought, and activism in time and place. The majority of images in *The AIDS Crisis Is Ridiculous* are of AIDS activists participating in direct action politics, as documented in Bordowitz's work with the AIDS activist video collectives (Testing the Limits and DIVA TV) and in his own filmmaking. There are also images from the work of others, including from feminist artist/activists Zoe Leonard, Martha Rosler, and Yvonne Rainer, as Bordowitz does that rare thing for a male artist: connecting his work to the work of women artists. The schematic image of image production is placed in the middle of the final essay, "More Operative Assumptions," from 2003, which also includes diagrams of the structures of two of Bordowitz's films, *Fast Trip, Long Drop* (1993) and *Habit* (2001). *The Order of Image Production* is a metadiagram that attempts to locate visually all of the aspects of image production. In a note Bordowitz writes that the "method used to draw this figure was derived from" Susan Buck-Morss's *The Dialectics of Seeing*, a text that itself seeks to diagram the complexity of Walter Benjamin's thought on the image and image production. Bordowitz's diagrams hint at a desire to find a way to freeze the complexity—structural, technical, emotional, political—of artist/activist work. In "More Operative Assumptions," Bordowitz surrounds the image of *The Order of Image Production* with words that further explain the diagram and its components, extending the analysis in a verbal unfreezing of the complexity of this "snapshot of a constantly moving phenomenon."[2]

This dual (some might say dialectical) process of freezing and unfreezing complexity operates throughout Bordowitz's work. In *The AIDS Crisis Is Ridiculous*, written some ten years before "More Operative Assumptions,"[3] Bordowitz pays tribute to queer theater icon Ludlam and his Ridiculous Theater Company. That essay opens with epigraphs from Ludlam and Gertrude Stein, creating a very queer, ridiculous even, coupling meant to suggest other, less direct, historical and creative lineages for Bordowitz's work in particular and for AIDS activist art more generally. The first epigraph is Ludlam's "Manifesto: Ridiculous Theater; Scourge of Human Folly," quoted in its entirety, including its aim ("to get beyond nihilism by revaluing combat"), seven axioms (for example, "The theater is an event not an object"), and "instructions for use" (for example, "Treat the material in a madly farcical manner without losing the seriousness of the theme").[4] The second epigraph is a quotation from Stein's "Composition as Explanation," which makes the rather obvious but important point that ways of seeing, doing, and making differ from one time to another. The process of explaining for Stein is, then, always already historical, a process of composing something anew in time. Here again, in the quotation from Stein used in Bordowitz, we have another example of echo as method-image: each explanation is a failed reproduction of the same, echoing incompletely and indirectly across generations.

These epigraphs are followed by Bordowitz's own narrative of a kind of reproduction in the section "Fantasy about a Father," which begins with a reference to Ludlam's death of AIDS on Friday, May 29, 1987, in New York City. Despite never having met Ludlam or seen him perform, Bordowitz feels this loss to queer community personally. He mourns Ludlam by fantasizing about a sexual and artistic connection with him: "This is a fantasy about lineage. I desire a link with Ludlam, a link with the past, a place in history. There must be some continuity between our lives, and if not our lives, the history and the forces that have shaped them."[5] Later, Bordowitz admits that the intimate relation he is trying to engender between Ludlam's theater work and activist video work is "implausible," and yet Bordowitz conceives of the relation "with Ludlam within what can be described as a psycho-geographic proximity. We exist in the same place at different times."[6] Through his "fantasy about lineage" and desired links—a fantasized fantasy echo, doubling Scott's phrase—Bordowitz provides me with another method-image for my project of historicizing illness, thought, and activism in the period just before and just after AIDS arrives in the United States.

Bordowitz shifts from his fantasy about lineage to a section in his essay entitled "Queer Structures of Feeling," in which he utilizes Raymond Williams's concept of structures of feeling to argue that "there are counter cultural strategies that belong specifically to queers. A queer structure of feeling shapes cultural work produced by queers."[7] Bordowitz contends that although these strategies are practiced by and for queers, they are not or not only about sex but rather can be used to reveal the material conditions of the production of events—artistic and political.[8] In his genealogy of queer structures of feeling, then, Bordowitz links contemporary AIDS activist video to queer theater of the seventies through a shared engagement with the ridiculous. The ridiculous is an echo of a camp sensibility, and Bordowitz argues that such a sensibility is brought forth into AIDS activism. At the same time, something else is at work. He notes that the experience of AIDS in queer communities, inflected as it is by the failure of the U.S. government to respond adequately to the devastation, has meant that the videos are "produced in a dialogue with the social movements to end government inaction. The documentation of protests is one form of direct action; distributions of these tapes are demonstrations."[9] Along with the ridiculous, then, documentation, direct action, and demonstration all fit under the rubric Bordowitz calls "queer structures of feeling."

I would argue, however, that this queer modification of the concept reduces rather than expands its uses. As with the freezing of the image of the order of image production, this may be a necessary reduction of a concept's complexity to make it useful in a time of crisis. "Structures of feeling" is, of course, probably the most well-known and taken-up concept from Williams, and it might be said to be one of the key keywords[10] in the emergence of the interdisciplinary field of cultural studies, which Williams helped to bring into being in the period just before AIDS. Through this concept and his articulation of it,[11] Williams wants to think about how cultural productions (for Williams, most particularly, literature) capture forming and formative processes without making them into formed wholes.[12] How do we grasp something as it is forming, not once it is already formed? By making the concept explicitly queer, Bordowitz would seem to overly concretize it into an already-formed identity mold, even if queer itself is a forming or re-forming concept in the moment Bordowitz is writing. This concretizing is apparent when Bordowitz discusses two factors in the formation of a specifically queer structure of feeling: "how heterosexist oppression attempts to contain queer sexualities, and how queers fight oppression by forming communities." He goes on to explain that "a queer structure of feeling is a set of cultural strategies of survival for queers. It is marked by an appreciation for the ridiculous, and it values masquerade. Mockery is its form; posing is its strategy."[13] Although the ridiculous, masquerade, mockery, and posing might be aspects of a structure of feeling, there is nonetheless, in Bordowitz's overdetermined definition, a problem of temporality: he condenses the present with the past and collapses emergent feelings into specific survival strategies. This is the emergency time of crisis not the emergent time of prehistory.

By turning a structure of feeling into a strategy, Bordowitz overinstrumentalizes the term and the cultural work it does. In doing so, he would seem to demonstrate, unwittingly, what Williams describes as "the basic error" of much materialist analysis: "the reduction of the social to fixed forms."[14] In Williams's attempt to delineate the concept, he notes that it is meant to suggest a "social experience which is still in *process*, often indeed not yet recognized as social but taken to be private, idiosyncratic, and even isolating."[15] In some sense, then, all structures of feeling are a little queer— that is, "out of sorts; unwell; faint, giddy," as in one of the definitions of the word in the *OED*. This is not so much *queer* as a category of identity or as political consciousness ("We're here. We're queer. Get used to it.") but *queer* as ill feeling.

If I take his definition of the concept "queer structures of feeling" as overdetermined and overdetermining, I think we can nonetheless discern structures of feeling in Bordowitz's own writing. We don't necessarily find these in the direct action strategies of the production and distribution of AIDS activist video, important as these strategies most certainly were in the early days of the epidemic and as documents that help us to historicize that moment in the present.[16] Rather, we find them in the many indirect actions described in Bordowitz's less polemical writings, like "Boat Trip" and "Dense Moments," which are concerned with the affective experience of living with an emergent illness and the embryonic practical consciousness that attempts to make sense of a crisis as it is taking shape. One example from "Boat Trip" will illuminate the distinction I am making between a survival strategy and a structure of feeling. "Boat Trip" is a diary-like record of a vacation to the Virgin Islands that Bordowitz took in 1992 with five other members of his HIV support group: David Barr, Spencer Cox, Mark Harrington, Derek Link, and Peter Staley,[17] all of whom would become key players in the Treatment Action Group (TAG) that would spin off from ACT UP in 1992, the same year as the boat trip. This significant development in the history of AIDS activism and of health activism more generally makes only a fleeting appearance in Bordowitz's account of the trip as a conversation among them in which "each gave his version of what went wrong with the AIDS movement."[18] In a brief introduction to the piece, written ten years afterward for the publication of his collected writings, Bordowitz notes that "the group was an extraordinary example of self-care emerging out of the democratic principles and methods of our activism" and that it was formed to address "fears about death and to lay the groundwork for the future when each of us would die."[19] "Boat Trip," then, is a story of a group engaged in self-care not, or not only, treatment activism.

The timing of the trip is bittersweet: the group sets off from New York on November 9, the second anniversary of the death of Ray Navarro, an active member of ACT UP, cofounder of DIVA TV, and Bordowitz's "very dear friend." Still, Bordowitz describes the trip, hopefully, as a "new line of flight toward something living rather than away from something dead."[20] Onboard the boat, far from the epidemic's epicenter in New York, Bordowitz comes to understand something about HIV/AIDS when he sees the same rash he has on the bodies of two of his traveling companions. He writes:

> My doctor told me that the rash on my arms and back is caused by my infection. I never believed that HIV was the cause, until now. The fact that each of us is infected with the same kind of virus is astonishing. My awareness of this fact is unconsciously mediated, managed, so that the full emotional weight doesn't register. I feel embarrassment when my denial is momentarily revealed to me. The sad reason for our group's existence is made present to my mind.[21]

What is revealed to Bordowitz in this moment of seeing a likeness of his rash on the backs of his fellow boaters is that he would not be in this place with this group of people if not for the illness they share. Although he wants them to be more and different to each other than simply a support group, what he will discover on the boat trip is that such relations between them may no longer be possible, and it is this realization that makes him both sad and desirous of more. What Bordowitz captures in this image of shared illness is not quite or yet about "how heterosexist oppression attempts to contain queer sexualities, and how queers fight oppression by forming communities." Rather, it is about embarrassment, sadness, and unease about relations in the present moment and yet also about hopefulness for the future: a structure of feeling rather than a fully realized strategy for surviving AIDS.

Bordowitz ends his brief introduction of the piece with the following simple statement: "All the members of the group are still alive."[22] Less than ten years later, this statement would no longer be true. In December 2012, twenty years after the boat trip and the formation of the Treatment Action Group and shortly after the release of the documentary *How to Survive a Plague,* which features all the members of Bordowitz's support group as key players in the struggle against AIDS and which I will discuss at greater length in my conclusion, Spencer Cox would die of AIDS-related causes at the age of forty-four. In an article for the *New York Times* entitled "Surviving AIDS, but Not the Life That Followed," Jacob Bernstein discusses the shock and grief that many fellow AIDS activists felt when they learned that Cox most likely died because he stopped taking the drugs that he had fought so hard to make available and had also acquired a destructive crystal methamphetamine habit. Bernstein notes that many questions arose among activists in the aftermath of Cox's death about "pill fatigue" and noncompliance and about the debilitating and disfiguring side effects of the drugs.[23] In another article about Cox's death, John Voelcker, who worked with Cox in ACT UP and cofounded the Medius Institute at the Gay Men's Health Crisis with him, argues that Cox was prescient about the need to "look in a cross-disciplinary way at all the factors affecting the physical, mental and emotional health of a set of men who had lived through the AIDS epidemic, come out the other side and were too often doing startling, illogical and very dangerous things."[24] I end this first snapshot with a glimpse of the shadow cast by the recent death of Spencer Cox in order that this image of future illness remains inside the frame of this project as I trace back to the period before AIDS.

2

Que(e)rying the Clinic, circa 1970

In "AIDS, Activism, and the Politics of Health" for the Sounding Board section of the *New England Journal of Medicine* published in January 1992, Robert M. Wachter, at that time professor of medicine at the University of California in San Francisco and a frequent commentator on health policy, begins his look at the impact of AIDS activism on health policy and on movements fighting other diseases by looking back at the "roots of AIDS activism."[1] Wachter's narrative relies heavily on what I discuss in chapter 1 as the "origin story of AIDS activism," a story repeated so frequently it is now the de facto "authorized" version. This origin story of AIDS activism provides a neat and tidy narrative arc: a period of passivity—what Wachter calls "a tragic period of hesitation"—is replaced, finally if belatedly, by activism with the founding of the AIDS Coalition to Unleash Power (ACT UP) in 1987.[2] The passivity-to-activism narrative arc can be discerned even in the way Wachter formulates one of his article's key questions: "What are the roots of AIDS activism, and why was the epidemic six years old before the movement crystallized?"—as if social movements have a normal period and manner of gestation.[3]

Wachter acknowledges in the opening paragraph that "trends toward empowering patients and questioning scientific expertise antedated" the AIDS epidemic, noting increasing patient involvement in health care organizations and policy decision making from the late 1960s and an even longer tradition of advocacy by charitable groups devoted to raising money and awareness to fight particular diseases and counter the stigma often associated with them.[4] Still, for Wachter AIDS activism brought something qualitatively different to "the health care scene"—"a jarring new dimension to what was previously a genteel dialogue between patient advocates and clinicians, researchers, and policy makers."[5] As I will show in this chapter, Wachter's memory of a "genteel dialogue" covers over a much more contentious—and queerer—challenge to the discourses, practices, and institutions of medicine by feminist and community mental health activists, among others, in the period immediately prior to the emergence of AIDS.

I begin with Wachter's discussion of the emergence of AIDS activism in the *New England Journal of Medicine* to provide an image of how medicine sees itself before and after the arrival of AIDS. In Wachter's account, written primarily for a medical audience, just ten years into the epidemic and five years after the emergence of ACT UP, what has already crystallized is a memory of AIDS and the early response to it founded on a forgetting of an other-than-genteel activism around health during the two decades prior to the arrival of AIDS. Wachter does mention the modern gay liberation movement, whose origin he dates, as many historians do, to 1969 and the riots at the Stonewall Inn in New York City, and he also states quite explicitly that AIDS activism "evolved directly" from gay liberation. In Wachter's account, however, this particular lineage proves more detrimental than beneficial to the queer species when AIDS arrives. According to Wachter, the emphasis on sexual freedom in the 1970s "had two disastrous consequences when a new virus entered the gay community in the late 1970s": the first consequence was that "the promiscuity in the community facilitated the rapid spread of the new sexually transmitted pathogen," and the second was that many in the gay community were unwilling to change their sexual behavior and, relatedly, were uninterested in "political militancy," presumably because they were distracted by sex.[6] The gay liberation movement of the 1960s and 1970s, as well as its challenges to intimate, social, and political relations, is not then a resource for AIDS activists, in Wachter's formulation, but a stage that had to be and, thankfully, was outgrown. For Wachter gay liberation was a kind of prepolitical adolescence preceding the political maturation that came with the sobering experience of AIDS and the activism that eventually emerged from this experience.

In his analysis Wachter also suggests that sexuality is a domain separate from politics and that the struggle for sexual liberation is wholly personal and not political. Wachter's analysis fits into a general rhetoric of depoliticization—or, we might say, neoliberalization—of personal experience that gained momentum in the 1990s in a climate of increased deregulation and privatization under Reagan in the United States and Thatcher in the United Kingdom. Already in Cindy Patton's work from the late 1980s "The AIDS Service Industry," we see an awareness and analysis of diverse models for responding to AIDS within the gay community and beyond in the early years of the epidemic, as well as a concern with what she calls "the political economy of AIDS work."[7] This is to reiterate the historical point I made in the introduction and chapter 1 that Patton was worrying, around 1990, about complicating the history of the response to AIDS because a reductive cultural memory of AIDS was already beginning to sediment. I take Wachter's account as emblematic of this problem. As I showed in my discussion of doing queer love in chapter 1 and will show in my discussion of feminist self-help clinics, interpretations of the feminist practice of "personal politics,"[8] a condensation of the phrase "the personal is political," have changed since the 1970s and are now most frequently used to describe an individual rather than a structural critique. My point is that AIDS activism was hardly unprecedented in its militant personal politics in general and sexual politics in particular, and yet this is not the story that tends to get told. While certain sexual practices (rather than promiscuity) facilitated the spread of AIDS in the gay community and, of course, other communities, other sexual practices invented in the gay community, like safe and safer sex, also very quickly facilitated a response to AIDS that would in time successfully slow the spread of the disease in and beyond the gay community.[9]

Queer Clinics

In order to uncover some of the forgetting that an analysis like Wachter's enacts, I am interested in attempting to discern some of the underlying—or preexisting—conditions in medicine and politics in the period before AIDS. While I am sympathetic to a desire to understand AIDS as representing a rupture in the practice of both medicine and queer politics, as well as in the everyday affective experiences of gay community formations, I want to resist this interpretation by thinking more about what gets brought forward into AIDS activism from the health movements of the 1960s and 1970s and what doesn't. Or we might ask, echoing and extending a question Julian Bourg asks about the ethical and political legacies of May 1968 in France, what aspects of the social movements of the 1960s and 1970s did and did not make it into the 1980s?[10]

The clinic is one place to look to help discern the "present field of possible experiences of medicine" and the interconnectedness between illness, thought, and activism in a particular historical moment. In her introduction to a recent collection of essays that revisits Foucault's *Birth of the Clinic* as a jumping-off point for a variety of ethnographic and historical treatments of "the clinic," Patton provides a genealogy of sorts of Foucault's own thought, suggesting the importance of the clinic to his later disciplinary and biopolitical formulations:

> Before Foucault treats the research-science disciplines of biology, economics, and linguistics (as he does in *The Order of Things*), he launches his argument about the emergence of modernity in the messy, deeply experiential space installed *by* and *as* "the clinic." Fifteen years before Foucault describes the panopticon and its extension as the carceral society, he elaborates "the clinic" and its extension as a relationship between science and people, between medical practitioners and patients, and between all of these elements and the state.[11]

In this spirit, in this chapter I want to offer my own treatment of "the clinic" in time, in particular by thinking about how the clinic—as concept and space—might be que(e)ried, that is, both questioned and made queer. I present two historical case studies that might be said to queer clinical thought and practices in the period before AIDS and, for that matter, before the full-blown arrival of queer theory on the Western theoretical landscape.[12] These two cases—the practice of self-help developed in and beyond the women's health movement in the United States and the practice of transversality developed in and beyond the institutional psychiatry movement in France—challenge the practice of medicine in the prehistory of both AIDS and queer theory, yet as Wachter's history of AIDS activism demonstrates, they are not generally seen as precursors, or related in any way, to AIDS activism. In a sense, then, I also want to question and make queer the history of AIDS as we conventionally know it today by extending that history backward and outward to earlier queer critical and clinical practices, including especially, though not exclusively, self-help and transversality.

Self-Help

A glaring omission from Wachter's presentation of the roots of AIDS activism is his failure to mention the importance of the women's health movement in transforming medicine in the 1960s and 1970s. Such an omission is clearly necessary to sustain the portrait of a pre-AIDS "genteel dialogue between patient advocates and clinicians, researchers, and policy makers." In Wachter's essay feminists do appear, but only belatedly in the section "Does the Model of AIDS Activism Apply to Other Diseases?," in which he describes the potential influence of AIDS activism on breast cancer activism. Here, Wachter connects the emergent breast cancer lobby of the 1990s to "the earlier development of the feminist movement, which had been urging women for years to take control of medical decisions affecting their bodies."[13] In Wachter's genealogy AIDS activism and feminist activism precede the organization of a potent breast cancer lobby, but there is seemingly no connection between health feminism and AIDS activism, and relatedly, the earlier feminist impact appears to be solely on individual women and their bodies and not on medicine more broadly.

I realize that my close reading of Wachter's genealogy may seem like little more than semantic quibbling or may appear to privilege a now little-read piece that presents bad history by a doctor who is neither a scholar nor an activist, but I contend that Wachter's history of health activism is a useful example of a long tradition of trivializing women's complaints, personal and political, in medicine in general and in medical journals like the New England Journal of Medicine in particular. As Wachter's essay also demonstrates, the forgetting of feminist activism in and on medicine before AIDS will echo a forgetting of feminist health activism after AIDS, as I have already shown in chapter 1. The process of forgetting is not simply an absence of a memory of activism in part or in whole but has political effects that echo beyond the moment of activism and its forgetting. I try to unfold this process in the text of Indirect Action by returning not just to memories of activism but also to repeated forgettings. Wachter's forgetting has repercussions, and I think these repercussions are apparent in the later forgetting of Pius Kamau and of the commenter on the women's studies listserv I discuss in chapter 1. My point is not that we can finally now remember all that has been forgotten but that we must try to account for the how of remembering and forgetting by discerning both the diversity and the range, the ecological breadth and historical depth, of the prehistory of AIDS.

Perhaps not surprisingly, the women's liberation movement is mentioned only very occasionally in the pages of the New England Journal of Medicine, and the women's health movement is mentioned even less frequently.[14] Two articles, one published in late 1974 and the other in early 1975, however, do take seriously the attempts by health feminists to transform medicine. The first is the text of a talk given by Mary C. Howell, a physician and associate dean for student affairs at Harvard Medical School, at the Harvard Medical School Alumni Day in 1974 on a panel entitled "What It's Been Like," to celebrate the twenty-fifth reunion of the first Harvard Medical School class to include women. The second is a contribution from Howard M. Spiro of the Yale School of Medicine to the Visceral Viewpoints section entitled "Myths and Mirths: Women in Medicine."[15] I point briefly to these articles to show how feminists figure in the *Journal*, which exemplifies how they figure in medicine more generally, before I take up the self-help clinic as one feminist remedy for the unsatisfactory treatment of women in and by medicine.

The page that includes the first half of Howell's article for the Sounding Board section of the *Journal* tells us just about everything we need to know about how women figure in medicine. The page begins with a direct quotation from an interview with Dr. Estelle Ramey in *Perspectives in Biology and Medicine* from 1971, which Franz J. Ingelfinger, longtime *Journal* editor, uses to introduce his own editorial, titled "Doctor Women," in which Ramey notes, "Cultural biases never change rapidly. Stereotypes are bred in the bone of a society and the stereotype of a woman doctor is a horse-faced, flat-chested female in supphose [support hose] who sublimates her sex starvation in a passionate embrace of the *New England Journal of Medicine*."[16] Ingelfinger identifies Dr. Ramey as a professor of physiology at Georgetown and an "articulate feminist" who "helped to harry off the market that textbook which illustrated anatomy with Playboy-type bodies."[17] With this auspicious opening, Ingelfinger offers a statement of support for women in medicine and even challenges those damaging stereotypes that suggest intelligent women are not attractive by noting that the four "married ladies with M.D. degree" who participated in the Harvard Medical School Alumni Day program were "handsome in countenance, dressed with elegant simplicity, far from shapeless."[18] We might call this a rhetorical form of supphose, *New England Journal of Medicine* style!

Ingelfinger explains that three of the four speakers, including Howell, discussed the difficulties they had encountered in being "recognized as professionals no different from their male counterparts, that they should be thought of as doctors, not women doctors."[19] Ingelfinger admits, however, to favoring the presentation style and approach of the final speaker, a Mrs. Garrison, a fellow in psychiatry at the McLean Hospital, who had anticipated a more informal discussion and so, as Ingelfinger tells it, "spoke in simple, unrehearsed words." In contrast to the overly earnest and prepared equality feminist arguments of her three fellow panelists, Garrison offers what we would now call a difference feminist argument in a different, less threatening manner: women are "different in their spiritual, attitudinal and emotional make-up" from men, but these "feminine traits" make them better doctors than men. And oh so much more appealing to Ingelfinger or, as he identifies himself, "this unregenerate and perhaps porcine bearer of the Y—chromosomally rather than collegiately speaking."[20] I know, I know—"unregenerate" and "porcine" attitudes are not particularly remarkable for an old guy writing in the *Journal* in 1974. I point them out not simply to take a cheap shot at Ingelfinger, one of the most influential voices in the *Journal*'s history. What is remarkable about Ingelfinger's editorial, even today, is the masterful way it personalizes a structural problem. I can picture him crossing his legs as he is forced to listen to Mary Howell and her ilk complain about not being treated like men (taking themselves and each other so seriously), and I can feel his relief when Mrs. Garrison offers a prettier picture—literally and figuratively—of women in medicine.

If, consciously or not, Ingelfinger sought to undermine Howell even before she began, his editorial becomes a perfect example of the problem Howell seeks to understand. Her article is a fascinating assessment of the practices of professionalization and what she argues are mostly unconscious habits of discrimination against women in the field of medicine. Sounding almost Erving Goffman–esque, Howell begins:

> The process of professionalization includes learning attitudes about work, about relations with colleagues, and about patients or clients. Along with the learning of information and skills, the adoption of these "approved" attitudes brings the novitiate into full membership in a profession. In medicine, as undoubtedly in every profession in society, these attitudes are strongly colored by a demeaning regard for women. How could it be otherwise? In the first place, such attitudes about women are pervasive in society, and, secondly, the medical profession has been virtually a male province.[21]

Howell utilizes interviews with women medical students to diagnose the treatment of both women patients and women physicians in training, and despite many advances by women in medicine since the time of Howell's article, these comments still resonate today. For example, one informant tells Howell that she had been told by a surgeon that "a 25-year-old female with abdominal pain was *by definition* an 'unrealiable historian.'"[22] Again, in Howell's analysis discrimination is not, or not only, about personal behavior but, more importantly, about structures that exclude women from spaces of learning, including, for example, "the discussion-review of a surgical procedure" in the men's dressing room after surgery.[23] The women's liberation movement is mentioned at the end of Howell's article in a section on possible remedies to the problem of discrimination against women in medicine. Howell highlights two positive effects of the women's liberation movement: changes to the law brought through implementation of Title IX of the Higher Education Amendments of 1972 and changes to attitudes of both doctors and patients as a result of the women's health movement.[24]

Whereas Howell ends with the effects of the women's liberation movement on medicine and the law, Spiro begins there: "Of all the revolutions of the past few years, the one that seems most likely to have the longest life is that in sex, simply because people have a vested or, as appropriately, a 'bloused' interest. 'Women's lib' in medicine bids fair to be as permanent as any revolution can be."[25] What follows is a sympathetic assessment of the difficulties for women in medicine and an even-handed approach to the complex relationship between biology, psychology, and culture, an approach that allows Spiro to arrive at sensible assertions like this one, which echoes somewhat the difference feminism of Mrs. Garrison and preferred by Ingelfinger, though with perhaps more nuance and less romanticism: "Regardless of whether they are culturally or biologically determined and regardless of whether society is mistaken in calling them womanly virtues, what are generally seen as psychic characteristics of women should be just what American medicine needs at present."[26] Yet although Spiro expresses unequivocal support for "women's lib," the portrait of women's lib, nonetheless, relies on what in 1975 were already well-worn clichés, including that it is a movement "occasionally shriller than it need be" and that it "sometimes has a relentlessness that excludes humor."[27] And so Spiro ends with this rather bizarre hope: that "women will laugh at jokes men make about women, or even that men physicians will laugh at the jokes women doctors make about men patients," which makes me wonder whether there will ever be any jokes about men physicians to laugh at.[28] I point to Spiro's trivial conclusion to an otherwise serious take-up of women's liberation to suggest some of the reasons that, by 1992, the feminist challenge to medicine had been largely forgotten as a precursor to AIDS activism. At the risk of sounding like a shrill person who can't take a joke, it seems important to point out that such people are not generally perceived as having a positive impact on others, and for women the impact—or perceived impact—on others is always key.

Although not mentioned in the *Journal,* feminist self-help clinics were up and running at the time of these articles, created across the United States beginning in the early 1970s as a structural response, of the sort Howell's interviewees sought, to the problem of the absolute authority of doctors, the objectification of women's bodies in health care, and the increasing specialization, technologization, and dehumanization of medicine, touched on in chapter 1 in my discussion of Dreifus's *Seizing Our Bodies.*[29] In some instances the clinics created were formal institutional spaces with permanent staff and funding, as in the case of the network of Feminist Women's Health Centers, while in other instances these clinics were more informal and transient spaces for consciousness raising around issues relating to women's often negative experiences of their bodies and the institution of health care. As Michelle Murphy notes in her discussion of early feminist self-help practices in Los Angeles, "*Self help clinic* was the official term used for events—not places," a point that resonates with my own description of illness as a multiplicity of experiences and events.[30] Some informal groups eventually became more formal, like the Boston Women's Health Book Collective, which began as a consciousness raising group but would become increasingly influential with the publication of *Our Bodies, Ourselves,* the most widely read articulation of the theories and practices of feminist self-help.[31] What happens when the collective becomes co-opted into mainstream institutional forms? Do vestiges of older practices of politics and medicine remain?

In a typical statement promoting the practices of self help, the pamphlet *A Self-Help Manual for Women,* jointly authored by Louise Marshall, Valerie Vogel, and Aida Bogas in 1978, introduces the concept in this way, using "self-health" and "self-help" interchangeably:

Self-health, in its broadest sense, means people educating themselves about their bodies and taking responsibility for their own health care. To us (as well as many other members of the women's health movement) self-help means groups of women getting together to share knowledge, to do research, to physically examine themselves for health maintenance, and to support each other. A self-help group can be any number of women of any age who are committed to working together, and to enjoying the excitement and power which comes with knowledge and self-awareness.[32]

The authors explicitly link the practices of self-help to the political transformation of women that began in the United States in the 1960s, and importantly and somewhat paradoxically, they explain that *self*-help is practiced most effectively in a group. Through group work on their selves and bodies, women created a critical and clinical method that challenged the exercise of medical sovereignty.[33] The state and medicine took this challenge seriously, calling into question the legitimacy of those leading the self-help workshops and founding the self-help clinics. In several celebrated cases the women leading the movement were arrested for practicing medicine without a license—that is, they were arrested for being, in the eyes of medicine and the law, medical pretenders.

In an article in the *Medical Tribune* from 1973, Carol Downer, who founded the Feminist Women's Health Center in Los Angeles and was one of the women arrested for practicing medicine without a license, is quoted as stating, matter-of-factly, "Physicians have not yet realized how angry women are about the treatment they've been getting and that we are working to change the situation."[34] This assessment seems to be confirmed by the lack of coverage of the women's health movement and its critique of and challenge to the conventional practice of medicine in the *New England Journal of Medicine.* The short article in the *Medical Tribune* ends with a comment from Dr. Mary E. Costanza, who is identified as an instructor in medicine at Tufts University Medical School and as "herself active in a woman's self-help group." Because her identity seems to bridge the binary established in the article's title, "Physicians and Feminist Patients: Conflict Grows," her comments can be taken as at once sympathetic and authoritative, giving greater credence to her ultimate dismissal of the possibility of change coming to medicine from the outside.[35] Dr. Costanza notes that self-help groups are useful in "making people aware of better kinds of communication between patients and professionals" and that "what is learned will be incorporated into existing institutions." Nonetheless, she believes the medical usefulness of self-help groups is limited because they "aren't funded, and depending on volunteers to provide comprehensive medical care is a pipe dream."[36] With the assurance of an impeccable professional logic, Costanza describes a powerful dynamic through which medical sovereignty is maintained and even extended through a dual process of both delegitimation and incorporation of alternative practices of health. This comment also echoes forward to the point made by Sarah Schulman, Maxine Wolfe, and other feminist AIDS activists that what changed with AIDS activism was the combining of the economic power and sense of entitlement of gay men with the political know-how of lesbians and feminists.

Precisely this kind of professional logic is challenged in handouts from self-help clinics, in which women are addressed as practitioners and given step-by-step instructions on how to do a particular medical examination or procedure. The handout *How to Do a Pelvic Examination* from 1976, for example, is addressed to the woman doing the exam in the hope that a new approach will make the experience better—less traumatic, for the examiner as well as the woman being examined. The handout encourages a relaxed attitude and pedagogical approach; the examination becomes an opportunity for teaching and learning to happen across the practitioner/patient binary.[37] The reduction of trauma and its psychologically and physiologically damaging effects is key to a successful exam.

Many of the pamphlets advocating the self-help clinic as a practice of health point to the joy and wonder many women felt in discovering new knowledge about their bodies and themselves. The new knowledge is important, but so too is the "transmission of affects"—both positive and negative—that happens in these clinics.[38] It is through the facilitation of the transmission of affect between and among women that we might consider the feminist self-help clinics as queer. Adapting Foucault's "two great procedures for producing the truth of sex"—*ars erotica* and *scientia sexualis*—I want to think about a clinical *ars erotica* as a practice that contrasts with a clinical *scientia medicalis*, or put slightly differently, we might say the clinic is a domain where these two procedures for producing the truth of health are brought together and sometimes into conflict through different clinical practices, despite the fact that the increasing hegemony in the twenty-first century of a clinical *scientia medicalis*, in which laboratory tests and imaging technologies predominate, can hardly be disputed, a point I will make with regards to articulations of generalist and ecological counternarratives in chapters 3 and 4.[39]

In a newsletter from 1972 entitled *The Self Help Clinic*, Colette Price describes what I consider a kind of queer clinical *ars erotica* of the self-help clinic:

For all practical purposes, men have probably had more intimate contact with, and certainly far greater accessibility to the vagina than women ever had. The male organ, on the other hand, has always been exposed. The male organ, you see, is external and we really do seem to feel that seeing is believing. Thanks to the (Women's Liberation) Self-Help Clinic of Los Angeles, however, the same possibilities are now available to women.[40]

Likewise, the handout *How to Do a Pelvic Examination* encourages the practitioner to help her patient see her own body as part of the examination because, as the handout intones in quasi-romantic though hardly heteronormative language, "it is a really exciting experience to see one's cervix and vagina, especially for the first time."[41] For Price and other self-help practitioners, the vaginal speculum becomes a technology of the self, allowing women to get "in touch" with themselves by viewing their own vaginas. Looking at the self intimately becomes a way of deobjectifying the self because this process of looking happens in a group of women and creates both a public health and a public sexuality. Or put another way, a public is created in the practice of looking at one's body in a group of other women also looking at their bodies and in the feelings of excitement produced as a result of this intimate—yet public—activity.[42]

Price and others, however, acknowledge one criticism of the practices of self-help: they displace a structural analysis with a potentially solipsistic focus on the individual and advocate a "do-it-yourselfism" that encourages, first and foremost, greater consumption of health care.[43] On the one hand, I think it is clear that feminist health activism in general and the practices of self-help in particular effectively challenged medical sovereignty and influenced from the outside some of the key transformations occurring within medicine in the 1970s, including the formation of the new subfields of family practice, bioethics, and medical humanities. On the other hand, I also contend that health feminism's initial challenge ends up in many ways extending medicine's biopolitical and sovereign modes of power, as medicine appropriates one of health feminism's key tenets—that our relationship to our bodies and health must be an active, even vigilant one. What happens when a collective vigilance becomes a personal vigilance—or we might say, what happens when the self-help book replaces the health collective? The active, or activist, patient—or what I called the "politicized patient" in *Treatments*—morphs in the 1990s and 2000s into the consuming patient, who is most adept at negotiating the seemingly limitless choices of Healthcare, Inc.

In her analysis of the transformations and travels of the self-help manual *Our Bodies, Ourselves* (*OBOS*), Kathy Davis diagnoses a "shift in how knowledge and feminist knowledge practices are viewed in *OBOS*," leading to an assumption, in later editions of the feminist classic, that women are "first and foremost, 'informed consumers.'"[44] We can also see this shift from activist to consumption practices in the final section of Wachter's article on AIDS activism, which begins:

> Because AIDS activists have demonstrated the degree of influence that a well-organized, highly motivated advocacy group can have, we can be certain that the empowerment of patients will be a major part of the American social landscape of the 1990s. In this new order, some health professionals will view a powerful consumer movement as a direct threat to their competence and power.[45]

In the new order that Wachter presents, the rather vague notion of the "empowerment of patients" of the first sentence narrows to a "powerful consumer movement" in the next. As Annemarie Mol argues, the logic of choice now dominates the contemporary practice of medicine in the West. "As if it were a magic wand," Mol notes, "the term 'choice' has ended the discussion. All the possible advantages and disadvantages of . . . [a] treatment, all its goods and bads, have been turned into private concerns."[46] Mol offers an alternative to the logic of choice—the logic of care—noting that "care is not a limited product, but an ongoing process."[47] It seems to me the promise of the self-help clinic was in offering a space for the ongoing process of care—of the self and of others and to the self through others. Within the context of a medicine dominated by the logic of choice, this counterlogic of care is decidedly queer.[48] I am interested in these competing logics in relation to illness experiences and events, therapeutic thought and practices, and clinical and caring spaces and institutions. How a logic of choice has come to dominate over and against a logic of care is one of the questions I explore in my analysis of the conjunction illness-thought-activism in the period just before and after AIDS.

Transversality

The second queer method I explore in this chapter is the practice of transversality, a term utilized by Félix Guattari, who is best known for his long collaboration with the French philosopher Gilles Deleuze, in particular on their two-volume magnum opus, *Capitalism and Schizophrenia.*[49] Guattari's contribution to *Anti-Oedipus* and *A Thousand Plateaus* is often diminished or sometimes even overlooked entirely, yet his ongoing experience working with Jean Oury at the La Borde clinic in the Loire Valley of France and his many radical political interventions were key inspirations for the theoretical, methodological, political, and aesthetic innovations that came out of his collaborations with Deleuze.[50]

One formative influence on Guattari's critical and clinical interventions was the institutional psychiatry movement, which emerged in France out of the French experience of occupation during World War II. The theories and methods of institutional psychiatry—or what Guattari preferred to call "institutional analysis" or, sometimes, "institutional pedagogy," in order to indicate some of the deauthorizing of conventional psychiatry at work in these practices—would eventually migrate into other domains in conjunction with the protest movements fomenting in France around May 1968.[51] As Bourg notes, the Saint-Alban clinic in the south of France became an "incubator" for creative thought and therapeutic methods, bringing together a diverse group of individuals—including communists and Christians, surrealists and psychoanalysts, the healthy and the ill—who took refuge in the clinic and resisted the Nazi occupation.[52] After the war both Frantz Fanon and Jean Oury interned at Saint-Alban in the 1950s, and they exported and extended the thought and practices they learned at Saint-Alban's to, in Oury's case, the La Borde clinic in central France and, in Fanon's case, to the Blida-Joinville Psychiatric Hospital in Algeria, as I will discuss further in snapshot 4. I focus here on the clinic at La Borde and what I take to be its queer method of transversality, which Guattari developed out of and in relation to the experimental clinical practices he participated in there from the 1950s until his death in 1992. Guattari is another important relay across the terrain *Indirect Action* traverses: extending practices that began during the resistance to occupation to the Algerian war of liberation against colonialism to the uprisings during and after May 1968 to the radical ecological movements of the 1980s to, even less directly, the political and aesthetic response to AIDS in New York City in the

1980s, as I will show in the snapshot that follows this chapter.[53] Guattari is also one of my key generalists; his preoccupations are many and diverse. Guattari describes transversality as a theory and practice of ranging across identities, disciplines, concepts, and milieus in order to keep open the possibility of desire. In an important genealogy of Guattari's use of the term, Gary Genosko explains that "transversality was not a philosophical but a political concept, and one never loses the impression, despite the heavy Freudianism of the early Guattari, that the idea was to use it imaginatively in order to change, perhaps not the entire world, but institutions as we know them, beginning with analytic method."[54] The concept and practice of transversality developed out of the psychoanalytic concept and practice of transference: transversality was a group form of transference that allowed for an impersonal love through an analysis of the institution. In an interview in 1973, Guattari suggests transversality as a means to get out of the trap of psychoanalysis and its habit of confining desire to the "small, secret domain of the couch."[55]

In the same interview, he then demonstrates transversality by making connections beyond and outside psychoanalysis: "The problem of psychoanalysis is the problem of the revolutionary movement, the problem of the revolutionary movement is the problem of madness, the problem of madness is the problem of artistic creation. Transversality is, at heart, nothing but this nomadism."[56] The equation Guattari sets up—psychoanalysis plus revolutionary movement plus madness plus artistic creation—is both conjunctive and disjunctive: the autonomy of each practice is problematized when placed in relation to the other practices of thought and desire. Guattari's concept derives from one of the definitions of *transversal*, now rarely used, according to the *OED*, as something "lying athwart" or, figuratively, a "deviation" or "digression." A more common current use of the term comes from geometry and refers to "a line intersecting two or more lines, or a system of lines."[57] Transversality activates and puts into motion a transversal, a line that deviates, digresses, and/or intersects across multiple lines, planes, and plateaus, in the terminology developed by Deleuze and Guattari.

All of these processes suggested by the concept of transversality will become key to the thought created in the collaboration between Deleuze and Guattari. Indeed, their thinking and writing together is infused with the spirit of a complex transversality between them and between institutional analysis, philosophy, and politics. As they themselves have described it, the collaboration brought together a psychoanalyst influenced by Lacan but interested in overturning the orthodoxy in both the theory and the practice of psychoanalysis and a philosopher interested in concepts and the means by which new concepts might be created rather than in expressing a proper deference to the history of philosophy.[58] Transversality leads away from the dead-end familialism of psychoanalytic and philosophical thought and practice and toward many of the key concepts demonstrated in *Capitalism and Schizophrenia*: deterritorialization, the body without organs, nomad thought, lines of flight, and assemblages, to name just a few. In a conversation with Deleuze and Catherine Backès-Clément on *Anti-Oedipus*, Guattari explains that at the start of his collaboration with Deleuze, he had "too many 'backgrounds,'" including leftist political work, Lacan's seminars, the institutional analysis practiced at La Borde, and working with schizophrenics. He describes these backgrounds as more than just discourses, as "ways of life," and says he is "to some extent torn between them."[59] Guattari's emphasis on (political-conceptual-therapeutic) "ways of life" that may be in conflict with each other anticipates Foucault's later turn to ethics or arts of existence, which itself anticipates a queer way of life or ascesis as opposed to a gay identity, as discussed in chapter 1 in relation to AIDS activism. For Guattari these diverse ways of life—combined with his writing with Deleuze—bring into being a "logic of multiplicities" that counters reductive logics, especially, in Guattari's experience, oedipal, Marxist, and scientific ones.

Both Deleuze and Guattari were interested in the how not the what or essence of an object, and Guattari especially understood the clinic as a space in which one might explore how psychological, social, political, and institutional discourses and practices work. Deleuze and Guattari's challenge to psychoanalysis, philosophy, and politics, then, was not simply a theoretical exercise but also a therapeutic and political one. They argued that psychoanalytic thought and practice failed to be therapeutically effective because it did not go beyond the analytic scenario of a person on a couch talking about his or her childhood—the couch becoming a metonym for therapy as a reduction of desire and creative thought. In this conventional analytic scene, transference does not open up the machinic productivity of desire but drives desire back into the nuclear household and the past. The problem was "the reduction of the social investments of libido to domestic investments, and the projection of desire back onto domestic coordinates," as Deleuze puts it in conversation with Guattari and Backès-Clément.[60]

In his essay "La Borde: A Clinic Unlike Any Other," Guattari presents some of the background for the experiment in institutional analysis that began at La Borde in the 1950s and continues to this day. The adjective Guattari uses to capture the treatment at La Borde is *baroque*, which he glosses as "always in search of new themes and variations in order to confer its seal of singularity—i.e., of finitude and authenticity—to the slightest gestures, the shortest encounters that take place in such a context."[61] Both Deleuze and Guattari were interested in what I would describe as the queerness of the baroque understood in two senses: both as a historical period that "could be stretched beyond its precise historical limits" and as a conceptual apparatus that "invents the infinite work or process."[62] Deleuze begins his book on Leibniz and the baroque by noting that "the Baroque refers not to an essence but rather to an operative function, to a trait. It endlessly produces folds."[63] Deleuze emphasizes the mannerism and fluidity of Leibniz's baroque, arguing, "The spontaneity of manners replaces the essentiality of the attribute."[64] Such spontaneity of manners would come into play in the day to-day operations of the clinic at La Borde.

If the feminist self-help clinic queered the clinic by extending knowledge and power to women in relation to their doctors and by highlighting rather than downplaying the transmission of affects within the clinic, La Borde queered the clinic by "treating the institution as a whole"[65] and transforming the interactions between doctors and patients even further. At La Borde distinctions between the "presumably 'noble' tasks of the medical staff and the thankless, material tasks of the service personnel" were eliminated.[66] All staff—medical and service—performed all tasks in rotation, upsetting the doctor's usual position at the top of the institution's structure of authority by turning decision making into a horizontal not vertical process. Guattari explains the logic of La Borde as follows:

> What we aimed for through our multiple activities, and above all through the assumption of responsibility with regard to oneself and to others, was to be disengaged from seriality and to make individuals and groups reappropriate the meaning of their existence in an ethical and no longer technocratic perspective. . . . The institutional machine that we positioned didn't simply remodel existing subjectivities, but endeavored, instead, to produce a new type of subjectivity. The supervisors created by the "rotations," guided by the "schedule," and actively participating in the "information

meetings," gradually became, with training, very different people from what they had been upon arrival at the clinic.[67]

The clinic becomes a space for the production of new subjectivities, not just among the patients but also among the medical and service staff as well, and this inventiveness transforms—queers, we might say—the institution of psychiatry. More than this, the clinic becomes a kind of laboratory out of which "a collective critique of the power relations in society as a whole" is produced.[68] In this way the therapeutic effects go well beyond the boundaries of the clinic (never mind the couch) and out into society at large.[69]

Although Guattari's methods were often associated with the antipsychiatry movement led by R. D. Laing and David Cooper in the United Kingdom and by Thomas Szasz in the United States, he found that movement's sometimes "demagogic exaggerations" and overdetermined familialism to be reductive rather than productive of new subjectivities. Indeed, one of the problems with antipsychiatry, as formulated by Laing, Cooper, and Szasz, was that it was decidedly heteronormative in its analysis of family relations. In *Psychiatry and Anti-psychiatry,* for example, Cooper focuses exclusively on the male child unable to establish an autonomous identity within his family, who then becomes schizophrenic—all because of an overbearing mother. In Cooper's assessment it is often the case that families themselves are psychotic (and, in Cooper's formulation, mothers are the main culprits within the family), and "the identified schizophrenic patient member by his psychotic episode is trying to break free of an alienated system and is, therefore, in some sense less 'ill' or at least less alienated than the 'normal' offspring of the 'normal' families."[70] On the one hand, Cooper is critical of normalization, but on the other hand, his critique relies on a gender normativity in which boy children must break free of their mothers to become autonomous selves. I will return to the heteronormativity of antipsychiatry—and other doctrinaire medical logics and practices—in chapter 5.

We might say, then, that much of antipsychiatry presents, in the terminology of Eve Kosofsky Sedgwick, a paranoid critical practice in relation to psychiatry, whereas La Borde and Deleuze and Guattari offer a reparative critical practice. In his review of Guattari's use of the concept and practice of transversality, Genosko shows that Guattari contrasts what he calls the "coefficient of collective paranoia" with the "co-efficient of transversality," and according to Genosko "the latter is connective and communicative, and the former is restrictive and reticent."[71] I want to conclude my attempt to que(e)ry the clinic in the prehistory of AIDS with a brief discussion of Sedgwick's essay on paranoid and reparative readings, already mentioned in the introduction, because like Wachter's piece in the *New England Journal of Medicine*, one of the things it does is look back at the early days of AIDS from a position in the 1990s. As literary critic, poet, teacher, and one of the most creative and influential forces in the emergence of queer theory in the 1990s, Sedgwick obviously approaches the 1980s from backgrounds different from Wachter's. I think it is useful, therefore, to add Sedgwick to Wachter in order to multiply the logics circulating in the early years of the AIDS epidemic and infuse my own analysis of AIDS activism and its clinical and critical prehistory with a reparative not paranoid sensibility.

Sedgwick opens with a story about a conversation she had, "sometime back in the middle of the first decade of the AIDS epidemic," with a friend, scholar/activist Cindy Patton.[72] Sedgwick asks Patton about the "sinister rumors of the virus's origin"; she wonders whether Patton believes any of the conspiracy theories about the making of the virus. Was it, for example, a biological weapon concocted in a U.S. military laboratory and tested on certain populations deemed expendable, or even worse, was it invented to kill those populations, including Africans, African Americans, and homosexuals? In Sedgwick's presentation of the conversation with Patton, she hopes Patton's expertise in the field will provide her with evidence for what she thinks must be true: that the U.S. government is somehow behind the spread of AIDS. And yet Patton's response surprises Sedgwick. Although she doesn't deny that there could be a conspiracy, she tells Sedgwick she is uninterested in spending her energy determining whether such theories are true, and this unexpected response, for Sedgwick, "open[s] a space for moving from the rather fixated question—Is a particular piece of knowledge true, and how can we know?—to the further questions: What does knowledge *do*—the pursuit of it, the having and exposing of it, the receiving again of knowledge of what one already knows? *How*, in short, is knowledge performative, and how best does one move among its causes and effects?"[73] Sedgwick realizes that the paranoid practice of exposure often becomes an end in itself, forgetting or ignoring the important, further questions about what knowledge does. Sedgwick returns to her surprising conversation with Patton in the mid-1980s to problematize what she sees as a "paranoid imperative" in criticism and politics in the mid-1990s. Although she acknowledges that "queer studies in particular has had a distinctive history of intimacy with the paranoid imperative," she worries that by the 1990s it has become *the* queer methodology rather than one of many possible critical positions.[74] She hopes to unfixate queer studies by offering a call for other critical practices—reparative ones as well as paranoid ones.

We might consider, then, as another example of Sedgwick's paranoid critique the important work of the antipsychiatry movement in exposing the horrors of many psychiatric institutions and practices. And yet we also might—indeed, must—ask what have been some of the negative effects of antipsychiatry on the mentally ill, especially as a result of the massive deinstitutionalization that was first promoted by antipsychiatry activists and later became a cornerstone of the state's progressive neoliberalization of mental health care in the 1970s and 1980s. Deinstitutionalization was a, sometimes literal, exposure of the mentally ill on the streets of U.S. cities. For Sedgwick the problem of the paranoid practice of criticism is that it is "averse above all to surprise," preventing us from glimpsing the "lineaments of other possibilities"[75] that might arise when we deviate, digress, or intersect. These lineaments of other possibilities were what the clinic at La Borde tried—and tries—to open up for both its patients and staff. The desire was not simply to deinstitutionalize patients but to create alternative spaces for "a therapeutic social life" to happen.[76] In the contemporary neoliberal logic of medicine, a "therapeutic social life" is difficult to imagine. Yet I contend that it helps our clinical imagination to look back to earlier experiments—not necessarily as offering a one-size-fits-all model of the future but as visions of the past that open up other logics in the present. We que(e)ry the clinic of the past in order to denaturalize the clinic of the present and to produce new therapeutic sites of the future.

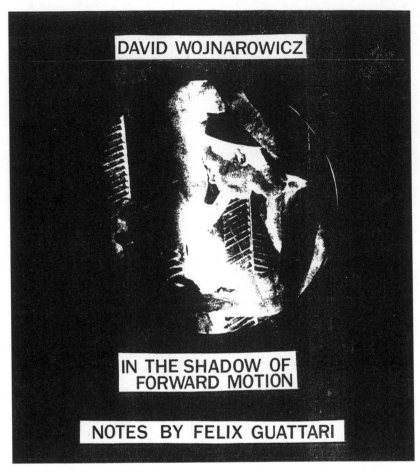

Figure 2. In 1989 Félix Guattari contributed a foreword to a xeroxed catalog for a show of David Wojnarowicz's In the Shadow of Forward Motion *at the P.P.O.W. gallery in New York City. The cover image on the catalog, a detail from Wojnarowicz's Sex Series, is a copy of an x-ray photograph of a sexual encounter as if viewed through a microscope or pinhole. Courtesy of the Estate of David Wojnarowicz and P.P.O.W., New York.*

Félix Guattari's "David Wojnarowicz" (1989)

*History has been written and preserved by and for a particular class
of people so in my work I want to rewrite or give new meaning to
the histories that exist in textbooks using present day experience as a
departure. For example, in a painting about the American West, I focus
on the steam engine; the train that carried white culture through the land
inhabited by the Indians. Obviously, judging by the current state of Indian
affairs, there was intense exploitation and eradication by white people of
anything or anyone that resisted their cultural expansion. Given that I
wasn't born at that time, I can only speak of these elements in terms that
exist today—I gather them by traveling, or from written works, images in
popular culture, dreams and other symbols that will help me construct a
discourse about this reality rejected or hidden by the white culture.*

—David Wojnarowicz quoted in Félix Guattari, "David Wojnarowicz"

*One day, I asked David if he would like somebody to write a foreword
about his work. He was always complaining that nobody really wrote
about it. And he was so attracted to all these philosophers, like Baudrillard
and Guattari. At the time I was living at Félix's place in Paris, so I
suggested to David that I could ask Félix to write a text for the catalogue.
In order to get him interested, we put together a slideshow and wrote a text
in French that you translated. So we ended up having a foreword by Félix
Guattari in this cheap Xeroxed catalogue. David was very proud of it.*

—Marion Scemama interviewed by Sylvère Lotringer in *David Wojnarowicz*

In 1989 Félix Guattari contributed a foreword of sorts to a photocopied
exhibition catalog for David Wojnarowicz's *In the Shadow of Forward
Motion* at the P.P.O.W. gallery in New York City. Nestled in the middle
of Guattari's short notes on Wojnarowicz's work is a long quotation from
Wojnarowicz himself, a quotation that appears to be a Guattarian articulation of a Wojnarowiczian articulation—that is, "articulation" in Stuart
Hall's double sense as both a form of expression and a linkage between

multiple expressions, concepts, and objects. Guattari collages into a single and singular quotation several of Wojnarowicz's exhibition notes to help him express the transversality of Wojnarowicz's work, which gathers elements encountered on his travels, in words and images, dreams and nightmares, about history, machines, and nature. Wojnarowicz's words become the literal and figurative link between Guattari's statements about Wojnarowicz's singular visual and verbal statements about creative work as a way of life in the face of death.

The cover image on the catalog, a detail from Wojnarowicz's Sex Series, is a copy of an x-ray photograph of a sexual encounter as if viewed through a microscope or pinhole (Figure 2). What we see is difficult to discern, and we must peer closely at the image to see there are two men in the scene; as microscoped, x-rayed, and then photocopied fragment, sex is not simply *im*personalized but *de*personalized. The sex is both there for all to see and difficult to discern. Our own voyeuristic desire is captured in the pinhole's structuring call to look. The image vibrates eerily on a black background while the text boxes—"David Wojnarowicz," "In the Shadow of Forward Motion," and "Notes by Felix Guattari"—float in white rectangular blocks above and below the image. The catalog materially and conceptually links the names, words, and ideas of Guattari and Wojnarowicz, even though the two men never met.

A name not on the cover of the catalog is that of the photographer, Marion Scemama, who collaborated with Wojnarowicz and was a friend of Guattari's; it was Scemama who brought the two men together at the very end of the first decade of AIDS, in 1989, three years before both of their deaths, only weeks apart, in 1992. In an interview with Sylvère Lotringer, the founder of Semiotext(e), a cultural theorist, and an archiver of French theory in the United States, Scemama describes how Guattari's involvement in the catalog came about and the pleasure Wojnarowicz felt in having his work linked with Guattari's.[1] Because Guattari couldn't come to New York to meet Wojnarowicz or see his work in person, Guattari's "David Wojnarowicz" is, Scemama believes, a "little superficial" but nonetheless important as "a gesture."[2] "Gesture" is a key word and concept in Wojnarowicz's work and features frequently in his diaries. Wojnarowicz's concept of the gesture emerges not only from his practices of art and writing but also from his practices of sex. For Wojnarowicz the gesture is a link between word and image, writing and painting, sex and intimacy. For example, in a diary entry in September 1981, Wojnarowicz describes picking up a guy in a park in the East Village and going for coffee with him.

As they make "slow spare conversation," Wojnarowicz explains, "I knew I wanted to lie down with him but nothing was mentioned. I wondered how it would be approached, if at all. What words, what gestures."[3] Or as Agamben puts it in his "Notes on Gesture," "The gesture is the exhibition of a mediality: it is the process of making a means visible as such."[4] The snapshots in my project are meant to function like gestures: they are intertexts and interimages that make a means visible—in this snapshot, linking sex, illness, art, and politics before and after AIDS.

Thus, I want to both extend and incorporate the moment of the gesture that Guattari's forward to Wojnarowicz's exhibition catalog performs by reconnecting Wojnarowicz and Scemama and Guattari, not only in the interest of recovering queer friendships and creative collaborations that might otherwise be forgotten but also as a means of trying to make visible the mediality of how things work on both a small, intimate scale and on a world-historical scale. My terminology intentionally echoes Scemama's interpretation of Wojnarowicz's Sex Series, which she describes as "looking behind or on the reverse of what is not shown: the negative. In Photography," Scemama continues, "you never show the negative side, you only show the positive, so it's more like revealing something that you can't see. It's also the idea of the microscope, looking through a microscope—all those little holes—at how things work."[5] Ways of seeing from the front and back, positively and negatively.

In his superficial gesture, Guattari argues that Wojnarowicz reinvents the "inspiration of the great 60s movements" in order to "transcend the style of passivity and abandon of the entropic slope of fate which characterizes this present period."[6] A superficial gesture, then, links Wojnarowicz back to the social movements of the 1960s and forward or, perhaps we should say, in the shadow of a forward motion to "a singular message that allows us to perceive an enunciation in process," as Guattari puts it.[7] The enunciation in process catalogs macroevents, like the worldwide devastation of AIDS, the detritus of capitalism, and the expropriation and exploitation of land once inhabited by the Indians. In his writing and visual art, Wojnarowicz demonstrates the metamorphosis of all things—rusted-out factories, defunct machines, and insect shells are placed side by side as images of "what history means reached through the compression of time."[8] We might say that Wojnarowicz figures the ecoontological in his work, drawing connections across historical genocides and between humans and nonhumans via a visual rhetoric of "material immortality," to use a phrase of Rachel Carson's, which reminds us of the persistence of organic and inorganic substances and which I will discuss in more detail in chapter 4. In an essay about animals in Wojnarowicz's work, Mysoon Rizk notes that the perspective is often extraplanetary, and from such a great distance, the human is imagined as an "infinitesimal speck in an infinitely broad stratum [that] dissolves the demarcations that might otherwise separate one species from another, or human animals from non-human human animals."[9] A speck is a kind of gesture in space. This comparison between the infinitesimal speck and the infinitely broad stratum seems to me to demonstrate well the problem of scale and movements between the very small and the very large in size and the very long and the very short in duration that I work to transverse in this book.

The broad canvas of Wojnarowicz's enunciation in process gives form to microexperiences, expressions of intimacy across differences, both molecular and molar, like what Scemama calls "the strange love" between her and Wojnarowicz, a heterosexual woman and a gay man: "A love beyond genders, beyond the restrictive and reductive definition of what it is to be a woman or a man in this 'pre-invented' world, and what part is assigned to each person, whether homosexual or heterosexual, queer or female, breeder or sucker. We dreamt of breaking these frontiers. We just wanted to be human beings, detached from genders, or being all genders at once."[10] For Wojnarowicz and Scemama, the love beyond genders is expressed not so much interpersonally as impersonally, not heteronormative reproduction but a sex series—history reached through the compression of time as glimpsed through a peephole cut into the fabric of the world.

My own superficial and small gesture here redraws a line between Guattari and Scemama and Wojnarowicz. The redrawing of the line is not meant simply as a reminder that politics is about the personal, in the sense that through personal relationships we make politics, although of course personal relationships are an important aspect of the practice of all politics. Rather, what I want to think about are those figures who act as relays between people, places, ideas, and entire movements: Scemama between Guattari and Wojnarowicz but also Guattari between the radicalism of May 1968 and forms of AIDS activism in the 1980s. Like Wojnarowicz, I am interested in "what history means reached through the compression of time," a snapshot or a xeroxed catalog linking two names, word and image, sex and love, art and politics. Doing politics is about all kinds of further gestures: personal and impersonal, large and small, profound and superficial.

3

Enacting Clinical Experience, circa 1963

In a chapter in *The Birth of the Clinic* entitled "The Old Age of the Clinic," Foucault argues that the history medicine likes to tell of itself has at its center an unchanging idea of the clinic. "Medicine has tended," Foucault writes, "since the eighteenth century, to recount its own history as if the patient's bedside had always been a place of constant, stable experience, in contrast to theories and systems, which had been in perpetual change and masked beneath their speculation the purity of clinical evidence."[1] Like all of Foucault's work, *The Birth of the Clinic* attempts to challenge this age-old and seemingly fixed idea by investigating the clinic as a multiple and complex object that emerges at a particular moment in history and gets enacted in and through various practices. For Foucault that moment of emergence is between 1769 and 1825.[2] By exploring the moment the idea of the clinic first emerged, Foucault demonstrates how one very particular historical "truth" of the clinic comes into being and covers over multiple other "truths" of the clinic. Foucault argues this ideal account of clinical medicine must be historicized in order that it may "be understood in relation to the . . . establishment of clinical institutions and methods," which then present this ideal account "as the restitution of an eternal truth in a continuous historical development in which events alone have been of a negative order: oblivion, illusion, concealment. In fact, this way of rewriting history itself evaded a much truer but much more complex history."[3]

The Birth of the Clinic is as much a history about how we tell history in a particular present as it is a history of a particular object. This practice of double description is what I want to attend to in relation to illness, thought, and activism in the prehistory of AIDS. For Foucault what matters is the form of thought as well as the context or milieu out of which thought forms. While Foucault's archeological methods help him to glimpse and describe the domain of clinical experience and "the structure of its rationality,"[4] he is also aware that it is only "because a new experience of disease is coming into being" making possible "a historical and critical understanding of the old experience."[5] The particular historical moment in which he writes—the early 1960s—provides him with a changing discursive framework that he utilizes in diagnosing the conditions of possibility that resulted in the birth of the clinic two centuries earlier. We can explore a particular medical experience and its "types of discourse"[6] only if that experience and those discourses are not still our own. A new experience of disease is a conceptual and affective apparatus through which an old experience comes into view. Foucault's *Birth of the Clinic* not only becomes, then, a diagnosis of the condition of the old age of the clinic but also participates in the enactment of a new age of the clinic and a new experience and event of illness emerging in the 1960s and 1970s.

In order to extend Foucault's history into the present of the archive out of which he writes in the 1960s, I read *The Birth of the Clinic* alongside John Berger and Jean Mohr's *A Fortunate Man: The Story of a Country Doctor*, from 1967.[7] Foucault's analysis takes us back in time, while Berger and Mohr's brings us forward into the present of the 1960s. In chapter 1, I utilized Foucault's discussion of "friendship as a way of life," articulated just before the first media coverage of a new illness that would become AIDS, in order to help me think more about the affective and effective response to AIDS in the gay and lesbian community in the United States. In chapter 2, I que(e)ried the clinic before AIDS, exploring some continuities and discontinuities between two clinical practices—self-help and transversality—that emerged before AIDS. In this chapter, I want to take another small step back, comparing two texts that consider the event of the clinic in history, paraphrasing Tani Barlow's grammar of distillation in her evocative analysis of the "event of women" in Chinese feminism.[8] By doing so, I hope to undermine the inevitability of a hegemonic clinical experience in the present that privileges specialization over generalism, a logic of choice over a logic of care, and emergency time over indirect action.

Berger and Mohr's text is a remarkable sociohistorical document, a hybrid form that combines reportage, memoir, social and psychoanalytic theories, and photographic images to present the story of an individual, John Sassall, the fortunate man and country doctor of the title, and a community of "foresters" in rural England. Although I have no evidence that Foucault was familiar with *A Fortunate Man* or the extensive critical and literary work of John Berger, the more prominent of its two authors, I think it is fair to say this is the kind of work that would have interested Foucault as an exemplary artifact of a particular historical moment. It is in this spirit that I look back at both *The Birth of the Clinic* and *A Fortunate Man* as exemplary artifacts of the event of the clinic of the 1960s.

I have written elsewhere about what I call the multiple practices of witnessing,[9] and here I want to think in terms of doctoring itself as a practice of witnessing[10] that gets demonstrated in and through words and images in Berger and Mohr's account.[11] In considering witnessing as a practice, I move away from a focus on the subjectivity of the witness. My concern is less with who sees what than with how seeing happens in practice and with how subject positions are constituted through particular "ways of seeing," a phrase that of course echoes the title of Berger's BBC documentary and companion book from 1972, key texts that diagnose and treat the conditions of cultural production and consumption in postmodernity.[12] My approach also shifts the question from one concerned first and foremost with discerning the accuracy or authenticity of the account of a particular witness to one concerned with the constitutive effects of witnessing. The key question in this chapter, as well as throughout this project more generally, is, What do we bring into being through our practices of witnessing? In taking up medical perception and experience as a practice of witnessing, I am extending the concept beyond a specifically psychoanalytic understanding of the term, which tends to fixate on individual encounters between doctors and patients within the privatized space of the psychoanalytic clinic. Instead, to use terminology that echoes Foucault's work, especially his work in the 1960s, I want to consider the conditions of possibility that constitute a particular experience of seeing—in the case discussed in this chapter, the particular experience of a doctor seeing illness in rural England in the 1960s.

While it is certainly true that *A Fortunate Man* might easily be (and has been) read as a humanist text that presents Sassall as an ideal model of a compassionate doctor (and, as I will discuss, one who reads and is changed by his intellectual encounter with Freud),[13] I think such a reading misses the formal, theoretical, and methodological complexity of Berger and Mohr's text. And although it may strike some as odd to read *The Birth of the Clinic* with and against *A Fortunate Man*, in reading these texts together I am attempting to follow Foucault's own method of historical analysis by juxtaposing—"present[ing] side by side," as he says in *The Order of Things*[14]—various practices, figures, and "forms of finitude"[15] of the old and new ages of the clinic. Foucault is known to have dissuaded scholars from writing *about him*, but he did encourage scholars across various disciplines to make use of and transform his methodological "gadgets" to explore domains beyond—in time and space—the ones to which he had already applied his methods.[16] By reading *The Birth of the Clinic* and *A Fortunate Man* as historically situated texts and in relation to each other, I show the ways in which they each enact a method for analyzing a kind of experience, in this case clinical experience, in a particular time and place. My point is not that these texts are simply about the clinic in the 1960s but rather that they participate in the event of enacting the clinic in the 1960s. This distinction matters, I think, in that it allows a conceptual shift from an approach concerned with representations to one concerned with historical ontologies of the clinic—what different clinics bring into being in different times and places.

I also want to read them together as a means to consider the function of literature and the literary critical in Foucault's work in order to think, more generally and indirectly, through some of the methodological questions that emerge out of my analysis of the conjuncture illness-thought-activism in time. Foucault frequently turns to literature to provide exemplary texts of particular kinds of thought, and this is especially true of his work of the early 1960s. As Pierre Macherey has noted, in one of the few works to discuss Foucault and literature, "Foucault does more than reflect *on* literature. He works *with* literature; he is preoccupied with making theoretical use of it rather than elaborating a theory of literature."[17] Macherey doesn't find it simply happenstance that Foucault should have published his one book-length work on literature, on the early twentieth-century French writer Raymond Roussel's somewhat obscure modernist fiction, the same year as he published *The Birth of the Clinic*.[18] Taking up Roussel and the figure of writer as madman allows Foucault to consider the relationship between language, experience, illness, and death, which is also the complex relationship enacted throughout *The Birth of the Clinic*. Macherey describes Foucault's reading of Roussel's literary method as "exemplary because, thanks to his rigorous work on the forms of language, it results in a questioning of the order of things. We can speak here of an ontological question. What is a thing?"[19] By manipulating language, by dissecting it, Roussel reveals its hidden disease, what Macherey calls the "sickness of language."[20] Macherey explains that Foucault reads Roussel's work with and in language as demonstrating "that things themselves are sick, or in other words not quite as we see them."[21]

If words and things are sick, then how do we treat them? How might this revelation from the domain of literature on the sick condition of language help us investigate the domain of medicine and the being of illness? Or put another way, why this detour into literature and Foucault's work with literature in a discussion of the historical event of the clinic? I make this detour because I want to suggest here that *A Fortunate Man* is a work of literature that is exemplary in its work on forms of language—including visual forms—that also results in a questioning of the condition of things. I want to make theoretical and methodological use of *A Fortunate Man* in an attempt to discern the beginning of a shift in the ordering of clinical experience in the 1960s. In *A Fortunate Man,* Berger, Mohr, and indeed Sassall together enact both an old clinical experience and the possibility of a new one. I organize my discussion of their enactments of doctoring in a shifting clinical order of things around four general domains: space, time, theory, and politics, which are also the main coordinates of Foucault's method demonstrated in *The Birth of the Clinic.* The questions that frame my discussion in this chapter are, then, as follows: What are the spaces of the clinic and the temporalities of doctoring? How do various theories inform or transform medical practices? How is politics brought into or excluded from clinical experience?

Becoming Clinical

In *The Birth of the Clinic,* Foucault explores how medicine became clinical. If we consult the *Oxford English Dictionary* for its definition of *clinical,* we discover that Foucault's archeological account of clinical medicine is backed up by the history of the word itself. The first use of the word in English is from 1780, for the newly elected "Clinical Professor to the Radcliffe Infirmary at Oxford," and its earliest meaning was "of or pertaining to the sick-bed, specifically to that of indoor hospital patients: used in connexion with the practical instruction given to medical students at the sick-beds in hospitals."[22] In the nineteenth century, the word would also take on an ecclesiastical meaning, referring to baptisms administered at the bed of someone ill or dying. By the time Foucault is writing *The Birth of the Clinic* and Berger, Mohr, and Sassall are enacting *A Fortunate Man,* the word has acquired a new meaning: "coldly detached and dispassionate, like a medical report or examination; diagnostic or therapeutic, like medical investigation or treatment; treating a subject-matter as if it were a case of disease, especially with close attention to detail; serving as part of a case-study."[23] "Coldly detached and dispassionate" refers here to clinical spaces, discourses, and practices, and these might be said to be the culmination of the shift in medical experience Foucault describes in *The Birth of the Clinic*, a shift other commentators have described as from bedside medicine to hospital medicine to laboratory medicine,[24] from practices of generalism to increasingly narrow specializations. We also see in the definition an extension of the term to other, nonmedical case studies and forms of treatment that are attentive to detail—*clinical* as word and practice becoming critical, a becoming I argue then transforms how we might do clinical medicine.

Looking back to the 1960s, we can now see this moment in which Foucault writes as creating the conditions of possibility for a movement away from this rarefied clinical mode and toward a practice of doctoring that once more takes the patient as subject of her experience of illness rather than simply or only as object of disease. This movement away from a rarified clinical mode requires another look back, and this is demonstrated explicitly in Foucault's work, if less explicitly in Berger and Mohr's. The look back is not motivated by a desire to restore an older medical experience but rather by a desire to inspire a different future of the clinic from the one that appears to be an inevitable culmination of a history always already conceived of as progressive. These histories of the clinical present of the 1960s anticipate changes in medical experience of the 1970s, some of which I discuss in chapter 2, and I argue that we can read Foucault's text as continuous with those intellectual, social, and political movements that would seek to transform medicine in the late 1960s.

Although the rhetoric and practices of specialization and scientization would dominate medical experience in the 1960s, a counterrhetoric and counterpractices of generalization and narrativization would emerge at this same time. One prefiguration of the counterdiscourse of generalism can be found in Joseph S. Collings's study "General Practice in England Today: A Reconnaissance," published in the *Lancet* in 1950.[25] The Collings report is fascinating as much for its approach as for its findings. Roland Petchey argues, in a revisiting of the study for the Education and Debate section of the *BMJ* in 1995, that it "merits recognition as a pioneer of ethnographic research at a time when it was largely unknown elsewhere in British social research."[26] The Collings report is also a fascinating example of employing qualitative social science methodologies as tools to help do medicine better. As Petchey notes, Collings, an Australian who had practiced in New

Zealand and Canada and was at the time a fellow in public health at Harvard, had never visited the United Kingdom and "so was unfamiliar with the health system and conditions there."²⁷ This lack of familiarity didn't prevent Collings from condemning what he found; indeed, it may well be the case that only an outsider could have been so brutal in his assessment of the state of general practice in Britain in the late 1940s, a time when the country was recovering from war and, as a cornerstone of that recovery, the National Health Service was being put into practice. In an attempt to present a "mosaic" of the "general picture," Collings observed fifty-five English practices, which he classified as "industrial," "urban-residential," or "rural."²⁸ Along with comparisons between locations across England and the implicit cross-class analysis this comparison allowed, Collings also added appendices on general practice in Scotland and New Zealand to encourage further transnational comparative research into alternative models of medical practice in general and general practice in particular.

Collings opens with an assertion that would be impossible to make now in our current era of specialization: "General medical practice is a unique social phenomenon. The general practitioner enjoys more prestige and wields more power than any other citizen, unless it be the judge on his bench."²⁹ Although he is not at all nostalgic for the country doctor of lore, Collings does make several important points about what was good about the old age of the clinic, as well as some recommendations for the transition to a new age. According to Collings, one of the key differences between rural and industrial or urban-residential practices is that the country doctor has the time to examine his patients and to "know them intimately"; thus, "his judgment is usually based on a greater knowledge and a deeper consideration, both of the person and of the ailment, than his city colleagues can compass."³⁰ Collings adds that the rural doctor fulfills a function "in the psychological as distinct from the organic field," and he notes as well that the therapeutic practices of the rural doctor are more diverse than the practices of city doctors, who tend to rely exclusively on the anticipated quick fix of pharmaceutical treatments. Although he does not use the term, Collings seems to be calling for a more holistic approach to doctoring, as well as encouraging a broader and deeper curiosity about the well-being of people across the life cycle. He is most impressed by a rural group practice whose four doctors had an "attitude of mind [that] was different from that of the average doctor: they were constantly trying to improve their equipment and to widen the scope of work, and they were interested in children and old people to a degree not usual in the general practitioner."[31] Collings worries that the "trend towards more and more hospital and specialist care" will lead to the disappearance of the general practitioner and the "breaking of the one remaining link which gives the patient some continuity of care, and the removal of a focal point for dealing with the non-organic problems—the psychological, economic, and social worries of the people."[32] Collings calls for the immediate creation of more group practice units to do "experimental work" on the clinic.[33] For in Collings's diagnosis, the clinic itself is chronically ill, and the problem requires structural not individual remedies.

Collings's structural approach means that he doesn't pay much heed to patients' stories, although, interestingly, it is patients' stories that lead him, conceptually and rhetorically, to his diagnosis of general practice as chronically ill:

> An account of some of the patients who passed through surgeries I visited would make quite dramatic reading. . . . However, I do not believe that such stories, however striking in themselves, would contribute anything to the analysis or solution of the problems of general practice. When an individual error is pointed out, the usual reply is "we can all make mistakes." This is certainly true in general practice, and the individual mistake pales into insignificance beside the predisposing factors which make serious mistakes not only possible but in some circumstances highly probable. I have concerned myself throughout with these causes and predisposing factors and not with collecting examples of errors. I regard the errors as merely symptoms of the chronic illness of general practice today.[34]

In Collings's critical medical study of the general practice clinic in England in 1950, the patient's experience makes a fleeting appearance, only to be marginalized as providing the stuff of drama—the errors of individual doctors affecting the lives of individual patients—not analysis. The Collings report interests me both for its emphasis on the "predisposing factors" of the event of the clinic before 1960 and for its not entirely successful attempt to exclude the experience of the patient from its purview. General practice in 1950 is diagnosed as in need of more (clinical) analysis and less (patient) drama. Yet as David Armstrong has argued, following Jewson, by the 1960s the "sick man" [sic] has reemerged in medicine. I contend that both *The Birth of the Clinic* and *A Fortunate Man* demonstrate and, indeed, help to enact this reemergence.[35] I turn now to Foucault's later account of an earlier event of the clinic in history.

Spaces of the Clinic

The Birth of the Clinic begins: "This is a book about space, about language, and about death; it is about the art of seeing, the gaze" (ix). After this statement Foucault presents his readers with two descriptive images. The first is an image of a body and its treatments, which is meant to shock us as we read it in the twentieth and twenty-first centuries. The image is taken from Pomme's mid-eighteenth-century account of treating and curing "a hysteric by making her take 'baths, ten or twelve hours a day, for ten whole months'" (ix).[36] The hydrotherapeutic treatment for hysteria that Pomme describes results in "membranous tissues" peeling away "like pieces of parchment" and causing "some slight discomfort" to the hysteric (ix). As presented by Pomme, the treatment apparently works as a result of the sloughing phenomenon caused by the hysteric's lengthy immersion. She is cured because her disease literally sloughs away from her internal organs, restoring them and her to health. Although the narrative structure of this cure is somewhat familiar to readers in the present moment—what's a little discomfort on the road to recovery?—the particular method of cure seems fabulous—and simply wrongheaded—to our twenty-first-century discernment.

Foucault's second image is from less than one hundred years later and is of an anatomical lesion on the brain of a patient with "chronic meningitis," a term Foucault places in quotation marks, signaling the crucial observation that all diagnoses are historical events. A particular diagnosis like "chronic meningitis" does not simply identify a thing that is chronic meningitis; the disease is constituted in the act of diagnosis. Diagnosis might be thought of, therefore, as a kind of performative, in Austin's sense of the term, and I will return to diagnosis as performative in later chapters on epilepsy and schizophrenia as two exemplary disease performatives. The later shift from GRID (gay-related immune deficiency) to AIDS (acquired immune deficiency syndrome) demonstrates this performative point again in what I described in the introduction as the precipitation of AIDS as a substance in history. Despite the de-gaying of the diagnosis in the move from GRID to AIDS, the association remained, which meant women were often simply not diagnosed with AIDS.

According to the historical disease performative Foucault discusses, meningitis causes "false membranes" to form in the brain, and these membranes are described in detail and in a tone that sounds measured to our (Western) ears, especially in contrast to the hysterical-sounding description of the hysteric's peeling internal organs. We are told, for example, "This matter often displays different shades in different parts of the same membrane" (x), which seems to be an unembellished and matter-of-fact assessment to us even now of a discernible (with instruments) physiological change. Foucault anticipates that his readers will apprehend the two images as in sharp contrast to each other:

> Between Pomme, who carried the old myths of nervous pathology to their ultimate form, and Bayle, who described the encephalic lesions of general paralysis for an era from which we have not yet emerged, the difference is both tiny and total. For us, it is total because each of Bayle's words, with its qualitative precision, directs our gaze into a world of constant visibility, while Pomme, lacking any perceptual base, speaks to us in the language of fantasy. But by what fundamental experience can we establish such an obvious difference below the level of our certainties, in that region from which they emerge? How can we be sure that an eighteenth-century doctor did not see what he saw, but that it needed several decades before the fantastic figures were dissipated to reveal, in the space vacated, the shapes of things as they really are? (x)

For Foucault our ability to perceive the shapes of things as they really are is hindered by a historicist certainty that we perceive better now than we did then. Foucault challenges this historicist attitude by juxtaposing two historical images in order to demonstrate two different arts of seeing illness. He suggests that we can perceive the artifice—fantasy even—that structures the first art of seeing because we no longer perceive in this manner, whereas the fantasy or artifice behind the later image is harder, if not impossible, for us to discern.

Medical perception is always shaped by discourse, by the words we use to describe what we see medically. Foucault delineates the emergence of the clinic as a particular mode of discourse governed by exemplary exchanges between doctors and patients. The new structure that emerges at the beginning of the nineteenth century, of which the clinic is a sign, "is indicated—but not, of course, exhausted," Foucault argues, "by the minute but decisive change whereby the question: 'What is the matter with you?' . . . was replaced by that other question: 'Where does it hurt?,' in which we recognize the operation of the clinic and the principle of its entire discourse" (xviii). In this new discourse of the clinic, the experience that matters is not the experience of the patient, who must remain silent,[37] but the experience of the doctor, who alone is capable of perceiving and speaking the truth of disease. The change in question reflects a change in authority (from patient as authority on the subjective experience of illness to doctor as authority on the objective experience of disease), and it also signals a change in the spatialization and temporalization of disease. "What is the matter with you?" is a question that asks for a response that situates the body of the person who is ill in a larger world and longer history, while "Where does it hurt?" is a question that already assumes that the answer can and must be localized and located in the body that the doctor examines here and now. The first question moves from the individual patient and her particular embodied experience out into the world and back into history, while the other moves in from world to body to tissue to diseased lesion. The clinic is a space where the internal spaces of the body can be made visible through the doctor's supposedly objective practices of examination and his interrogation of the patient. The emergent instantiation of the clinic that Foucault delineates is as a space in which the body is isolated from history and the outside world in order that disease may be objectified, made visible to and by the doctor. The clinic is the space of that isolation of the body from its environment.

A Fortunate Man is also a book about space, language, and death, and it too uses images to demonstrate a particular medical experience and its art of seeing illness. Like The Birth of the Clinic, A Fortunate Man brings together writing, philosophy, and doctoring in order to problematize the relationship between words, images, and practices in a particular historical moment. The book opens with two of Mohr's black-and-white photographs, both of which cover two pages. The first image is of a narrow road bordered on either side by hedgerows and curving its way through an idyllic-looking English countryside (Figure 3). The landscape is dense with trees, except for a field that enters the picture's frame on the right. There are at least three built structures, two in the background, which appear to be houses, and one in the foreground, which may be a barn. A tree branch jutting from the foreground into the upper half of the left side of the photograph both obscures our view of the scene and directs our gaze toward the right side of the photograph and, in particular, toward the small, white car making its way along the country lane. The significance of the car in the scene will become clear once we begin reading Berger's written narrative. On first glimpse of this photograph, before we are provided with a narrative that will contextualize, at least in hindsight, the image for us, we might read the car as a sign of movement through space and as indicating that this particular place, though perhaps idyllic, is not isolated from but connected to a larger world.

Turning the page, we are presented with another image, this time of a man going either in or out a partially opened door. He appears to pause at the threshold, looking slightly downward, and is perhaps speaking to someone who is not visible to the viewer, suggesting what is absent from view will still be significant to this story. It appears we are looking from within a hallway or an entryway to a door that leads farther into a house. Our gaze is directed by the angles of the walls of the hallway and by the light that slips out from behind the door and shines on the face of the man, who we can see is carrying a leather bag, which we gather is a medical bag from our knowledge of the book's subject matter. This is the title page, and the names of the book's authors, John Berger and Jean Mohr, are above the door, and the title is written across the door and below the man's head. The front cover of an early edition of the book published in the United Kingdom uses a cropped version of this image (Figure 4), further framing the doctor at the door with a border of words—the authors' names at the top and bottom and the book's title on either side, written from top to bottom on the left and from bottom to top on the right. Words serve literally as a frame for the image of the country doctor. From the cover image, we sense we will have a glimpse into the country doctor's experience, but we are also made to see him as a liminal figure, who moves between certain spaces and who embodies a hinge moment in history, a moment marked by a shift from one type of doctoring to another, a shift that the Collings report both diagnosed and attempted to treat.

I describe both of these images in detail because they are meant to tell us something about the spaces of clinical experience that the book investigates. Berger's written narrative begins in the midst of two more photographs that also cover two pages. His words help us to read the photographs, but not in a conventionally illustrative way; they are not simply captions that serve to explain the photographs. Berger and Mohr have

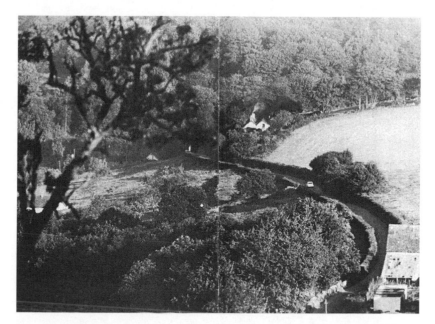

Figure 3. This particular place, though perhaps idyllic, is not isolated from but connected to a larger world. John Berger and Jean Mohr, A Fortunate Man: The Story of a Country Doctor (New York: Pantheon Books, 1967), 1–2. Reprinted by permission of the authors.

placed the opening words of the book in the top right-hand corner of another idyllic scene, this time of a river running through a rural landscape. A small wooden rowboat with two men—one fishing, the other rowing—sits on the river, with fields and then shadowy hills rising in the background. Berger's text begins: "Landscapes can be deceptive. Sometimes a landscape seems to be less a setting for the life of its inhabitants than a curtain behind which their struggles, achievements and accidents take place" (13). This photograph appears to have been taken at dawn; a mist hangs over the river valley, somewhat shrouding the dark mountains in the background and creating a ghostly light and painterly effect.

The next image is similarly ghostly and painterly, though this time the scene appears to be at dusk. A heavy darkness descends from the top and rises from the bottom of the photograph, squeezing a band of light between black clouds and mountains. A dozen or so houses glow in the darkness of the mountains but are otherwise dwarfed and obscured by the landscape of which they are a part. In white typescript across the dark, somewhat

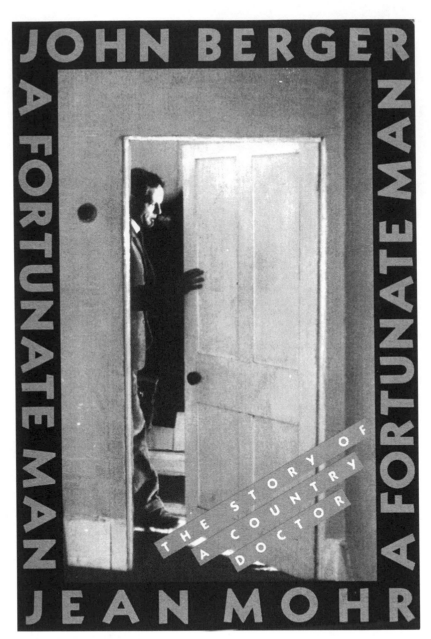

Figure 4. Doctor as liminal figure, moving between certain spaces and embodying a hinge moment in history, a moment marked by a shift from one type of doctoring to another. John Berger and Jean Mohr, A Fortunate Man: The Story of a Country Doctor (New York: Pantheon Books, 1967), front cover. Reprinted by permission of the authors.

foreboding landscape, Berger and Mohr have placed the following words: "For those who, with the inhabitants, are behind the curtain, landmarks are no longer only geographic but also biographical and personal" (15). Berger and Mohr's archeology of medical perception will attempt to look behind the curtain to discern the geographic, those larger environments that frame and sometimes obscure experience, and the biographical, those personal stories that are embedded in those larger environments. But like Foucault, they will also try to bring the curtain itself into view to expose those structures that determine what and how we see.[38]

After the opening sentences about landscapes as curtains and landmarks as geographic, biographical, and personal, Berger's narrative opens with the story of an accident in the forest: "One of them shouted a warning, but it was too late. The leaves brushed him down almost delicately. The small branches encaged him. And then the tree and the whole hill crushed him together" (17). In Berger's account the man is literally crushed by the landscape, which we have up to this moment come to perceive as simply beautiful or, in my already overused term, "idyllic." The doctor is called to the scene of the accident, and we are told that "as he drove through the lanes he kept his thumb on the horn the whole time, partly to warn oncoming traffic, partly so that the man under the tree might hear it and know that the doctor was coming" (17). The story Berger tells makes us look back at the photograph of the car on the lane and see that too as part of the record of a doctor on the way to the scene of an accident. Combined with the photograph of the doctor on the threshold, these are the opening images of John Sassall, and importantly, both images are of him being called. He is called to the forest to administer to a man crushed by a tree, and he announces his coming as a means to give comfort to the man even before he arrives. The horn echoing across the landscape signals the doctor's coming, and this echo and its offer of comfort are Sassall's first treatment. Or in less humanistic terms, Sassall is interpellated as doctor in the moment he is called and responds to that call. His practice of doctoring is incumbent upon his interpellation as doctor by the people of the forest community.[39]

In the images and words gathered together to remember this scene, we are given a glimpse behind the curtain, but we are also made to think about the construction of the story and to problematize the evidence of experience. Berger demonstrates the constructedness of experience by telling us that one of the witnesses to the accident "would tell the story many times, and the first would be tonight in the village. But it was not yet a story" (17–18). What are the discursive conventions that will transform an event that is "not yet a story" into a story? Such a question must be asked about the accident in the forest and the story of the accident but also about the doctor's treatments and the story of those treatments. In its form and content, A Fortunate Man demonstrates medical experiences as enacted through both treatments and the story of treatments and in the space between the thing and the story of the thing. We might read A Fortunate Man, therefore, as anticipating the emergence of a kind of "narrative medicine" not simply by acknowledging the need for better communication between doctors and patients but also by attempting to delineate those discursive practices—including the discursive practices of examination, diagnosis, and treatment—that bring clinical experience into being.

As the event of the accident in the forest makes clear, the spaces of Sassall's treatments are not limited by the four walls of his clinic, which is close to but separate from his house. A photograph of the clinic shows it as part of the rural landscape, and Berger's narrative situates it for us: the clinic "is on the side of the hill which overlooks the river and the large wooded valley. From the other side of the valley it is almost too small to be visible" (43). There are several other photographs of the interior spaces of Sassall's clinic, including one of the waiting room and another of what appears to be Sassall dispensing pills to one of his patients. The small window of the dispensary frames the face of one of his patients, and Sassall is a blur as he consults what might be an appointment book. The small window through which we see the patient is itself framed by neat rows of medical charts, suggesting that each patient's experience of illness is framed by and in the particular knowledge recorded in those charts and case histories, reminding us again that medical perception is shaped by discourse. There are other photographs of Sassall in his clinic: in some he is examining patients, and in others, performing minor surgery, but such images of the practices of surgery and examination are not at all predominant in the text. Instead, they are interspersed among photographs of landscapes, of community gatherings, in which Sassall is often present, and many more portraits of the people of this rural community. There are no captions to tell us exactly what we are seeing; both Mohr's photographs and Berger's narrative must be read and interpreted. Sassall and his clinical practice are integrated into the fabric of the community, and his practices of doctoring are extended beyond the four walls of his clinic. In order to give us a fuller image of Sassall as doctor, Berger and Mohr present him in relation to the people and environment of the community in which he works. The text demonstrates the possibility—necessity even—of doctoring as extending out from the doctor at the patient's bedside to the doctor in and of the community. There is something both old and new about these images; they conjure a hallowed figure of the rural general practitioner and a futuritial figure of the specialist in family medicine.

Temporalities of Doctoring

If the spaces of the clinic are extended in *A Fortunate Man,* so too are the temporalities of doctoring. In his essay "Space and Time in British General Practice," David Armstrong provides a genealogical account of the shift in the spatial and temporal organization of the experiences of British general practitioners (GPs) from the interwar years to the 1960s. Armstrong's rendering of this shift in spatial organization echoes Collings's findings and recommendations, showing a movement from domestic to public spaces, from clinics in the GP's own home to clinics, like Sassall's, "constructed as a separate annexe of the GP's own home" to the "specifically designed or built separate surgery premises," those health centers or "group practice premises" that are established beginning in the 1960s.[40] One of the explanations for this shift in the spatialization of the clinic is that these newly designed clinic spaces were considered more efficient than earlier ones, as a result of increasing specialization, as well as the increasing concentration in one place of various outpatient health care services and procedures.[41] This is also the moment when doctors become less likely to make house calls, and this change in the spatialization of the event of illness is rationalized in terms of the necessity of saving the doctor's time, which begins to be understood as limited and thus in need of constant and close monitoring.

Armstrong connects the new spaces of the clinic with an emergent "time orientation" of medicine in the 1960s. But he also suggests that this "reconstruction of space and time within British general practice" was not enacted in the same way everywhere in Britain, again echoing Collings's earlier diagnosis. He argues that the "perception of time pressures and constraints were mainly found in urban practices" and that the "different time perceptions of some remote, rural, single-handed GPs might also represent the vestiges of an older regime of general practice."[42] These vestiges of an older regime of general practice, with time oriented not toward efficiency in any simple sense, are revealed in *A Fortunate Man.* Yet I also want to read these vestiges as more than just traces of the past. They reverberate into the future and will be heard in later conceptions of clinical experience.[43] When we encounter *A Fortunate Man* today, we will miss the force of those echoes from the past into the present of the 1960s and beyond if we simply take it as evidence of a bygone form of medical experience.[44] *A Fortunate Man* is evidence of a past medical experience, but it also calls for a new temporality of doctoring, from one based on efficiency and emergency to one based on what I have elsewhere called "health and the emergency of the long term."[45] This new temporality of doctoring requires that we reconceive the relationship between health and illness. Rather than treating health and illness as essentially dichotomous conditions and mutually exclusive categories, we must consider the frequently chronic character of illness, as well as the fact that the cellular changes that may eventually lead to illness often take place long before there are symptoms or other signs of illness. In many cases, the time of disease is extended well beyond a clear-cut and acute temporality, and if we are to understand the complexity of disease, then a new temporality of doctoring seems called for, a point I will develop further in the next chapter in my discussion of ecological theories and practices of health.

Sassall himself describes discovering a new temporality of doctoring as he is forced by his own experience to think about illness and its treatments in the long term. He explains to Berger that when he first started his practice in the forest community, initially assisting another older doctor, he "had no patience with anything except emergencies or serious illness." Berger writes of Sassall:

> When a man continued to complain but had no dangerous symptoms, he reminded himself of the endurance of the Greek peasants and the needs of those in "very real distress," and so recommended more exercise and, if possible, a cold bath before breakfast. He dealt only with crises in which he was the central character: or, to put it another way, in which the patient was *simplified* by the degree of his physical dependence on the doctor. He was also simplified to himself, because the chosen pace of his life made it impossible and unnecessary for him to examine his own motives. (54–55)

This is a telling comment from Sassall, revealing one of the key problems that I take up throughout this book—the problem of simplification or reductionism in the practices of doctoring, as well as in the practices of thought and politics. Sassall's comment also suggests other important relationships, which I will engage with in more detail in the next chapter: between direct and indirect actions and between clinical and ecological practices. While direct action is often a necessary response in the emergency time of crisis, illness, thought, and activism also operate in other temporalities.

In his midthirties, Sassall's approach to doctoring begins to change, and his own transformation comes about when he begins to see his patients as complex individuals whose lives are constantly in flux and impossible to simplify. We might think of Sassall's new temporality of doctoring as enabled by a change in his disposition toward his immediate environment, over time, and in relation to others, again, over time. His new interest in the long-term situations of his patients required that he develop different practices of doctoring. He realizes that although "emergencies always present themselves as *faits accomplis*" (55), if we trace back far enough, we will likely discover a moment before the emergency became inevitable. As he lived among the same people over a longer and longer period of time, Sassall "began to notice how people developed. A girl whom three years before he had treated for measles got married and came to him for her first confinement. A man who had never been ill shot his brains out" (55). The long-term view of health and illness necessarily deheroicizes his interventions; rather than coming to the rescue from outside the community, he is of it, which allows him to anticipate problems better, to be in a position to try to understand why, for example, a man who has never been ill might shoot his brains out. The key is not the discovery of some final, complete understanding of the meaning of such an act but a new disposition that takes the time to comprehend even as one realizes one will fail to know with certainty why someone has done something so drastic or desperate or . . . what? Questions always remain.

One story of diagnosis and treatment in particular helps Sassall explain the shift in his time orientation and practices of doctoring. He is called to the cottage of a couple of old-age pensioners who had lived in the forest for thirty years, and when he examines the wife, he discovers something completely unexpected: "'She' was a man. . . . The trouble was severe piles. Neither he nor the husband nor she referred to the sexual organs which should not have been there. They were ignored. Or, rather, he was forced to accept them, as they had done according to their own reasoning which he would never know" (56). In this moment, doctoring becomes something more than simply the examination of a patient and the diagnosis and treatment of a condition. Here, the drama of a man passing as a woman is presented undramatically. Doctoring is characterized not by the certainty of knowing a diagnosis or the heroism of offering a treatment; rather, it is based on an awareness "of the possibility of his patients changing" and that, as a result, his knowledge of them and their bodies will always be only partial.

Berger explains that Sassall's patients, "as they became more used to him, sometimes made confessions for which there was no medical reference so far as he had learnt. He began to take a different view of the meaning of the term crisis" (56). In order to be better able to handle a crisis in the present, his knowledge of his patients must extend beyond the spaces of the clinic and the immediate moment of examination. He must see his patients not in isolation but in relation: to their own past, to their family history, to their changing bodies and environment, and to the future, but also in relation to all that is unknowable. The art of seeing that Sassall must cultivate is a bifocal one; it must be able to focus both inward with a magnifying lens on his patients' bodies and outward with a wide-angle lens on his patients in the world and in history. With its ever-increasing cultivation of expert knowledges and specialized practices, medicine and its mode of perception at the time of the making of *A Fortunate Man* are becoming more and more microscopic, but Sassall is a figure of a doctor who struggles with, though not entirely in opposition to, this reduction of the practices of doctoring. It isn't that he doesn't utilize those technologies that help to better illuminate disease within the patient's body, but he recognizes that these technology-based practices cannot entirely define the contours of the task of doctoring. This brings up again the methodological question I have asked throughout: How do we approach an event like illness?

Theories of/and Medical Experience

This bifocal art of seeing enacted in and by *A Fortunate Man* challenges the dominant idea of the clinic that Foucault diagnoses in *The Birth of the Clinic*. Foucault argues that the clinic emerged as a result of certain exclusions. In "Signs and Cases" and "Seeing and Knowing," two chapters at the center of his archeology of medical perception, Foucault investigates what the "conceptual transformation" of clinical medicine excluded as it emerged: theories, experimentation, and imagination.[46] According to Foucault's rendering of the history of the clinic, "eighteenth-century doctors had used and abused the notion of 'complication'"[47] because they had not yet mastered the art of the clinical gaze, which required opening up "to investigation a domain in which each fact, observed, isolated, then compared with a set of facts, could take its place in a whole series of events whose convergence or divergence were in principle measurable."[48] Within the spaces of the clinic, theories, experiments, and imaginings were seen as obstacles that could insinuate themselves between the doctor's observing gaze and "the sensible immediate" of disease, which was the object of the clinical gaze.[49] The clinic becomes a neutral domain in which a "pathological fact" can appear "in its singularity" in order that it may be observed and described in exhaustive detail by the doctor.[50] The clinic, then, is a space in which it is possible to set aside that which is deemed "extrinsic" to medical experience: theories and systems, anticipatory knowledge, and uncertainty and complexity, all of which require cultivating the practice of imagination.[51]

The "great myth" that structures clinical thought and its methods is, according to Foucault, "a speaking eye," which combines a pure gaze with pure language and which is "the servant of things and the master of truth."[52] A concept of vision, as well as the relationship between seeing and knowing, is also at the center of *A Fortunate Man,* and somewhat eerily, Sassall's eyes figure prominently in Berger and Mohr's account rendered in both words and pictures. Berger recounts a story of Sassall having to perform a procedure on one of his patients, which disturbed the patient in the intimacy of its violation of his person. When Sassall inserts a syringe deep into the man's chest, the man explains to Sassall that it makes him feel not so much pain as revulsion, because, he says, "that's where I live, where you're putting that needle in." Sassall replies, "I know. . . . I know what it feels like. I can't bear anything done near my eyes, I can't bear to be touched there. I think that's where I live, just under and behind my eyes"(47, 50). Berger understands that Sassall's belief that he lives just under and behind his eyes tells us something about Sassall's identity as a doctor, but I think it also tells us something about becoming through a kind of desubjectification—after all, it is not at all obvious what it might mean to be touched under or behind the eyes, though the intimacy of such a gesture feels obvious, to me at least. Sassall becomes his eyes and his eyes become him in certain moments of practicing doctoring. Again, I am suggesting that *A Fortunate Man* shows something about witnessing not just in relation to the subjectivity of the person who witnesses but in terms of what a particular way of seeing brings into being historically. And also, perhaps, *A Fortunate Man* reveals the alienation and anxiety that often accompany witnessing, a point that I will explore in more detail in the two chapters on witnessing epilepsy and schizophrenia. Eyes will figure prominently, and uncannily, in those discussions, too. Later in *A Fortunate Man*, Sassall's eyes come up again. When Sassall tells a story about himself, Berger explains, he often makes himself appear absurd, as a "comic little man." Berger interprets this habit as part of Sassall's method of seeing and knowing; his comic performance provides him with a position from which "he can then re-approach reality once more with the entirely un-comic purposes of mastering it, of understanding it further" (84). Berger continues, "You can see this in the difference between his two eyes: his right eye knows what to expect—it can laugh, sympathize, be stern, mock itself, take aim: his left eye scarcely ever ceases considering the distant evidence and searching" (84). Sassall's bifocal vision allows him to concentrate on both the here and now and that which is distant in space and time. His seeing combines the ability to feel in the present as well as to ask questions of the past and future. Berger tells us that the only time Sassall's left eye stops "considering the distant evidence and searching" is when "he is occupied with some relatively minor surgical task" (84). The concentration required for such a task brings him relief because "for a moment there is certainty" (84). This certainty is expressed not through exhaustive description in the sense of Foucault's speaking eye but in and through surgical practices. In these moments in his clinic, Sassall's is a doing eye. But those moments of doing, of relief and certainty, are only one aspect of Sassall's practices of doctoring, only part of his method of seeing and knowing. Several of Mohr's photographs make visible Sassall's bifocal vision. A close-up of Sassall's head reveals that one eye appears focused on what is immediately in front of him, while the other is focused farther afield (Figure 5). Another captures the moment of concentration on a surgical task and perhaps even a sense of the relief and certainty Sassall feels (Figure 6). In that photograph Sassall wears a magnifying lens over one eye, and the other is squeezed shut as he leans closely over the skin of a patient, who is otherwise out of view. By closing one eye, biological binocularity is prevented, reducing the perception of depth in space. The prosthetic eye both extends his vision and depersonalizes his doctoring, but this doesn't so much dehumanize him as it seems to shield that place where Sassall can't bear to be touched.

As Sassall, Berger, and Mohr present them, Sassall's practices of doctoring explicitly incorporate the theoretical, and theory offers a line of flight away from simplification and reductionism. For Sassall, including the

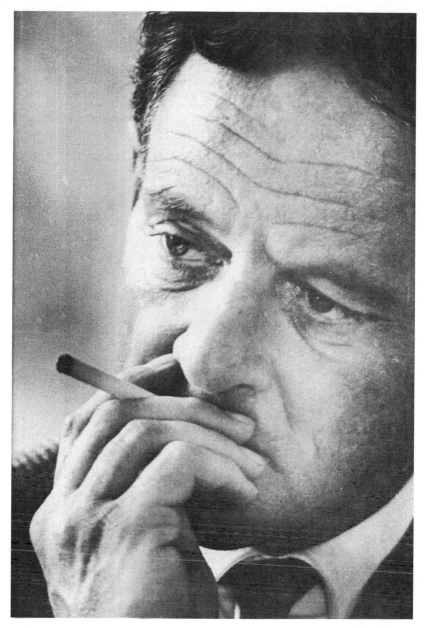

Figure 5. Several of Mohr's photographs make visible Sassall's bifocal vision. A close-up of Sassall's head reveals that one eye appears focused on what is immediately in front of him, while the other is focused farther afield. John Berger and Jean Mohr, A Fortunate Man: The Story of a Country Doctor *(New York: Pantheon Books, 1967), 59. Reprinted by permission of the authors.*

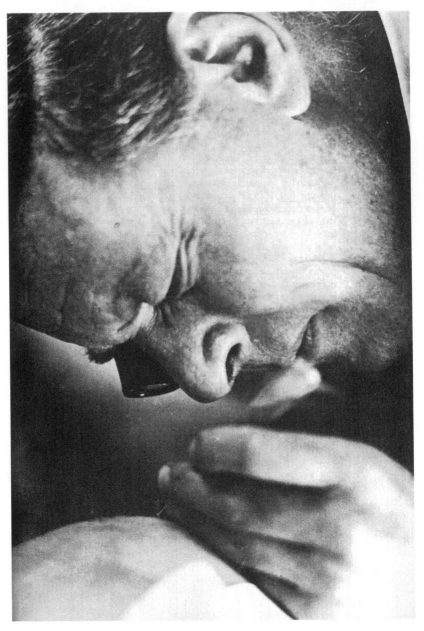

Figure 6. *The prosthetic eye both extends his vision and depersonalizes his doctoring, but this doesn't so much dehumanize him as it seems to shield that place where Sassall can't bear to be touched.* John Berger and Jean Mohr, *A Fortunate Man: The Story of a Country Doctor (New York: Pantheon Books, 1967), 51. Reprinted by permission of the authors.*

theoretical in his practices means that he must observe closely and broadly not just his patients but also himself and each—patient and doctor—as always in relation to others. Berger and Mohr's text extends this method of observation not to fix once and for all and with certainty Sassall's identity as a country doctor but to reveal the uncertainty—the knowing that he can never know enough—that drives Sassall's curiosity. In order to learn more about himself, his patients, and illness but also as a recognition of all he will never know, Sassall begins to read. In particular, Berger tells us, Sassall reads Freud (60). Berger describes Sassall's period of reading Freud as a time of self-analysis and isolation, and he compares this to the period of crisis that "precedes in Siberia and African medicine the professional emergence of the *shaman* or the *inyanga*" (60–61). The doctor studies Freud, and this encounter with the theories and practices of psychoanalysis leads to a transformation of Sassall's practices of doctoring from "the life-and-death emergency" to "the intimation that the patient should be treated as a total personality, that illness is frequently a form of expression rather than a surrender to natural hazards" (62). As Berger warns, this meandering "is dangerous ground, for it is easy to get lost among countless intangibles and to forget or neglect all the precise skills and information which have brought medicine to the point where there is the time and opportunity to pursue such intimations" (62). At the moment that an idea of the clinic as a space for seeing and knowing unencumbered by theories, especially social and psychological theories, is seemingly secure in its dominance, at that very moment complication returns.

Both Sassall and Berger were influenced by the work of Michael Balint and others at the Tavistock Clinic in London in the late 1950s and 1960s.[53] Along with the practices of self-help and institutional analysis discussed in chapter 2, the Tavistock Clinic is another example of an alternative therapeutic space. At the same time as these therapeutic experimentations are happening, psychoanalysis will begin to lose its dominant position in psychiatry, replaced by a psychiatry that is increasingly scientized and codified, concerned with accuracy in diagnosis, and reliant on pharmacological treatments.[54] In the same moment that psychoanalysis loses its hegemony in the domain of psychiatry, it also gains authority in critical theory in particular and humanities scholarship in general. This is an odd displacement that Freud himself might have found fascinating, if also, perhaps, a disturbing reaction formation against the claim that psychoanalysis is a science. In *A Fortunate Man*, but also in *The Birth of the Clinic*, the simplification and biological reductionism at the center of clinical experience is problematized, and through this problematization of what is taken for granted as foundational to a particular clinical experience, the possibility of other ways of doing the clinic appear.

Politics of/and Medical Experience

Foucault ends *The Birth of the Clinic* by bringing together and demonstrating the affinities between medical, philosophical, and lyrical experience at a particular historical moment. "This form of experience, which began in the eighteenth century, and from which we have not yet escaped," Foucault argues, "is bound up with a return to the forms of finitude, of which death is no doubt the most menacing, but also the fullest."[55] In order to examine the "changes in the fundamental structure of experience" that took place at the end of the eighteenth and beginning of the nineteenth centuries and that still structure our experience to a great extent today, Foucault takes as his object the "formation of clinical medicine."[56] In *The Birth of the Clinic,* he demonstrates "a vertical investigation of this positivism," and his method uncovers "a whole series of figures—hidden by it, but also indispensable to its birth—that will be released later, and, paradoxically, used against it."[57] In the early 1960s, Foucault's vertical investigation releases some of these figures in history so that they might be used against the established structures of medical experience in the present of the 1960s and echoing forward to today. While Foucault's method is vertical, Berger and Mohr's method is horizontal, but like Foucault, they also demonstrate the structures that connect medical, philosophical, and lyrical experience—illness, thought, and narrative. Berger and Mohr, however, extend the weblike structure of *A Fortunate Man* into another domain—politics—which is implied in Foucault's text if we read it as a history of the present and in relation to the rest of Foucault's oeuvre. Taken together, Foucault's work can be read as extending politics into domains not previously perceived as domains of struggle. Politics is made explicit in *A Fortunate Man* because Berger and Mohr describe the structural violence of poverty and isolation that constrains the choices of the foresters who Sassall treats.[58] *A Fortunate Man,* then, connects politics with clinical experience, even though, as Berger asserts, Sassall himself does not or cannot within the particular historical a priori that structures his medical perception. Sassall represents a kind of threshold figure not just with regards to his medical practices of doctoring but also with regards to his nascent and only partially realized political practices of doctoring. Sassall acknowledges a feeling of inadequacy in relation to what he can and cannot do for his patients. He asks questions—social as much as medical—about his patients' lives. He comes to realize that they deserve better, and he understands that an important aspect of the treatment he can offer is to recognize them not just for who they are but for who they might become. Sassall's ability to recognize his patients in this way requires "continually speculating about, extending and amending his awareness of what is possible" (142). This speculating, extending, and amending requires, according to Berger, that Sassall combine three practices: "theoretical reading of medicine, science and history; . . . his own clinical observation[; and] his imaginative 'proliferation' of himself in 'becoming' one patient after another" (143). These are Sassall's practices of doctoring, and they are also practices of witnessing,[59] but still, Berger admits, "it is easy to criticize" Sassall for "ignoring politics" and for "practicing alone" rather than in a group practice or health center, making explicit a link between politics and the restructuring of clinical practice. Recognizing his own failures, Sassall tells Berger, "I sometimes wonder . . . how much of me is the last of the old traditional country doctor and how much of me is a doctor of the future," and he asks, "Can you be both?" (147). It seems Sassall can be both traditional doctor and a doctor of the future in and through A Fortunate Man, which becomes a space for the politicization of medicine—a textual, conceptual, methodological domain of struggle—in the 1960s. In that text Berger and Mohr uncover a complicated figure: the country doctor who is both the present Sassall of A Fortunate Man and future Sassalls, both a vestige of the past and a sign of the future.

By reading A Fortunate Man with The Birth of the Clinic, I use the figure of one Sassall against the other not in order to say once and for all what medicine is or should be but to propose an alternative therapeutic genealogy that problematizes and, indeed, struggles against a totalizing discourse of the progressive scientization of medicine.[60] Foucault's insistence in the preface that The Birth of the Clinic "has not been written in favour of one kind of medicine as against another kind of medicine, or against medicine and in favour of an absence of medicine" does not render the practices of medicine outside political critique. Rather, what Foucault wanted The Birth of the Clinic to do in the early 1960s is still relevant today: to open medicine up to the task of transformation.

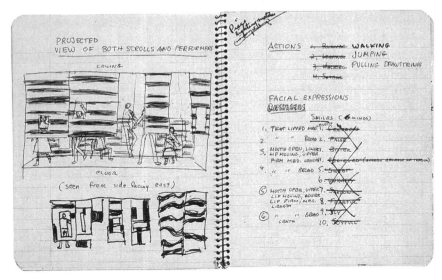

Figure 7. At the first staging of Kaprow's happening, an eighteen-year-old Samuel R. Delany happened to be in the audience. Delany would record his impressions of his experience of that event, first in his own notebook that he always carried with him at the time and later in his memoir, The Motion of Light in Water. Allan Kaprow, 18 Happenings in 6 Parts, *notes, 1959. Allan Kaprow papers. Reprinted by permission of Getty Research Institute, Los Angeles (980063)

Samuel R. Delany's Happening (1959)

An image of an open spiral-bound notebook provides a glimpse into the prehistory of an art/cultural event that took place in 1959—the first "happening," Allan Kaprow's *18 Happenings in 6 Parts*. On the left-hand page, rough sketches are drawn of the event of the "happening," which Kaprow has labeled "projected view of scrolls and performers," the slightly larger top sketch in blue ink and the smaller bottom sketch in black ink. In the top sketch, four scrolls hide much of the scene behind them; rectangular cutouts frame the disembodied heads of performers behind the scrolls on the left, and larger gaps between two narrower scrolls show the almost whole bodies of performers on the right. Because the scrolls do not hang all the way to the floor, the bottom third of the scene is not screened, making the legs of the performers also visible. The right-hand page of the notebook image presents two lists: the first, "actions," and the second, "facial expressions." The phrase "facial expressions" has replaced the word "gestures." The rejected word can just be made out beneath waves of blue ink that almost disappear its trace. The two lists are in blue ink, but some of the writing in blue is struck through with black lines or marked out with large black X's. The image from the notebook provides a glimpse of what we might call a becoming-happening, complete with appearing and disappearing gestures and "gestures"—the word itself and the things themselves.

At the first staging of Kaprow's happening, an eighteen-year-old Samuel R. Delany happened to be in the audience. Delany would record his impressions of his experience of that event, first in his own notebook that he always carried with him at the time and later in his memoir, *The Motion of Light in Water*, which attempts to capture Delany's "experience," as a "black man," a "gay man," and a "writer," in the sexual, literary, and artistic subcultures in New York City in the late 1950s and early 1960s.[1] I put the term "experience" in quotes, along with the identity categories "black man," "gay man," and "writer," to echo Delany's own questioning of categories throughout *The Motion of Light in Water,* as exemplified starkly in section 42.7, which, in its entirety, asks these three identity questions:

A black man . . . ?
A gay man . . . ?
A writer . . . ? (356; ellipses in original)

Delany will repeat these three lines as statements later in the text; the full stop acting to foreclose, both visually and verbally, the open-ended ellipses–question mark configuration. Later still, indicating the ongoingness of these identity formulations/formations, Delany will amend the second and third editions of the memoir to include a Woolfian statement of citizenship via negation, a statement open at both ends by ellipses: ". . . you are neither black nor white. You are neither male nor female. And you are that most ambiguous of citizens, the writer . . ." (398). Although Delany's memoir occupies a prominent place in a poststructuralist genealogy of queer theory,[2] I want to also situate it here in the prehistory of AIDS, not only for its ethical treatment of sexuality but also for its ethical treatment of madness or, put another way, for its linking of the experiences and events of both sexuality and (mental) illness to questions of queer subjectivity and historical method.

Before turning to Delany's snapshot of the historical happening of sexuality and mental illness, I want to first look briefly at Joan W. Scott's "The Evidence of Experience," an essay first published in 1991, which begins and ends with divergent readings of Delany's memoir as a means of problematizing the category and concept of experience as the foundation of historical knowledge of difference.[3] Scott opens her essay with an image from Delany that has become hypostatized as an image of gay visibility and queer becoming and that in its hypostatization echoes, for me, the resounding citational effect of Foucault's diagnosis in *The History of Sexuality,* volume 1, of the emergence of the figure of the homosexual in the nineteenth century.[4] The freezing of Delany's image of gay visibility and queer becoming, I argue, comes about, paradoxically, because of a frequent misreading of Scott's reading of Delany.[5] By the end of her essay, Scott disavows her earlier reading as an incomplete, perhaps even outright wrong, reading not only of Delany's image of visibility but also of the metaanalysis of historical evidence his text enacts. That Scott's first reading of Delany is so often taken as the kernel of her argument, despite her subsequent disavowal of it in the text itself, suggests to me something about the enduring authority of practices of visibility in politics, even queer politics, that I want to challenge in this book in general and via the snapshots that cut up the text in particular. The image from Delany with which Scott opens her essay is of a scene at the St. Marks Baths in 1963 in which Delany saw before him "an undulating mass of naked bodies, spread wall to wall."[6] Scott quotes further from Delany as he attempts to describe what he apprehends—seizes upon and embraces but also fears—in his seeing of this mass grouping of people who are, ostensibly, like him:

> But what *this* experience said was that there was a population—not of individual homosexuals, some of whom now and then encountered, or that those encounters could be human and fulfilling in their way—not of hundreds, not of thousands, but rather of millions of gay men, and that history had, actively and already, created for us whole galleries of institutions, good and bad, to accommodate our sex.[7]

I echo Delany's words and Scott's citation of them here because I want to suggest something about the double practice of hypostatizing an image and dissolving and dispersing that image back into its multiplicity that seems to be key to doing both conceptual and political work. Heeding Scott's own methodological imperative to read for the literary, by reading Scott herself for the literary, I return briefly to Delany's text and its contexts: the New York of his remembered past, in the late 1950s and early 1960s, and the New York of his writing present, in the mid-1980s. Delany's *Motion of Light in Water* provides a snapshot of the prehistory of AIDS, or perhaps it is more accurate to say that it provides multiple, flickering snapshots, as well as a method for documenting them, that disappear in the glare of the recuperated and recuperating image of the illuminated bathhouse scene.

In her essay on the evidence of "experience," Scott discusses Delany's method-image, an image of parallel narratives in two columns with a gap between them. The image of the parallel narratives, explicitly in Delany's text and echoed in Scott's reading of Delany's text, is meant to capture the separation of the material column from the column of desire. In *The Motion of Light in Water*, the double narrative is presented not literally, in parallel columns, but sequentially, which temporalizes the spatial concept or, we might say, historicizes the conceptual. Yet it is important to also note that Delany includes a third narrative, which he calls parenthetical and oblique and which comes in the form of his rendering of someone else's recollection of the same past events that he records in the present[8] or, in some cases, as a kind of holding gesture to our desires for the future encoded in our recollections of the past. In Delany's text parenthetical narratives both draw together and separate the material column from the column of desire.

In a parenthesis between materiality and desire, AIDS appears. Delany brings AIDS into the text in a long paragraph set off from the main narrative, a parenthetical gesture that in both content and form suggests the future anterior of what I am calling the prehistory of AIDS:

> (What is the reason, anyone might ask, for writing such a book as this half a dozen years into the era of AIDS? Is it simply nostalgia for a medically feasible libertinism? Not at all. If I may indulge in my one piece of science fiction for this memoir, it is my firm suspicion, my conviction, and my hope that once the AIDS crisis is brought under control, the West will see a sexual revolution to make a laughing stock of any social movement that till now has borne the name. That revolution will come precisely because of the infiltration of clear and articulate language into the marginal areas of human sexual exploration, such as this book from time to time describes, and of which it is only the most modest example. Now that a significant range of people have begun to get a clearer idea of what has been possible among the varieties of human pleasure in the recent past, heterosexuals and homosexuals, females and males will insist on exploring them even further. I sincerely hope this book—not as nostalgia but as possibility—helps. Indeed, as Harvey Fierstein has already said: the AIDS situation and our accommodations to it *are* that revolution, nascent and under way.) (294)

In "The Evidence of Experience," Scott also quotes from the middle of this long paragraph and glosses it as Delany's imagining, "even from the vantage of 1988, a future utopian moment of genuine sexual revolution,"[9] but surprisingly, the parentheses are not included in her citation, nor does she mention the formal elements of this future anterior aside, in which AIDS appears for the only time in the text, not to signal the death of desire but as a revolution-in-the-making in 1988, as a reminder that Delany's prehistory of sexual revolution is also a history of the present of AIDS and the possibility of new social, sexual, and political forms of belonging.

If science fiction is Delany's literary form of choice for imagining new social forms, it is his "experience" of Allan Kaprow's "happening" that provides a method-image to help him articulate the historical eventfulness of the late 1950s and early 1960s from the vantage point of the mid-to-late 1980s. Delany introduces his description of 18 *Happenings in 6 Parts* by noting that historians had settled on the year 1956 as marking the "transition from America's 'Industrial Period' to its 'Postindustrial Period,'" because that year white-collar workers numerically exceeded blue-collar and agricultural workers combined (200). This sociohistorical "fact" leads into Delany's discussion of Kaprow's happening, and Delany notes that Kaprow's piece has also "been cited by art historians as the (equally arbitrary) transition between the modern and the postmodern in cultural developments" (201). What interests Delany, then, is the way history—and the "situation of the subject in history" (208)—is cut up in order to represent and analyze it.[10] What Kaprow's happening gives Delany is a genealogical method-image that echoes Foucault's delineation, in "Nietzsche, Genealogy, History," of how history becomes "effective" by "introduc[ing] discontinuity into our very being—as it divides our emotions, dramatizes our instincts, multiplies our body and sets it against itself."[11] Kaprow's happening cuts up experience both spatially and temporally, and by utilizing Kaprow's happening as method, Delany's memoir provides evidence not only of his own experience of Kaprow's happening but also of a sociohistorical moment—an arbitrary historical cut dividing the industrial from the postindustrial, the modern from the postmodern.

Importantly, Scott and later Muñoz place Delany's work in a genealogy of queer theory and practices in the prehistory of AIDS, yet I contend that what is queer about Delany's work is not just his explicit writing about sexuality but also his writing about illness, in particular, his own mental illness. As Foucault understood well, it is not simply the "experience" of sexuality that "divides our emotions, dramatizes our instincts, multiplies our body, and sets it against itself" but also the "experience" of madness and the intersection between these two experiences historically. Along with new forms of sexual belonging, Delany also describes new forms of therapeutic belonging. Indeed, much of Delany's own metacommentary about the interpretation of experience as constitutive of subjectivity is punctuated by the phrase "in the hospital" because it is there—in the therapy program at Mount Sinai's Day/Night Center—where Delany first comes out publicly as homosexual and also where he realizes that the public language available to him for recounting his experiences of sexuality betrays him and the multiplicity of his experience (405). It is in the hospital that Delany arrives at his notion of parallel narratives, separated and joined by a gap, and the realization that the "flickering correlations between, as evanescent as light-shot water, as insubstantial as moonstruck cloud, are really all that constitutes the subject" (356). Delany's account of his hospitalization suggests that the space and time of mental illness and its treatments are potentially an opening and not a bar to the articulation of the sexual subject in history. For Delany, like the "galleries of institutions for sex," the hospital was another institution that cut up experience, making it impossible to apprehend in its totality. *The Motion of Light in Water* is Delany's happening, his staging of the experience and event of the institutions of sex and illness, art and therapy.

4

Thinking Ecologically, circa 1962 and 1971

As seen in chapter 3 in relation to the shifting clinical experiences of the 1960s, while this period is indisputably one of increasing specialization in the practices of science and medicine, most especially in the U.S. context, nonetheless various outsiders and insiders to science and medicine challenged the rampant technologization and ever-higher levels of specialization, arguing that such approaches took science and medicine in the wrong direction. Sassall and his clinic, as presented in Berger and Mohr's hybrid text, demonstrate how a generalist clinical counternarrative was thought and enacted in a period of increasing specialization. In this chapter I continue to explore the resistance to specialization and reductionism through what we might call "generalist tendencies" by taking up another key, if also minoritarian, concept in the prehistory of AIDS—"ecological thought" or, as I delineate it here to emphasize the dynamic, multiple aspects of the practice, "thinking ecologically."[1] Echoing the structure of chapter 3 and my attempt throughout to describe a multifocal art of seeing, this chapter also juxtaposes two texts published in the prehistory of AIDS that diagnose the condition of scientific and medical practice and offer a generalist alternative to the hegemony of specialization—these texts are Rachel Carson's *Silent Spring*, published in 1962, and Lewis Thomas's Notes of a Biology Watcher column, published in the *New England Journal of Medicine* from 1971 to 1980.[2] Carson's writing clears a path for later literary–scientific writing like Thomas's. Both become scientists as public intellectuals, another threshold figure that is both vestige of the past and sign of the future.

Of all the texts I take up, Carson's work is by far the most well known, even iconic, if perhaps not always the most read; on the fiftieth anniversary of its publication in 2012, the book and its legacies again garnered widespread, mostly enthusiastic coverage. The resurgence of interest in Carson's text, even fifty years on, indicates that it continues to provide a timely model for innovative practices of ecology and health in the contemporary moment.[3] Unlike *Silent Spring*, Thomas's work has mostly disappeared from contemporary commentary on ecology and health, and part of my purpose in pairing Carson with Thomas is not simply to recover Thomas's work for a critical medical studies in the present but, more importantly, to make a point about method by drawing attention to the relationship between the ecological and the clinical in some popular literary–scientific work of the 1960s and 1970s.

In her recent book *Ecological Thinking*, feminist philosopher Lorraine Code brilliantly delineates how Carson's *Silent Spring* is ecological in the broadest sense of the term: concerned with the multiple, complex, and changing relationships "of living organisms to their surroundings, their habits and modes of life," according to the *OED*'s definition.[4] In 1963, in the shadow of the publication of *Silent Spring*, the *OED* definition of *ecology* is expanded further to include explicitly political aspects: "the study of or concern for the effect of human activity on the environment; advocacy of restrictions on industrial and agricultural development as a political movement; (also) a political movement dedicated to this." Although Code is more interested in reading Carson's work as providing a model for "a way of knowing nature and human nature" than in historicizing it as I do here, she does note that Carson is "one of the most eminent precursors and catalysts of the new social movements fueled by the 1960s civil rights and women's movement in North America and in the aftermath of the events of 1968 in France and elsewhere in Europe [and beyond Europe]—movements energetic in their opposition to multiple, mutually enforcing injustices."[5] For Code these new social movements challenged "entrenched power structures and tenacious beliefs in the 'natural' (pre-1960s) order of things, both human and nonhuman," and she sees this "subversiveness prefigured, if sometimes tacitly, in Carson's work."[6] It is this prefiguration of subversiveness in Carson's work in which I am most interested, in relation not just to the more immediate emergence of social movements of the late 1960s but also to health activist movements that emerge still later. Or put differently, in this chapter I draw out the health activism in Carson's work.

The extension of the political into new domains is one of the important immediate and long-term effects of the publication of *Silent Spring*. This connects at least tacitly, to use Code's useful word, to the extension of the political into the personal through the emergence of second-wave feminism at this same time. It seems to me there is an eerie echo between Betty Friedan's diagnosis of the feminine mystique as the "problem that has no name" among white, middle-class, suburban American women and Carson's diagnosis of another hidden poison of suburban life: "The fact that the suburbanite is not instantly stricken has little meaning, for the toxins may sleep long in his body, to become manifest months or years later in an obscure disorder almost impossible to trace to its origins" (24).[7] There is what I would call a temporopolitics, along with the more obvious spatial politics, at work in both Carson and Friedan, which asserts the difficulty in discerning biopsychosocial cause and effect. By drawing out these connections, I also want to problematize the way the feminist and environmental movements, as will the AIDS movement, become remembered as white and middle class. That Friedan and Carson focused on the plight of recent mostly white migrants to the suburbs in their discussions of the literal and figurative toxicities of suburban life has meant environmental and feminist activism has tended to be read as emerging out of white, middle-class constituencies first and only later diversifying in terms of race and class. By showing multiple genealogies of health activism before AIDS, I work against this progress narrative while analyzing what this whitening does in relation to how health activism is practiced today. I also want to reiterate a point that came up in chapter 3 with regards to Foucault's historicizing diagnosis of the extension of the political into other domains at this time. The possibility of a new practice of the political that was problematized in Berger and Mohr's portrait of John Sassall is also already prefigured in Carson's work.

Carson as Outsider to Science

We should recall that among the widespread commentary on *Silent Spring* at the time of its publication was discussion of Carson's status as an outsider to science; as a woman and as a biologist, her thinking was always already suspect, her reasoning perceived by many as squishy and soft, impertinent and partial.[8] Never mind the pesticide industry hacks who derided Carson for everything from her supposed lack of intellectual qualifications to her "spinster" status, which suggested some monstrous femininity,[9] even in some commentary that supports Carson's main arguments about the dangers of indiscriminate pesticide use, there is a palpable anxiety over whether her case against pesticides is well reasoned or overly emotional, even hysterical. For example, one scientist, who favorably ends his review by proclaiming that "the book is must reading for all biologists," calls "Miss

Carson's devotion to nature's way . . . naïve in a world made so unnatural by the activities of man," as if the "unnatural . . . activities of man" were not precisely her point, and chastises her for choosing examples for their "emotional mileage" rather than their representativeness.[10] Here, science and nature are understood dichotomously, and Carson, in a not-very-subtle essentializing move, is placed on the side of nature and emotion. Although obviously an advocate for and lover of "nature," what we understand by categories like the "natural" and the "social" was denaturalized by Carson's ecological approach, which emphasized the importance of relations between animate and inanimate objects rather than their attributes.

Carson's approach to ecological questions was always emphatically scientific, yet the question of how one might best do science and communicate scientific information was a theme Carson explored in and through all of her work. As Frank Egler, a dissident ecologist and one of Carson's collaborators and loyal supporters, noted in response to some of the negative reviews of *Silent Spring,* if anyone was emotional about pesticides and nature, it was the scientists and advocates for the pesticide industry who sought to discredit Carson: "There has been defense and counter-defense," asserts Egler, "a focusing upon minutiae, distortion, innuendo, bias, claims of emotionalism themselves written with extreme and apparent emotion."[11] By focusing on the uses of emotion on all sides in this case, Egler challenges the commonsense view that emotions are something people have or don't have and suggests instead that emotions circulate socially and are at work in the processes of inclusion and exclusion necessary to the formation of groups, professions, and communities. Emotions, too, are ecological.

In a series of letters to Carson that began after parts of *Silent Spring* were first serialized in the *New Yorker* in the summer of 1962 and continued until her death in 1964, Egler offers a fascinating meta-analysis, itself ecological in its approach, of the response to *Silent Spring* by the scientific community, the pesticide industry, and the public. The iconoclastic scientist and early practitioner of what might be described now as science studies was also a harsh critic of those many scientists content to practice the "normal science" handsomely rewarded by government and industry grants in the immediate postwar and post-Sputnik expansion of science spending in the United States.[12] "I have just read the New Yorker installment of your silent spring," so begins a postcard from Egler to Carson in 1962, which continues with the highest praise for Carson and her work:

Superb—in its literary style, in its scientific data, in its significance for the wise use by man of his environment. A milestone, I predict, that future generations will praise as the turning point in the unwise use of powerful chemical tools which, due to promotion by American industry and silence on the part of those who should be watchdogs in the public interest, clearly threaten the fabric of our society.[13]

In later letters and postcards to Carson, Egler reports on both good and bad reviews of *Silent Spring*, explaining, "These reviews are extremely interesting to me. They themselves represent so much in the way of independent thinking, flabby thinking, sometimes just a front for industry (like the one in *Time*)."[14] He admits to Carson that since he is mentioned in the preface, it would be inappropriate for him to write his own review: "Like a husband testifying at the trial of a wife," he tells Carson, "I am 'prejudiced.'"[15] Instead, Egler suggests that he could write a "*review of reviews*," which he believes "would be an extremely interesting sociological document!"[16] Although Egler never writes the "review of reviews" of *Silent Spring*, he does contribute a hard-hitting piece to the *Atlantic Naturalist* critiquing the National Academy of Sciences (NAS) and the National Research Council (NRC) for their "defense of the pesticide industry." Egler's piece might be described as an ecological critique of the too close relationship between science and industry as demonstrated in two *NAS Bulletins* (920 A and B) and the review of *Silent Spring* in *Science* by Ian L. Baldwin, who was then chairman of the Committee on Pest Control and Wildlife Relationships of the NAS–NRC.[17] In a carbon copy of an unpublished letter to *Science* protesting Baldwin's review, Egler offers this critique of the science in the two bulletins:

The sleek hand of a Public Relations expert is seen on every page. With a change in cover—and I say this in complete seriousness— these bulletins could serve as promotional literature for the chemical industry. They show a remarkable avoidance of ecological sophistication. The thinking is on the level of "there are the bad bugs—let's kill 'em. If anything else gets in the way, that's their tough luck." A third bulletin, on needed research, was mysteriously dropped from the program, as "unnecessary." Try as I might, I cannot avoid the conclusion, as sober a scientific conclusion as I have ever drawn, that if broad ecologic competence had existed in the committee, it was either muzzled, or influenced.[18]

In later letters to Carson, Egler will call his critique of the *NAS Bulletins* his "NASty" piece, and it is clear he derived pleasure from taking on the scientific powers that be by linking the "pesticide controversy" to a "much larger social web," including the tobacco–cancer issue and the thalidomide scandal, all of which show scientists towing a profit-driven party line—a capitalist version, Egler contends, of Russian Lysenkoism.[19]

Through his specific analysis of the larger social web in which pesticide science is enacted, Egler generates a more general theory about what he calls the "Flow of Knowledge," and in an attempt to visualize his theory, he produces a fascinating chart showing how knowledge about pesticides flows or not between various stakeholders. As a result of his interest in scientific communication in general, Egler recognizes that Carson is a much more effective communicator of scientific information than he is. His letters express awe at her remarkable ability to challenge scientific dogma while presenting an ecologically sophisticated worldview to the public, making connections across disciplines, experiences, spaces, and times. Her appearance on *CBS Reports* with Eric Sevareid on April 3, 1963, in a program titled "The Silent Spring of Rachel Carson" garners a rave review from Egler, who describes the "theatricality" of the event that favorably pits Carson against Dr. Robert White-Stevens, described by Egler as "industry personified" and the "Villain in a Victorian melodrama."[20] Egler's reading of Carson's performance adds another dimension to his theory of the flow of knowledge and again anticipates later work in science studies exploring how science is enacted in and through popular culture.

In the preface to his important book on slow violence, Rob Nixon draws out the connections between three important twentieth-century thinkers—Rachel Carson, Edward Said, and Ramachandra Guha—whose work, Nixon argues, demonstrates "a communicative passion responsive to diverse audiences, indeed a passion that has helped shape such audiences by refusing to adhere to conventional disciplinary or professional expectations."[21] I contend that this new form of literary–scientific writing and communication, of which Carson was an exemplary practitioner in the prehistory of AIDS, would become prominent in the response to HIV/AIDS by both doctors and patients, especially in the early years of the epidemic. New methods and forms—scientific, political, aesthetic—emerge to respond to new problems—ecological and clinical—creating new tributaries in and redirections of the flow of scientific and medical knowledge.

Silent Spring as Ecoontological Critique

Silent Spring is a remarkable book not only for its unflinching critique of the powerful economic interests of science but also for its explicit challenge to what Carson called an "era of specialists," in which the specialist scientist only "sees his own problem and is unaware of or intolerant of the larger frame into which it fits" (13). Carson's is an early call for interdisciplinary and collaborative methods in approaching socioscientific problems, and she herself becomes a relay figure between these minoritarian interdisciplinary and generalist initiatives from within science and what comes afterward: new social movements around women's health and environmental justice, as well as new feminist theories of relation not simply between and among agentic subjects but between and among subjects and objects, animate and inanimate.[22] Most often, we perceive the practices of interdisciplinarity and collaboration spatially; we are required to move between departments and disciplines—literally, down the hall and across campus. But these practices also require new temporal registers. For one, it takes time to communicate across different disciplines because the discourses taken for granted in one discipline often don't translate easily to other disciplines, and for another, our objects of study multiply across time as well as space. In our practices of everyday life, objects tend not to hold steady long enough for us to examine them thoroughly or even at all. In its form and content, Carson's essay draws our attention to multiple and divergent temporalities: of science and technology, ethics and politics, and the materiality of chemicals and disease in the environment and the human body.

The text opens with "A Fable for Tomorrow," which presents "new kinds of sickness" and an old explanation—sorcery—that no longer serves. As Ralph H. Lutts demonstrates, Carson's fable of a dystopic future, though it employed a speculative rhetoric, was written in the shadow of real historical events that had made perceptible the power and long-term effects of certain substances initially perceived as innocuous or even beneficial—radiation and thalidomide, to name two substances that Lutts shows had been in the air, in the case of radiation quite literally, as Carson was writing.[23] Lutts argues that people in the United States and beyond had been "pre-educated" by the event of radioactive fallout to understand the imperceptible threat of pesticides Carson details in *Silent Spring*.[24] Lutts's notion of preeducation isn't just about foreknowledge; rather, it also suggests a pedagogy that works through emotion and embodiment and on the imagination. Through her literary–scientific enactments in the text of *Silent Spring* and beyond, Carson manages to tap into this potentially paralyzing environment, enervating a public response, which her critics liken to paranoia and mass hysteria. This complex relationship between the public, science and medicine, and particular articulations that use new idioms to produce new linkages is what I am trying to discern through an analysis of the nexus illness-thought-activism. What is the public in general and medicine in particular preeducated for (and not) in different times and spaces? My return to the health activism of the 1960s and 1970s is an attempt to show how knowledge flows or is stymied or redirected between various health/activist environments across time and space.

Carson's speculative opening gives way to a chapter entitled "The Obligation to Endure," which sets the temporality of endurance against that of compulsive modification: "The rapidity of change and the speed with which new situations are created follow the impetuous and heedless pace of man rather than the deliberate pace of nature" (7). Endurance does not readily translate into autonomous agency, but this may be precisely the point, as Berlant has articulated through her concepts of "slow death" and "lateral agency" and through her shift in focus from traumatic events to what she calls "temporal environments."[25] Conceiving of "slow violence" and "slow death" works to stretch and make viscous the spatial and temporal parameters that frame our analysis of multiple and complex structures and forms of agency. It seems to me that although we might see *Silent Spring* as making spectacular what before it had been invisible, Carson's unheroic "obligation to endure" and her undramatic taxonomy of indeterminate causality best explains why the text itself endures. As Nixon argues by echoing Carson:

> To address the challenges of slow violence is to confront the
> dilemma Rachel Carson faced almost half a century ago as she
> sought to dramatize what she eloquently called "death by indirec-
> tion." Carson's subjects were biomagnification and toxic drift, forms
> of oblique, slow-acting violence that, like climate change, pose
> formidable imaginative difficulties for writers and activists alike.[26]

In order to address "death by indirection" and the challenges of slow violence, one effective tactic is to practice a temporopolitics by indirection, articulating microlinks across time and space. What I am positing, then, is that we consider indirect action, as well as direct action, in our attempts to understand the practices of illness, thought, and activism before and after AIDS.

Carson offers a model for analyzing indirect actions across time and space. In doing so, she presciently prefigures some of the "alternative social projects" of the 1970s that feminist anthropologist Elizabeth Povinelli describes in her recent book *Events of Abandonment*. As Povinelli explains of her work with Indigenous activists in Australia, "We are not trying to become something different. We are instead trying to extend something over space and time that has no viable language outside this iteration of its persistence. We are trying to be within a social imaginary in which the substance of human life is cosubstantial with geological/geographic life."[27] Povinelli is interested in the "immanent geontological"—the being of geology—and Carson too offers an immanent geontological or, perhaps we might say, ecoontological critique that points to the problem of the persistence of pesticides in soil, in groundwater, in fat cells, and in genes but also to the "regimes of imperceptibility," in Michelle Murphy's terminology, that are produced by different disciplines, discourses, institutions, and interests.[28]

For Carson an ecological approach connects environments with bodies, exteriors with interiors, macrosocial with microcellular contexts, and near with distant times, and in the part of *Silent Spring* deemed the most scientifically speculative at the time of its publication, thinking ecologically includes thinking metabolically and reproductively in general and theorizing about the possible links between pesticides and cancer in particular.[29] The madness of Rachel Carson is that she not only accumulates evidence of things we do know about chemicals and their destructive potency but also accumulates a kind of evidence of the countless things we don't know, an evidence of the persistence of matter,[30] and by doing so she magnifies the complexity of biopsychosocial causes and effects. This notion that we might need to somehow accumulate evidence of things we don't know is also what I am grappling with here in relation to the history of AIDS and health activism.

How do we approach this methodological question? Carson gives us an indirect route. Her astute critique of the Food and Drug Administration's method for setting chemical tolerance levels is one example of her ecoontological analysis. She notes that the use of laboratory animals in controlled settings to establish maximum levels of contamination "ignores a number of important facts." "A laboratory animal, living under controlled and highly artificial conditions, consuming a given amount of a specific chemical," Carson writes, "is very different from a human being whose exposures to pesticides are not only multiple but for the most part unknown, unmeasurable, and uncontrollable." For Carson the problem is not so much clear as messy: "This piling up of chemicals from many different sources creates a total exposure that cannot be measured" (182). As Murphy has shown in regards to the postmodern and post-Carson conditions of sick building syndrome and multiple chemical sensitivity, the tools we use to study the effects of chemical exposures produce domains of both perceptibility and imperceptibility, ways of seeing and not seeing.[31] Existing toxicological technologies, which were developed to discern acute industrial exposures, have not been able to render visible "specific and predictable causal pathways" for most environmental illnesses. The nonspecificity of disease causation becomes not a challenge for science but an alibi for not seeking more and different data. To pursue the cause of a nonspecific health event is to tilt at windmills and risk encouraging mass hysteria.[32] Still, we don't have to look very hard to determine the very specific economic interests that directly benefit from the all-purpose alibi of nonspecificity.

Moreover, Carson's concern for the piling up of chemicals from multiple sources is also an early note of precaution in regards to other forms of chemical treatment rolled out in the postwar era: those psychotropic and chemotherapeutic drugs that were synthesized in the 1950s and were beginning to be prescribed widely in the period in which Carson is writing *Silent Spring*[33] and that, like pesticides, brought some measurable benefits and many immeasurable (and most often unmeasured) side effects. From her extensive correspondence with the radical doctor Morton S. Biskind, who wrote about the harmful effects of DDT on human health and advocated vitamin therapies to rejuvenate the immune system, we can see that Carson's skepticism about the healing potential of chemical poisons was directed at products for treating both external and internal ecologies.[34]

Carson's ecological approach emphasizes multiplicity, complexity, and indirection in terms of both the being of cancer and its causation. She notes that "cause and effect are seldom simple and easily demonstrated relationships"; often they are "widely separated both in space and time" (189). The problem is one of "inadequate methods for detecting the beginnings of injury" (190), and for Carson this problem of inadequate methods for detecting beginnings is itself the beginning not the end of health research and activism. Carson, of course, was taken up as a kind of patron saint of breast cancer activism in the late 1980s and early 1990s. Even in the three major scientific studies mandated by the U.S. government to look into possible environmental causes of the high incidence of breast cancer on Long Island first widely publicized in the 1980s, Carson's *Silent Spring* figures prominently in the scientists' presentation of the emergence of a narrative of concern about a possible connection between pesticides and breast cancer on Long Island.[35] All three articles published in 2002 begin by referencing Carson's book, which explicitly discusses both the adverse effects of widespread pesticide spraying on Long Island and the community activism that emerged as a response to that spraying. Gammon et al. do not discuss Carson's text in detail, nor do they mention her own death from breast cancer. Rather, her text figures in these scientific studies as a time- and placeholder for the emergence of health activism on Long Island. This longtime concern (represented in these scientific texts as vague and unfocused) was then coupled with knowledge of the high incidence rates of breast cancer on Long Island, and in Gammon et al.'s account, this knowledge was provided by New York State epidemiological studies rather than by the activists' own knowledge of breast cancer in their communities.[36] Although I don't have space here to go into detail about breast cancer activism on Long Island, I point to it now to retrace a line back from the scientific studies into breast cancer and potential environmental causes in the 2000s to the breast cancer activism in the 1990s to Carson and ecological activism in the 1960s. Like Egler, I am interested in the flow of knowledge spatially, but additionally, I am interested in the question of how knowledge flows temporally. In many accounts that describe the increasing politicization of the experience and event of breast cancer, politicization is most often not traced back to Carson, environmental justice activism, or feminist health activism; instead, the political tactics are given a more recent and direct origin: the breast cancer movement is said to have been directly influenced by AIDS activism.[37] All of which suggests to me the domains of both perceptibility and imperceptibility at work in histories of illness and its forms of activism.

This is the historical paradox I am trying to work through: the perception of a unidirectional movement from AIDS activism to breast cancer activism forgets a whole history of activism—feminist and ecological—that challenged the practices of medicine and science in the two decades before AIDS. For me the question becomes: How do we account for this multiplicity and indirection, and why is it crucial to do so in relation not only to how we do health and illness but also to how we do history, thought, and politics? Many have celebrated Carson as a heroic figure, courageous and undaunted, who changed the course of history through sheer force of will, even as she endured her own experience of breast cancer as she was forced to publicly defend her work. But I prefer to see her as advocating a less direct and more uncertain approach, one that might yet be useful in apprehending what Larry Kramer would later describe as the "enormous thing": the underlying conditions of AIDS.

Thomas as Biomedicine Watcher

One of my favorite photographs of Carson, taken by her close friend and collaborator Shirley A. Briggs on a trip to Hawk Mountain Sanctuary in Pennsylvania in 1946, shows her perched on the top of a mountain peering through binoculars (Figure 8). Wearing a brown leather jacket, heavy trousers, and hiking boots, she is framed by a vast landscape behind her, which her body blends into both because of the photograph's composition and because of its sepia tones and mixture of light and shadow. Her curly light-brown hair merges with a grove of trees in the distance, and her arm, holding the binoculars, appears to be extended by a scraggy, leafless tree behind her. The angle of the shot—Briggs is to her side and slightly above her; what appears to be the photographer's shadow darkens the bottom of Carson's right leg in the foreground of the shot—means we see Carson looking, but not her eyes nor what she sees through the binoculars. What we see is a way of seeing, not the thing seen itself.

Later photographs of Carson taken by the Magnum photographer Erich Hartmann in Southport, Maine, in 1962 also include her binoculars, but in these shots the binoculars hang on her shoulder and are ready at hand but not being used. In several of Hartmann's photographs, Carson is posed leaning against what appears to be a dead or dying tree, and she looks back directly at the photographer and the viewer. One of Hartmann's photos of Carson graces the cover of Linda Lear's excellent biography *Rachel Carson: Witness for Nature,* and the notion of *witnessing for* is illustrated by the photo and in the way Lear frames Carson's story as a call to witness. The cover photograph is also the one of Hartmann's series in which Carson

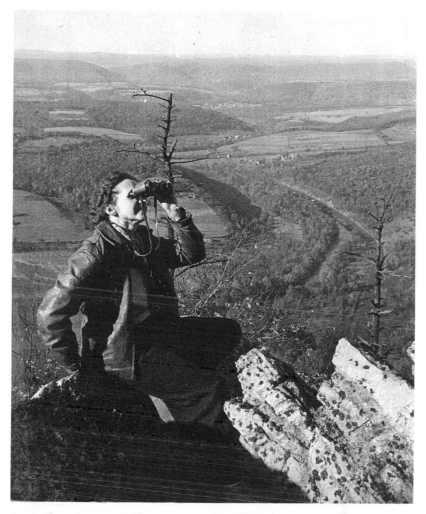

Figure 8. What we see is a way of seeing, not the thing seen itself. Photograph of Rachel Carson taken by her close friend and collaborator Shirley A. Briggs on a trip to Hawk Mountain Sanctuary in Pennsylvania in 1946. Image courtesy of the Linda Lear Center for Special Collections and Archives at Connecticut College.

is the most squarely facing her audience, unlike other photos shot from the side, in which she turns her head back. All these photos of Carson are affecting in that she looks somewhat frail physically (there is a visible tiredness around her eyes) but nonetheless utterly composed, with an unwavering gaze.

Like Briggs's earlier shot of Carson at Hawk Mountain, Hartmann also photographed Carson blending in and blended into a landscape—this time she is by the sea among rocks covered with seaweed, shells, and other shoreline detritus. Rather than looking up to the sky, here she is perched on her haunches and peering down at something that has clearly caught her eye—is it a bird? It is difficult to discern, which seems to be Hartmann's point. She appears unaware of or unconcerned about the photographer and us; instead, she is drawn to and completely taken with what she has spotted in the tide pool at her feet. It isn't unusual for Carson to be posed in nature, but Hartmann's shot, even more so than Briggs's, works to desubjectify her amid the environment she examines, which for me also suggests life as cosubstantial and ecoontological.

I use these images of Carson both as nature watcher and as nature itself to lead into my discussion of Thomas as biomedicine watcher. In contrast to the ecoontological images of Carson, Thomas begins the inaugural essay of his Notes of a Biology Watcher column with a commonplace image of "Modern Man" as detached from and in a position above nature:

> We are told that the trouble with Modern Man is that he has been trying to detach himself from nature. He sits in the topmost tiers of polymer, glass, and steel, dangling his pulsing legs, surveying at a distance the writhing life of the planet. In this scenario, Man comes on as a stupendous lethal force, and the earth is pictured as something delicate, like rising bubbles at the surface of a country pond, or flights of fragile birds.[38]

In economical language Thomas efficiently displaces humans from their position "above the rest of life," noting both the position and the hierarchy it enshrines are an illusion invented by man. Thomas states simply, "Man is embedded in nature," and he points out that recent ecological thinking in the biological sciences is undermining the "old, clung-to notions most of us have held about our special lordship" (3).

Thomas offers another minoritarian position in the era of ever-increasing specialization. Thomas was the son of a general practitioner who treated his patients across the span of their lives and often saw them in their home environments, not unlike John Sassall. By turning to Thomas, then, I return to questions about the changing spaces and temporalities of the clinic that I discussed in more detail in chapter 3, as well as to questions about the place of general practice in medicine in particular and the counterpractice of generalism more generally. In *The Youngest Science: Notes of a Medicine-Watcher,* a medical memoir of sorts, both doctor narrative and *doctoring* narrative, Thomas begins with a chapter that not only situates his father's practice in the family home but also provides us with an image of his father being "called out for patients who were dying or dead," not so much to do something for them but more simply to be with them in their homes as they lay ill and dying, echoing the image in *A Fortunate Man* of the doctor being called.[39] Thomas's father would frequently take his son along as he made these house calls, and the lesson Thomas learned from his father was that most often all the doctor has to offer is medicine as placebo, tonics that did no harm but "gave the patient something to do while the illness, whatever, was working its way through its appointed course" (15). Thomas would carry these early therapeutic lessons through a long and accomplished career as physician and researcher who also directed several clinical and research institutions before he began his column for the *New England Journal of Medicine.* The breadth of his topics—from entomology to etymology from symbiosis to cybernetics—provides an invigorating demonstration of the benefits of a generalist approach. In his opening foray into literary–scientific writing first published in 1971, Thomas uses the essay form to present new ways of seeing and thinking that not only do the macroecological work of embedding humans in nature but also do the microecoontological work of embedding all of nature and time in a single cell. We have another example of a bifocal art of seeing, coupled with a Spinozan-like monism where everything is contained in each thing.

In a passage striking for its capacity to both personalize and depersonalize the lives of cells, Thomas identifies a recent shift in feeling and thinking I would argue is another example of thinking ecoontologically:

We carry stores of DNA in our nuclei that may have come in, at one time or another, from the fusion of ancestral cells and the linking of ancestral organisms in symbiosis. Our genomes are catalogues of instructions from all kinds of sources in nature, filed for all kinds of contingencies. As for me, I am grateful for differentiation and speciation, but I cannot feel as separate an entity as I did a few years ago, before I was told these things, nor, I should think, can anyone else (5).

"Symbiosis" is a key term in Thomas's essays from the 1970s: he is interested in what he calls the "high technology of symbiosis" (8) across all levels of life forms, and he notes that symbiotic linkages and cooperative associations are biologically commonplace across species. Beyond a specific interest in symbiotic thinking, which recurs throughout the essays, what this passage also demonstrates is Thomas's methodological habit of embedding his own thought and feeling in the changing culture and politics of science and his attempt to reflect back on this embeddedness in a metadouble description.

It seems fitting that the edited collection of Thomas's writings should carry the same title as his first essay: the essay nests within the larger collection, and that collection contains multitudes and jumps between scales such that, for example, the essay "Germs," which argues that disease is the result of a symbiotic error, "an overstepping of the line by one side or the other, a biologic misinterpretation of borders" (76), is placed next to the essay "Your Very Good Health," which questions what we would now call the neoliberalization of health, described here as an emergent market fundamentalism that has turned medicine into "health-care delivery" (81). In this piece Thomas discusses with trepidation the transformation of patients into consumers and the invention of "new institutions called Health Maintenance Organizations, already known at that time familiarly as HMO's, spreading across the country like post offices, ready to distribute in neat packages, as though from a huge, newly stocked inventory, health" (82). In what follows, Thomas punctures this utopian picture, arguing that the obsession with health has turned into a kind of healthism, an ideology that is neither good science nor good politics, and anticipating later work against health as the basis for morality in postmodernity.[40] Thomas argues that we might learn something useful if we examined the health practices of internists and their families, and he even offers sample questions for such a study, about the number of physical examinations, x-rays, antibiotics prescribed, visits to doctors, surgeries, etc., in these families. His, admittedly unscientific, poll among his internist friends suggests such a study would show general practitioners and their families have health care delivered to them far less than the rest of the U.S. population. Thomas's point is that "most things get better by themselves," a simple truth known by most internists "but still hidden from the general public," and he believes it is a mistake to act as if, as well as design a system that acts as if, our health is in "constant peril" (85).

It isn't so much that Thomas believes that we can or should somehow go back to nature; rather, he is concerned with challenging medicine's interventionist ideology, which calls for direct and continual action to maintain health (86). Like Carson, Thomas emphasizes indirection and uncertainty as practices of health and crafts a literary–scientific form through which to communicate information about counterpractices of health, not just to doctors who read the *New England Journal of Medicine* but also to the general public. Yet of course, illnesses don't always get better by themselves, and many of us would be reminded of this simple fact with the emergence of AIDS around 1981, shortly after the publication of a second collection of Thomas's essays. By recalling these articulations of more indirect, passive even, counterpractices of health in the prehistory of AIDS, I am not suggesting that a better response to AIDS would have been a more indirect or passive one. Rather, my point is that the practices of direct action in relation to health and health care don't so much challenge earlier interventionist ideologies as continue and, perhaps, even strengthen them.

One of Thomas's preoccupations across his literary–scientific writings is the changing meanings and uses of particular words; he is especially interested in how and why certain words appear, disappear, and reappear—words like *superorganism*, which referred to the "collective intelligence" and adaptive potentiality of colonies of social insects and which was a key term in entomology from 1911 to the 1950s but then stopped being used or even thought as a new reductionism associated with an experimental ideology came into fashion in entomology (127). In a reading that provides a succinct image of the process by which knowledge becomes subjugated, Thomas explains that *superorganism*, word and concept-metaphor, "just sat there, in a way, and was covered over by leaves and papers" (128).

Similarly, in *The Youngest Science*, Thomas explores subjugated knowledges and practices of medicine by first drawing etymological links between *medicine, moderate,* and *modest,* arguing that the "root *med* has tucked itself inside these words, living as a successful symbiont and its similar existence all these years inside medicine should be a steady message for the teacher, the healer, the collector of science, the old leech" (54). This brief analysis of how words contain vestiges of older ways of thinking, being, and doing leads to a more lengthy discussion of the prevalence, at the time Thomas is writing in the late 1970s, of the desire for a return of the family doctor, a desire that Thomas notes resulted, paradoxically, in the emergence of "whole new academic departments"—including family medicine and preventive medicine (55)—dedicated to reproducing these figures of the old age of the clinic, but within the new technologized and bureaucratic field of contemporary medicine as key site of the exercise of biopower. Thomas also discusses the lost art of touching in medicine—with the hands and naked ear—and points to the phenomenon of doctors working more closely with the machines monitoring patients than with the patients themselves. In Thomas's writings, this lost art is not fetishized as so often happens in that other field—medical humanities—that emerges in the 1970s alongside family practice and preventive medicine; rather, Thomas enfolds this microstory of a doctor and her patient into other larger and more complex stories of medical professionalization and university governance, research practices and ethics, and political economies and ideologies.

What makes Thomas's work so compelling is what I have already described as his readiness to jump scales. In one of his columns, "The Planning of Science," Thomas describes the emergence of a "new kind of management" of scientific research that underlies a shift from, in the immediate postwar period, a blue-sky approach that emphasizes basic science to, beginning in the 1970s, a more targeted approach that emphasizes "mission-oriented" and applied research (116). For Thomas the "direct, frontal approach" of applied research requires "a high degree of certainty from the outset" and seeks to circumvent the possibility of surprise, which is often a desired outcome of basic research rather than its undoing. According to Thomas, what is needed to do basic research is a "high degree of uncertainty" and unpredictability, and the outcome may be little more (or no less) than the discovery of "connections between unrelated pieces of information" (118). In Thomas's stark contrast between the different spaces and temporalities of applied and basic research, we have another articulation of thinking and practicing ecoontologically that allows him to draw connections between the macrosocial and the microcellular environments.

These environments form, unform, and reform in space and time. Awareness of this fluid process means that Thomas is also attentive to the prehistory of medical treatments, "generations of energetic and imaginative investigators [who] exhausted their whole lives" on particular problems that didn't have obvious or immediate applications but were interesting simply as conceptual or methodological puzzles (117). Thomas's concerns about the increasing hegemony of applied approaches over basic science approaches appear to have been justified; since the time of the publication of Thomas's notes in the *New England Journal of Medicine,* the practices of research and medicine have become even more targeted and less open-ended. I return to Thomas's writings in the 1970s to point to the possibility that rather than representing a challenge to this hegemony, AIDS treatment activism becomes yet another event in a longer story of science becoming applied. Indeed, I would argue that the arrival of AIDS helped solidify the dominance of the applied approach. In the early years of AIDS, activists sought treatments, any treatments, to stop or slow the onslaught of so many deaths in so little time. That there was a need for drugs to put into bodies in the emergency time of the AIDS epidemic in the 1980s and 1990s is an unassailable truth. The repercussions of that truth are still being felt today.

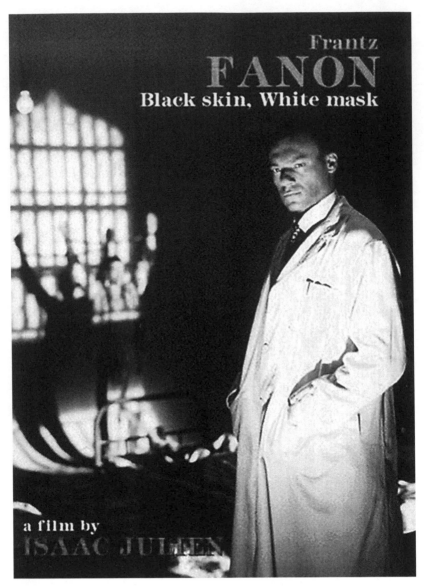

Figure 9. Inspired by his training in institutional psychotherapy at the Saint-Alban clinic in the south of France, one of the first things Fanon purportedly did at Blida Hospital in Algeria was to order that patients be freed from physical forms of restraint. Screen capture from Frantz Fanon: White Skin, Black Mask *(Isaac Julien, 1996).*

Frantz Fanon's "Colonial War and Mental Disorders" (1961) and Isaac Julien's "Fanon" (1996)

In 1953, just before the beginning of the Algerian war of liberation from France, Frantz Fanon took a position at Blida-Joinville Hospital, the largest psychiatric hospital in Algeria. Inspired by his training in institutional psychotherapy at the Saint-Alban clinic in the south of France, one of the first things Fanon purportedly did at Blida was order patients be freed from physical forms of restraint—straitjackets and shackles that kept them tied to their beds.[1] What has come down to us today is an image of Fanon at Blida that is an echo of what Foucault describes in *The History of Madness* as the key image of the "birth of the asylum": Pinel removing the chains from the mad at Bicêtre in 1794.[2] Many texts describing this scene at Blida, including Isaac Julien's film *Frantz Fanon: White Skin, Black Mask* (1996), reference the earlier scene at Bicêtre. In discussing the film, Julien and Mark Nash, the film's producer and Julien's partner, acknowledge that while the film presents an echo of the earlier image, it also immediately undercuts the accuracy of the image, though not its truth-effects. Julien and Nash explain:

> In our film we show patients in chains followed by an interviewee Alice Cherki who denies the "evidence" we have just put before the audience. Certainly patients were still in chains in psychiatric hospitals earlier in the century, but the historical evidence is inconclusive—the image of Fanon unchaining his patients has become a myth—a reinscription of the myth of Pinel, liberating patients at the Salpetrière hospital in Paris at the time of the French Revolution—overlaid with the Marxist and anti-colonial imagery of removing the shackles of oppression.[3]

Julien and Nash create an image of an image—a myth overlaying a myth. The scene the image depicts is both clinical and political, and what links these domains is a concept and practice of the therapeutic effects of liberation. This, then, is already a kind of snapshot of a snapshot, both clinical and critical, referencing an earlier historical image-event of a similar singular moment of chains being removed, what we might call the echo of a lie that haunts the event of revolutionary freedom struggles, struggles that are always already being appropriated by power. This snapshot, then, doubles again Julien's snapshot of a snapshot, connecting events of illness, thought, and politics across time and space.

Fanon also connects the events of illness, thought, and politics in the case studies of "Colonial War and Mental Disorders," published in *The Wretched of the Earth* after his death in 1961. Fanon demonstrates the many ways in which, in his words, "the war goes on" in the form of mental disorders that Algerian, as well as European, people carry with them as effects of colonialism and the war of liberation.[4] Fanon recognizes that this concluding chapter "will be found ill-timed and singularly out of place" in a book that articulates a theory of revolutionary violence (249). Following Fanon and self-consciously returning to what serves as a conclusion in another, earlier historical and critical context, I want this snapshot at the center of *Indirect Action* to suggest the ill-timed and out of place, as well as the ongoingness of events that we think are over and done with. Also following Fanon, who himself connected the critical and clinical in his work,[5] I explore the constitutive link between transnational experiences and events, like colonialism and war, and psychic and phenomenological experiences and events, like mental and physical illness. Bringing Fanon's essay together with Julien's later representation of Fanon demonstrates both the continuity and the discontinuity between colonial war and mental disorders and queer politics and theory, all of which I fold together in my analysis of the nexus illness-thought-activism in the prehistory of AIDS. Fanon's conclusion calls for new routes, not through what he describes as European "racist humanism" but via new inventions and discoveries— both revolutionary and therapeutic—that emerge out of the experiences and events of decolonization (315). By returning to the insight that the work of decolonization included the creation of therapeutic spaces and practices, in a book about health activism in the period before the emergence of AIDS, I want to demonstrate the myriad ways that health activism was practiced before AIDS not simply to draw out historical connections but as a resource for future clinical practices of healing through processes of decolonizing the mind, body, and social.[6]

Fanon brings the revolutionary and the therapeutic together because he sees firsthand the psychophysiological effects of colonization and decolonization. Even before the clinical final chapter, which draws together cases of mental illness among the French and Algerian populations in Algeria during the war of liberation from 1954 to 1959, Fanon diagnoses the negative affects—shame, anger, envy, fear, and terror are all mentioned—that emerge from settler colonialism, arguing, for example, that the native's struggle causes anxiety in the settler (43) and that the settler's violence against the native and the anger it causes are directed at least initially inward toward oneself and one's fellow natives (54). In Fanon's catalog of the nervous conditions of colonialism, the colonialist bourgeoisie is said to suffer from a narcissistic personality disorder, while the native becomes a "hysterical type" (46, 56–57). "Colonialism," according to Fanon, "forces the people it dominates to ask themselves the question constantly: 'In reality, who am I?'" (250) For Fanon the question is a sign of the disintegration of the personality under colonialism as well as a reaction formation against that disintegration. The "reactionary psychoses" that emerge are responses not only to evacuations, bombardments, and torture but also to a more generalized atmosphere of terror that permeates colonial society (252). Fanon's work offers an analysis that traverses the nervous conditions of individuals—settler and native—and of institutions—colonialist and revolutionary.[7] His important intervention, which is a tenet of institutional psychotherapy, as discussed in relation to the work of Guattari at La Borde in chapter 2, is to treat the clinic itself and its practices of diagnosis and treatment not as a refuge or neutral space in the colonial war but as a key site of struggle.

Julien's film is a collage of materials—newsreel footage of the French in Algeria; interviews, dramatizations, or what Julien and Nash call "visual reconstructions";[8] scenes from the fictional documentary *Battle of Algiers* (1965); and still photographs, to name just some of the visual and narrative elements in the film. The fictional materials are treated as factual, and the factual materials are fictionalized, a process that draws our attention to the production of truth in the fictional as well as the documentary. The British actor Colin Salmon plays Fanon in the visual reconstructions, but he doesn't so much act a part as act as relay for Fanon's words and ideas by voicing and embodying them.[9] "Restaging in this way," according to Julien and Nash, "avoids creating character or interiority as in the conventional fictional film. This enables the audience to project their own Fanon into the film, making 'Fanon' a more open sign."[10] Julien and Nash also work to transform materially the historical evidence they have gathered by, for example, making the newsreel footage "work differently—either by slowing it down, removing the voice over, reworking the sound track, or retinting the image" and by treating the *Battle of Algiers* "like other archive material . . . as part of a project of 'undoing the archive.'"[11] I am drawn to Julien's description of his film as part of a project of undoing the colonial archive as another method-image for my own project on the multiplicity of forms of health activism that seek to undo medicine's dominant diagnostic and treatment archive.

Julien's film treats most of Fanon's key ideas—from his analysis of the psychic life of racism to his dialectical theories of revolutionary violence to his romantic ideas of masculinity and conservative notions of femininity. One of the ways the film is able to draw all these themes together is by staging several scenes of therapy, what we might call therapeutic *tableaux vivants,* of some of the case studies from "Colonial War and Mental Disorders." The film cuts between newsreel images of war, reenacted scenes of torture, and scenes of Salmon as Fanon listening to a variety of patients tell their traumatic stories of war. In these scenes of colonial analysis, the patients speak the words that Fanon has recorded in the text of *The Wretched of the Earth,* but unlike Fanon's text, in which the case studies are presented sequentially, here the stories become intermingled, the images of the various patients speaking are intercut, and it is somewhat difficult to tell when one story ends and another begins, which works against fixed notions of national, ethnic, and gendered, as well as diagnostic, identity categories.

Through all these scenes of therapy, "Fanon" is a silent figure, listening closely but never speaking back to his patients. In a conversation with Coco Fusco about the film, Julien explains the specific filmic technique he used for these scenes: "In the scenes which we've dramatized from Fanon's chapter, 'Colonial Wars and Mental Disorders,' we used a split dioptre that brings the foreground and background into focus together—the image, so to speak, appears to have two planes of focus."[12] I'm fascinated by this technique, which creates an appearance of two planes of focus at once, as a method-image for the effect I want to create in this and other snapshots. Despite the fact that these scenes are structured similarly, there are subtle differences in the stagings of these therapeutic *tableaux vivants* that bring into focus aspects of the case studies not always apparent when reading them. Julien and Nash bring together several of the case studies, including of two French patients: the first is the case of a French soldier, who rather dispassionately describes administering torture, and the second is a French woman whose father was "highly placed in the civil service," who "threw himself into the Algerian manhunt with frenzied rage" and was eventually killed in a raid. The woman is traumatized by having heard the sound of her father torturing Algerians in their home, and rather than feel sorrow at his death, she confesses that she believes the "Algerians were right" and that if she were an Algerian girl, she would participate in the resistance movement (277). The final case is of an Algerian active in the resistance movement, diagnosed by Fanon as suffering from "marked anxiety psychosis of the depersonalization type after the murder of a [French] woman while temporarily insane" (261). In the scenes of therapy with the Algerian man and the French woman, Salmon as "Fanon" is seated in the background on the right side of the frame, his white doctor's coat visible as a sign of authority. The faces of the Algerian man and the French woman occupy the foreground and the left side of the scene; we see close-ups of their faces from the side as they speak, and the disembodied faces are almost grotesque in the way they intrude into the frame (Figures 10 and 11). In the scene of therapy with the French policeman, the positions are reversed, and Fanon's face dominates the left side in the foreground, and the French policeman is seated in the background, his uniform visible as a sign of authority that Fanon seems to have lost in this therapeutic *tableau vivant* (Figure 12).

The film stages another difference in these scenes of therapy: the space between Fanon and his patients is occupied by different objects—in the scene with the French woman, the object between doctor and patient is a white porcelain sink; in the scene with the French soldier, the object is a table; and in the scene with the Algerian man, the object is another man, whom I imagine to be an Algerian doctor or nurse translating for Fanon. I have imagined this scenario because interview evidence indicates Julien had been reading several thinkers who helped create a resurgence of interest in Fanon's work in the early 1990s—Homi Bhabha, Edward Said, Diana Fuss, Lee Edelman, and Stuart Hall are included in Julien's list, suggesting postcolonial and queer theoretical couplings were producing a new "Fanon" around 1990. In "Interior Colonies: Frantz Fanon and the Politics of Identification," the last chapter in her *Identification Papers,* Diana Fuss discusses "the subject of the translator in Fanon's clinical practice."[13] She notes that his "complete reliance upon translators to converse with his Muslim patients is nothing if not a powerful reminder, to both

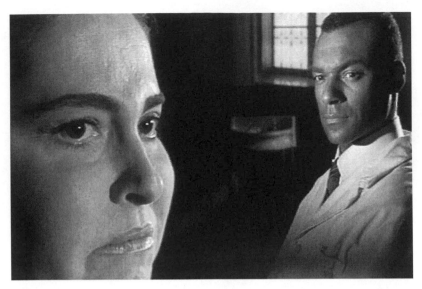

Figure 10. Julien stages several therapeutic tableaux vivants. Fanon with a French woman whose father was "highly placed in the civil service." Screen capture from Frantz Fanon: White Skin, Black Mask *(Isaac Julien, 1996).*

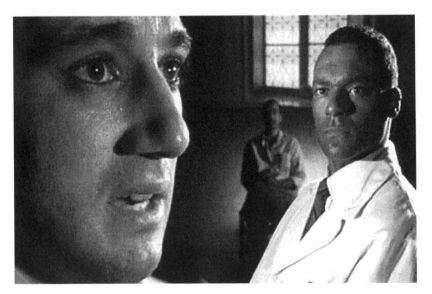

Figure 11. Fanon with an Algerian active in the resistance movement, diagnosed by Fanon as suffering from "marked anxiety psychosis of the depersonalization type after the murder of a [French] woman while temporarily insane" (261). Screen capture from Frantz Fanon: White Skin, Black Mask *(Isaac Julien, 1996).*

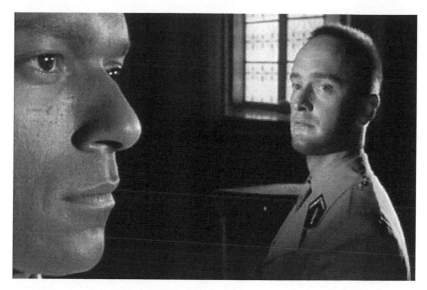

Figure 12. Fanon with a French soldier, who rather dispassionately describes administering torture. Screen capture from Frantz Fanon: White Skin, Black Mask *(Isaac Julien, 1996).*

doctor and patient, of the immediate political context in which the therapeutic dialogue struggles to take place."[14] Julien makes one of these nurse-translators visible—fleetingly, as background object to and relay between the scene of therapy in the foreground. Fuss argues that Fanon "was interested precisely in the linkages and fissures, the contradictions and co-implications, the translations and transformations of the theory-politics relation."[15] Although it is already implicit in Fuss's analysis, I would add the discourses and practices of the clinic to the relationship chain she describes—theory-clinic-politics.

Julien and Nash credit Donna Haraway with suggesting that their film visualizes critical theory, or as Julien puts it in the interview with Fusco, the film "made an act of visualization a form of theoretical production."[16] These two slightly different formulations—visualizing theory and making an act of visualization a form of theoretical production—are important to the illness-thought-activism counterarchive I draw on and draw together here. This snapshot attempts to literalize this process, while my next two chapters, on drawing epilepsy and witnessing schizophrenia, will work to visualize theory more figuratively.

5

Drawing Epilepsy

Throughout this book I have explored multiple sites of the conjuncture illness-thought-activism in the period just before and after the emergence of AIDS. I have been concerned not only with the content but also with the form of particular conjunctures, as well as with a metaquestion of method: of how to approach a particular conjuncture and with what tools. In this chapter I again explore the relationship between a specific illness experience and event in time—epilepsy, as drawn in David B.'s graphic narrative of his brother's epilepsy diagnosed in France in the 1960s—and a specific form, what has come to be called "graphic medicine."[1] In *Epileptic* David B. draws the experience and event of his brother's epilepsy as it emerges and evolves during the same period in which many—including Fanon, Foucault, Deleuze, and Guattari—are thinking critically about historical and contemporary practices of madness.[2] I am interested in *Epileptic* as a kind of historical heterotopia or, in Foucault's formulation of the concept, a space for the juxtaposition of multiple and contradictory sites.[3] In his 1967 lecture in which he introduces the concept of heterotopia, Foucault begins by describing a shift from a nineteenth-century obsession with history and temporality to a more recent interest in spatiality, simultaneity, and juxta-position. As in other chapters, I present a history of the present—here of madness/epilepsy in the 1960s and 1970s—by utilizing a form and method associated with that historical moment. As already discussed, the 1960s and 1970s was a period of upheaval in medicine, and because of radical changes coming from within and without, medicine seemed open to many possible futures, some of which came to fruition and others which did not. My goal in returning to this heterotopic moment of possibility in and for medicine and through both the form and content of *Indirect Action* is to open up other therapeutic spaces in the present.

One cultural symptom of the heterotopic turn that Foucault diagnoses as occurring in the 1960s and 1970s is the emergence of what Hillary Chute has called a "revolution in comics-making [that] developed out of the taboo-shattering and leftist politics of the 1960s, in which authors outside mainstream publication and distribution networks broke barriers in both radical content and form."[4] In *Epileptic* David B. makes visible the possibilities of the practice of radical juxtaposition by drawing together, literally and figuratively, many macro- and micromilieus—hospitals, homes, clinics, communes, dreamscapes, brain contours, frontiers between worlds, gardens, battlefields, rugged mountain terrains, etc.—in order to create spatial and temporal conjunctures and disjunctures on and beyond the page, even, potentially, into the domain of medicine itself. In my own work on graphic medicine, therefore, I am less interested in what the reading of graphic narratives does for the individual medical practitioners who read them than in what the form and practice of radical juxtaposition can provide for the practice of medicine more generally.

Comics are a kind of assemblage. As Will Eisner explains in his now classic instructional book *Comics and Sequential Art,* first published in 1985, through the varied mix of panels and frames, as well as the lines, borders, and gutters linking and separating panels and frames, comics encapsulate events through their form as much as their content: as Eisner puts it, the panel "is used by the artist to capture or 'freeze' one segment in what is in reality an uninterrupted flow of action."[5] In comics time becomes spatialized. Eisner is a realist, and thus, for him success "stems from the artist's ability (usually more visceral than intellectual) to gauge the commonality of the reader's experience," suggesting that comics present experience as self-evident rather than as always already an interpretation and open to further interpretation. Yet on a formal level, I would argue, contra Eisner, that many, if not most, graphic narratives work to re-present and interpret "experience" as a category of analysis by demonstrating both the desire to encapsulate an individual's "experience" and an event's eventfulness and the inevitability of never quite succeeding in doing so. The experience of illness is multiple, and tracking that multiplicity demonstrates that even as diagnostic categories, treatments, and illness narratives seek to contain and reduce—or to frame in the language of graphic medicine—an illness experience, the experience always also falls outside the frame, overspills the container, gets messy. Comics thematize, formally, boundaries and their leakiness—panels are breached, borders are dissolved, lines are drawn and undrawn, and boundaries are played with, on, and beyond.

Historically, the boundary between the diagnostic categories of madness and epilepsy is one of the most porous. In a lecture on the theme of psychiatric power, Foucault discusses the historical emergence of what he calls "the neurological body." In an echo of his earlier diagnosis of a conceptual and perceptual partition between two diseased bodies and their treatments in *The Birth of the Clinic*, Foucault argues in 1974 that from around 1820 to around 1870 to 1880 (when Charcot will appear on the scene), "the so-called convulsive illnesses—medically, clinically, no effective difference was made between epilepsy and others—were illnesses of the mind."[6] Foucault also refers to the hyphenated term "'hystero-epilepsy' to designate a hybrid form (composed of hysteria and epilepsy) marked by convulsive crises."[7] He then describes Charcot's "codification of the hysterical attack (*crise*) on the model of epilepsy. In this way," Foucault continues, "the huge domain of what before Charcot was called 'hystero-epilepsy,' the 'convulsions,' is divided in two,"[8] or at least this is the stated diagnostic and conceptual goal at the time.

Yet even one hundred years after Charcot, at the time Foucault is lecturing about shifting historical manifestations of psychiatric power, the diagnostic line between these two domains is still not established conclusively. The hybrid category remains operative conceptually and clinically, even if the term *hystero-epilepsy* is no longer favored in medical discourse. The abandoned diagnostic category hystero-epilepsy remains illuminating as an illness assemblage that confounds categories: Is it hysteria and/or epilepsy? Is it psychiatric and/or neurological? Is it mental and/or material? Deleuze and Guattari delineate the concept and practice of assemblage in *Kafka: Toward a Minor Literature*, noting that the "functioning of the assemblage can be explained only if one takes it apart to examine both the elements that make it up and the nature of the linkages."[9] The term and condition *hystero-epilepsy* is a strange combination that helps us to see illness in general as an assemblage of bodies, minds, diagnoses, treatments, and clinical, critical, and narrative discourses and practices. And thus, as Foucault's earlier reference to the hydrotherapeutic treatment for hysteria in his book about the changing experience of clinical medicine attests, the conceptual partition between organic and mental illness is precarious even to this day.

In order to consider the multiplicity of diagnostic categories and treatment modalities for epilepsy or, put more simply, in order to consider epilepsy itself as a multiplicity, I will juxtapose the clinical, critical, and graphic in order to demonstrate a method for approaching the complexity of the multiple experiences and events of illness. The act of drawing is key to the method I demonstrate in this chapter; the term itself, as utilized by

Deleuze and Guattari in *A Thousand Plateaus*, draws together the graphic, formal, and conceptual. As Brian Massumi explains in the notes on his translation, "To draw is an act of creation. What is drawn (the Body without Organs, the plane of consistency, a line of flight) does not preexist the act of drawing. The French word *tracer* captures this better: It has all the graphic connotations of 'to draw' in English, but can also mean to blaze a trail or open a road."[10] In *Epileptic* David B. draws epilepsy as a multiplicity and not a "pretraced destiny,"[11] and the text itself becomes an experimental treatment of experimental treatments. Thus, I explore some of the paths—graphic, narrative, and conceptual—that David B. opens up: paths through an endless round of doctors, diagnoses, and treatments for epilepsy and across multiple forms of epileptic expression as a means, perhaps, of becoming-epileptic. Again, I am less concerned with what graphic narratives can do instrumentally for medicine than with the graphic as method and form for capturing the multiple experiences and events of illness-thought-activism drawn together in the chapters and snapshots of this book.

Path 1: An Endless Round of Doctors, Diagnoses, and Treatments

In 1964, when Jean-Christophe is seven, Pierre-François[12] is five, and Florence is four, Jean-Christophe (also called Tito) has his first seizure while pretending to ride a motorcycle as his brother and sister look on. Pierre-François prevents him from falling off the motorcycle, bearing the weight of his brother until their father comes to help. "He's heavy. It feels like I've been holding him up forever," Pierre-François tells the reader. This is only the first of many images of the heaviness and burden of Jean-Christophe's falling disease, borne by Pierre-François and the rest of the family as much as by Jean-Christophe himself. Although his mother tells Pierre-François that Tito has "had a spell," Pierre-François is certain that Tito "got carried away by a typhoon" (10). These diagnoses become the first explanatory models for an epileptic seizure presented to the reader, and importantly, they are generated from within the family and without the input of outside experts. On the facing page, in a large square panel covering two-thirds of the page, David B. has drawn his mother, his father, and Jean-Christophe impassively standing in the middle of the panel surrounded by a ring of doctors who are holding hands and dancing some sort of expert's jig (Figure 13). The doctors are uniformly male, although they come in various shapes and sizes and sport different coat and hair styles, illustrating the

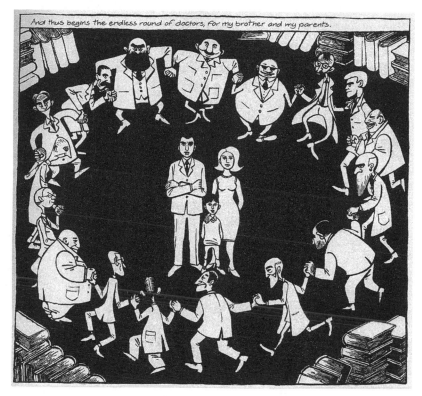

Figure 13. An endless round of doctors, diagnoses, and treatments. David B., Epileptic, *trans. Kim Thompson (New York: Pantheon, 2005), top panel, 11.*

range of their expertise. Piles of books are visible in the four corners of the panel; books become another layer in the rings of expertise that will engulf Jean-Christophe and his family (11).

Under this large panel, a row of three smaller panels at the bottom of the page shows Jean-Christophe's first encounters with doctors. In this sequence Jean-Christophe and his mother are passed from the family doctor to the family doctor's now-retired teacher to a Parisian neuropsychiatrist. The linear movement from generalism to specialization (family doctor to neuropsychiatrist) and from the margins to the center of knowledge production (Orléans to Paris) is in formal contrast to the "endless round of doctors" of the panel above, giving visual form to what will become one of the felt contradictions of Jean-Christophe's epilepsy: between, on the one hand, the seemingly endless cycle of hope and despair as various and sundry treatments are tried and believed in until they don't work and, on the other, the inexorable decline in Jean-Christophe's health and cognitive abilities, despite or, perhaps, partly because of the plethora of treatments. The not uncommon issue of the negative side effects of many conventional medical treatments—especially pharmacological ones—is important to consider in relation to questions about the efficacy or not of a particular treatment. In this chapter and the next, I highlight that in the cases of epilepsy and schizophrenia, "drugs into bodies" is the slogan not of the patient activist but of what we might call the practitioner activist. I will show in my concluding afterimage that the figure of the treatment activist will emerge as a kind of amalgam of patient and practitioner as activist.

The page grid denoting the passage from generalist to specialist ends with a diagnosis from the Parisian neuropsychiatrist and might be read as suggesting a progression from uncertainty to certainty in relation to the etiology of Jean-Christophe's problem. Yet the explicit mention of the doctor's economic incentives ("His diagnosis reflects his hourly billing," the narrator explains) along with his vague and patently inexpert diagnosis ("Ma'am, your son is a bad boy") counters this certainty and seems to indicate that expertise is a trap—economic and moral as well as medical—rather than an escape from illness and the stigma associated with it. The Parisian neuropsychiatrist's diagnosis also indicates that Jean-Christophe's illness will be perceived through multiple and sometimes contradictory lenses—physical, psychological, economic, and moral. Diagnosis is presented as heterotopic. Graphically, the diagnosis of Jean-Christophe's illness is spread across multiple and contradictory sites, across two pages and several juxtaposed panels, from family clinic to neuropsychiatric clinic, from Orléans to Paris. Although we read the panels from left to right and top to bottom, on the page Pierre-François's diagnosis, "He got carried away by a typhoon," faces off with the Parisian neuropsychiatrist's diagnosis, "Ma'am, your son is a bad boy." These two diagnoses also stand as visual and narrative bookends; they are the parentheses framing the endless round of doctors, diagnoses, and treatments. Through this heterotopic juxtaposition, David B.'s memoir becomes a visual and discursive counternarrative to expert knowledges and, through its composition as well as its content, challenges the authority of doctors. And yet I also want to note what is missing from this first heterotopic scene of diagnosis—Jean-Christophe's own interpretation of what is happening to him. He is the small, silent figure at the very center of the scene/page, flanked by his parents, his doctors, and the books of experts, and his silence during this scene of diagnosis will echo throughout the text (see Figure 13). I will return to the question of Jean-Christophe's silence in the final section of this chapter.

In this heterotopic scene of diagnosis, we already glimpse the contours of the family's long struggle to understand and best treat Jean-Christophe's illness—like the scenes of diagnosis, the scenes of treatment are heterotopic, too. The family's encounters with medicine occur at a time when at least two contrasting discourses and practices are vying for hegemony in medicine, as already mentioned in chapters 3 and 4. The first is the discourse of bioscientization and the practice of evidence-based medicine, and the second is the discourse of generalism and the practice of biopsychosocial medicine. In a now classic paper published in *Science* in 1977, George Engel presents what will become an influential argument for the general, holistic approach the family seems to need.[13] Though influential, Engel's argument was a minority position at the time and is even more so today, as scientization has become increasingly codified in medicine in the period since the 1970s. Engel coins the term *biopsychosocial,* inelegantly but effectively juxtaposing three huge domains.[14] Engel creates the clunky term in order to argue against psychiatry's attempts to become more "neat and tidy," as the rest of medicine was perceived to have become at the time, by adhering more closely to a model that reduces disease to biology, in particular to biochemical and neurophysiological processes. In his contrarian assessment of the condition of medicine at the time, Engel contends "that all medicine is in crisis, and further, that medicine's crisis derives from the same basic fault as psychiatry's, namely, adherence to a model of disease no longer adequate for the scientific tasks and social responsibilities of either medicine or psychiatry."[15] At a time when the thought leaders of psychiatry were attempting to move psychiatry away from a psychoanalytic past toward a biomedical future, Engel encouraged medicine to take a different course and turn away from an exclusively biomedical approach.

In order to diagnose the limitations of the biomedical model, Engel explores two conditions together: the first, diabetes mellitus, paradigmatic of a somatic disease, and the second, schizophrenia, paradigmatic of a mental disease. Engel insists that a better model would "account for the reality of diabetes and schizophrenia as human experiences as well as disease abstractions."[16] As Engel shows, the clinical expressions of diabetes and schizophrenia are incredibly variable, as is the individual's experience of these illnesses, which is affected by complex psychological, social, and cultural factors.[17] Engel's goal in putting forth a new medical model is "to neutralize the dogmatism of biomedicine" and to "provide a blueprint for research, a framework for teaching, and a design for action in the real world of health care."[18]

In David B.'s account the family tries just about everything, though it is clear they are drawn to alternative treatments like macrobiotics and various forms of esoterism because the conventional medical practitioners they encounter reflect precisely the sort of dogmatism in medical practice that Engel sought to counter. Jean-Christophe's parents' decision not to subject their son to a risky, experimental operation on his brain is received by the surgeon, Professor T., and his assistants with anger and derision (45). In a panel that covers the top third of a page, Professor T. and his coterie are presented as frightening black figures on a white background, like a group of judges at a religious inquisition, spewing vitriol: "WHAT? You're refusing Professor T's operation?"; "Get the hell out! There's nothing for you here!"; and, "Your son is doomed! It's criminal of you to refuse this operation!" (46).

In reaction to this dogmatic and unfeeling approach, the family turns to Master N., a follower of George Oshawa, the founder of macrobiotics, who is rendered graphically as a cuddly cat. As the narrator explains, "Macrobiology is presented as the remedy that cures everything. And I mean everything" (47). This statement is followed by a panel showing a happily heterosexual man testifying to Oshawa's successful treatment of his prior homosexuality through a no-sugar diet regimen—a panel clearly meant to poke fun at cures for everything. Following the unconventional teachings of Oshawa and his followers, David B. problematizes what we take to be disease, yet he also extends his skepticism regarding what does and does not constitute disease and who has the authority to make these determinations to the practitioners of alternative as well as conventional medicine.

This skepticism appears again in David B.'s graphic set piece of the family's eager participation in what the narrator describes as "the experiment of the macrobiotic commune" (63). Despite the commune's utopic promise, David B. renders the macrobiotic milieu as riven by power struggles over food and leadership styles that mimic conflicts in the world the family thought they had left behind. Or we might say, utilizing the terminology that Deleuze and Guattari were developing at the same time as the family's macrobiotic experiment, the family seeks experimental treatments as deterritorializing lines of flight out of the impasse of a reductive model of disease, but the desubjectification necessary for the deterritorialization of medical experience fails because the alternative treatments always seem to end up revolving around a guru/father figure who seeks to maintain or expand his influence over others rather than enlightenment.[19] Just as with Professor T.'s experimental surgery, the macrobiotic experiment is not a "path of escape in all its positivity"[20] but a reproduction or imitation of congealed social forms. And despite all the radical social experiments of the time, the tired figure of the powerful father keeps reappearing, the stalwart companion of another tired figure, the overbearing mother (as mentioned in chapter 2 and discussed later in this chapter).

As the family searches for the key to unlock the mystery of Jean-Christophe's illness, they receive advice from countless spiritual and medical practitioners. When a conventional doctor advises the father to "give [Jean-Christophe] enough medicine so you can get on with your lives," David B. asks, "Can we, in fact, get on with our lives?" He notes matter-of-factly that "it's not our choice to make. When the illness took up residence here it didn't seek our permission. It slumbers inside my brother and, upon awakening, it slithers out and insinuates itself into our lives" (79). The family understands that such a logic of choice, although seemingly offering a measure of control in a time of uncertainty, is inadequate for responding to the illness that has insinuated itself into their lives, like the serpent figure David B. draws to give form to Jean-Christophe's illness.[21] *Epileptic* shows the limits of this logic of choice and presents a counterlogic of care extended not just to Jean-Christophe but to the entire family.[22] The logic of care questions whether one can choose or not to get on with one's life where illness is concerned. In the family's holistic approach, the whole they seek to treat is the whole family as well as Jean-Christophe's whole person.

The family's holistic approach also fits with one of the main tenets of the antipsychiatry movement, which emerged during the years the family sought help for Jean-Christophe. Many proponents of antipsychiatry argued that an unhealthy environment at home led to mental illness in general and psychosis in particular. In much of the antipsychiatry literature, the unhealthy familial environment is exemplified by the figure of the overbearing mother, whose actions constrain her child (read: son) in his attempts to break free and become his own, autonomous person. David Cooper, for example, describes the "double bind" in which the child finds himself in relation to a mother whose statements and gestures contradict each other:

She tells her son, "Go away, find your own friends and don't be so dependent on me," but, at the same time, indicates non-verbally that she will be very upset if he does leave her, even in this limited way. Or, while signaling anxiety about any physical closeness, she says, "Come and kiss your mother, dear!" Unless her child can discover a ruthlessness, a counter-violence, in himself with which he can demolish the whole absurd interchange, his response can only be muddle and ultimately what is called psychotic confusion, thought disorder, catatonia, and so on.[23]

As this passage shows, Cooper's analysis remains caught in a reductive Oedipal logic, which Deleuze and Guattari sought to counter in their work together, as I discuss at greater length in chapter 2. In the entry "Schizophrenia and Society" of the *Encyclopédie universalis,* published in 1975, Deleuze expresses disappointment that "the effort to study 'schizogenetic' families, or schizogenetic mechanisms in the family, is a common trait shared by traditional psychiatry, psychology, psychoanalysis, and even anti-psychiatry."[24] Deleuze argues for an understanding of schizophrenia that escapes a narrowly familial discourse and that emphasizes schizophrenia as a process that creates "an eruption, a break-through which smashes the continuity of a personality and takes it on a kind of trip through 'more reality,' at once intense and terrifying, following lines of flight that engulf nature and history, organism and spirit."[25]

The creative process that Deleuze describes is given graphic form in *Epileptic*—the experience of epilepsy leads to "a kind of trip through 'more reality,'" at least for David B., if not for Jean-Christophe, a point I consider in more detail in the final section of this chapter. One of the affective engines for this trip is rage. Throughout *Epileptic,* David B. explicitly links a feeling of rage—his own and his brother's—to his brother's seizures, and he finds the only way he is able to mitigate this rage is through constant drawing (134). For David B. rage is felt and expressed not as individualizing but as massifying, not or not only as destructive but as productive. A kind of desubjectification happens on the page through the expression of rage: "I'm not any one person, I'm a group, an army. I have enough rage in me for one hundred thousand warriors" (20), and these one hundred thousand warriors are produced—almost literally—all over the pages of *Epileptic.* It is important to note, however, that David B.'s "ruthlessness" or "counter-violence," to use Cooper's terminology, is rarely directed explicitly at his mother. Indeed, in light of the pathologization of the mother in some of the antipsychiatry literature, it is interesting that in *Epileptic* it is Jean-Christophe's mother who is most hopeful her son will benefit from antipsychiatric approaches that understand disease as not or not only residing in the body or psyche of the individual. It seems plausible, however, that Jean-Christophe's mother's tireless search for a successful treatment for her son is at least partly motivated by a fear she is somehow guilty—the figure of the guilty mother occupying an equally prominent position as the figure of the overbearing mother in some of the "radical" youth movements of the time.

The events of May 1968 and the antipsychiatry movement are historically and spatially linked in *Epileptic,* as a single page draws together references to "riots" in Paris, striking teachers (we learn, for example, that although both Pierre-François's parents are art teachers, his mother but not his father is on strike), photographs of student demonstrations in *Paris Match,* and the only explicit mention of antipsychiatry in the text (36). After two panels depicting Pierre-François's nine-year-old self's understanding of the events of May 1968 as a war in Paris, David B. mentions the beginning of the antipsychiatry movement in the first of two panels across the bottom of the page. He explains that the movement is "propounded in France by people like Gilles Deleuze, Félix Guattari, Roger Gentis,"[26] and we see below this statement an image of Jean-Christophe's mother and father as they read in bed. In this domestic scene, the mother says to the father, "These are the kind of people Jean-Christophe should be seeing" (36). The father's ambivalent response, "You think?" along with the ambiguous image at the top of the page of mother facing left and father facing right under David B.'s comment, "My mother's on strike. My father isn't," positions the father as somewhat skeptical about the unconventional practices of antipsychiatry in relation to his son's condition and in opposition, perhaps, to the mother, who is more hopeful of the possibility of cure and less resigned to the fact of disease.

The last panel on the page shows Jean-Christophe and his mother at the "psychopedagogical institute," a newly opened clinic in Orléans (the father is notably not present in this scene) (36). In keeping with antipsychiatry's interests in the family origins of psychopathology, the teachers at the psychopedagogical institute test Pierre-François with art therapy exercises. When Pierre-François is told to draw his family on vacation, he finds himself unable to keep up normal appearances and hide behind a conventional family portrait. His drawing of an "enormous massacre" piques the interest of the teacher (37). Though we are not privy to the teacher's actual psychological assessment of Pierre-François and his family, we are told by Pierre-François that the teacher interprets his massacre drawing by writing words directly on top of his images. The grid ends with a panel in which a baffled Pierre-François exits a gate in the prison-like wall surrounding the institute, as the panel's caption notes, "Writing on a drawing! For a psychologist she's not very psychological" (37). Here, the words on the drawing are troubling because they attempt to delimit and fix the complex experience rendered in the drawing. In this grid David B. seems to suggest such delimiting and fixing of experience are not separate from but part of the problem of the experience and event of Jean-Christophe's epilepsy. In this scene, being psychological is contrasted with labeling a problem, or more succinctly, being is contrasted with knowing. Drawing is situated on the side of being, and writing, as interpretation, with knowing—and voilà, a messy scene is reduced to a few words that overwrite the mess on the page and in life.

As this scene at the psychopedagogical institute suggests, the family itself is constantly under scrutiny. As they lurch from one treatment regimen to the next, searching for a remedy and battling the stigma attached to the disease that has insinuated itself into their lives, it is as though the entire family has been diagnosed as epileptic. From the moment of his first seizure, Jean-Christophe endures the stigmatizing looks of others: in the eyes of the neighborhood kids, "Jean-Christophe is nuts" and becomes one of the many bogeymen—along with a mean old man and an Algerian immigrant day laborer—who are deemed to threaten the "normality" of the neighborhood. But as Goffman describes in his sociological analysis of the phenomena, stigma also operates by association.[27] We see this process in *Epileptic* as the family is subject to the normalizing gaze of others. Images of eyes are prominent throughout the text; sometimes, a single eye is positioned in the corner of a frame, highlighting the position of the spectator looking on at the events taking place in the frame, while in other frames numerous oversized, staring, animal-like eyes crowd the space of the panel, visually emphasizing the feeling that everyone and everything is watching the epileptic family—in these scenes, the eyes appear to be part of the landscape itself (Figure 14). Recall my discussion in chapter 3 of the doctor Sassall's eyes as described in *A Fortunate Man*. Sassall tells his patient, "I can't bear anything done near my eyes, I can't bear to be touched

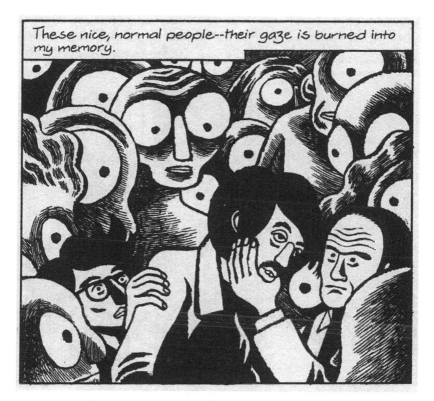

Figure 14. Eyes are drawn as creating a grotesque landscape of stigmatization. David B., Epileptic, *trans. Kim Thompson (New York: Pantheon, 2005), top right panel, 236.*

there. I think that's where I live, just under and behind my eyes."[28] One implication of Sassall's evocative description of living under and behind his eyes is that his eyes and the art of looking become a space of refuge for him that must be protected. In contrast, in David B.'s images eyes are drawn as creating a grotesque landscape of stigmatization.

David B. captures well the family's feeling that they are under surveillance in a sequence about a family trip to Switzerland. The family visits the sites along with other tourists, but soon they themselves become part of the "diversion" when Jean-Christophe has a seizure. The other tourists gawk and point as Pierre-François and his father try to help Jean-Christophe. When Pierre-François discovers that his mother has escaped the scene, he admits to feeling a similar dilemma in such moments: wanting to be elsewhere but feeling compelled to stay with Jean-Christophe. He believes the family owes his brother "this solidarity" but also understands his mother's "need to take a breather after working so hard to cure him" (238). What this public seizure scene reveals is how difficult it is for the family to simply be with Jean-Christophe when he has a seizure. On the one hand, this is because the outside world encounters as strange what is commonplace for Jean-Christophe and his family, reminding them that their normal isn't, and, on the other, because there is a fundamental contradiction between "working so hard to cure him" and being in solidarity with him in his experience of epilepsy. A stock image of the period looms up before us in David B.'s portrait of his mother: a disappointed mother who desires her son to be something he is not.

Path 2: "So What's It Like, a Seizure?"

The question of how best to be with Jean-Christophe during a seizure connects to the question of how Jean-Christophe himself experiences his seizures and the related question of how best to represent this experience. In the narrative and graphic terms set by David B., the experience question seems to condense into whether a seizure is one of two things for Jean-Christophe: either a trap or an escape. While David B.'s experience of his brother's epilepsy is a dense thicket of associations, affects, and desires, in contrast, Jean-Christophe's experience is reduced to the existentialist binary opposition between seizure as immanence and seizure as transcendence. Although motivated by a desire to give Jean-Christophe a way out of his epilepsy, David B.'s graphic treatment itself becomes, paradoxically, a kind of trap.

Toward the end of *Epileptic,* David B. goes to art school in Paris and begins to discover his calling as a graphic artist. Jean-Christophe also goes to Paris but, unlike his brother, apparently doesn't do much of anything, except continue to lose cognitive capacity and his ability to express himself to his family and the outside world. David B. describes the difficulty he has telling his new friends from school about his brother and his condition, and stigma is clearly one factor in this difficulty. This becomes especially apparent when he and his girlfriend contemplate having children, and she wants to know if epilepsy is hereditary (322). When David B. mentions this to his mother, he writes, "I glimpse the abyss this question opens up within her" (323). His mother, whom he has drawn as a mostly white and gaunt, ghostly and overexposed figure throughout the text, suddenly darkens, literally on the page, at the prospect of Jean-Christophe's epilepsy being hereditary. Yet for David B. the difficulty in telling is not only about the stigma associated with epilepsy but also about the failure of language to adequately capture the experience of epilepsy. He admits that the question he most loathes is, "So what's it like, a seizure?" because he knows it is impossible to satisfy the questioner's prurient desire to get a salacious inside story of seizure: "I feel my interlocutors hanging on my lips and I disappoint them," he writes. "It's hard to explain. Someday I'll draw it" (313). David B.'s concern here is with finding the right form in which to craft a representation that will not disappoint his friends. Jean Christophe's epilepsy becomes the thing that both resists representation and provokes a creative response from David B.—it both closes down and opens up the possibility of relationships for David B.

A page toward the end of the text exemplifies what I would call *Epileptic*'s graphic and narrative recursivity. The page is separated into two large panels that, despite a single horizontal line between them, are visually connected and seem to flow into each other. The top panel shows the family sitting within the contours of a white shadow horse whose head is an open book and who is in full stride, carrying the family along. The mother's long hair flows behind her, doubling as the horse's tail, as she tells a story to Jean-Christophe, Pierre-François, and Florence, who all sit at her feet eagerly listening. The family is surrounded by a landscape cluttered with story images, and the caption at the top reads: "I want to recapture what I loved when my father and my mother told us stories. I want to rediscover the delight and the strength that fairy tales give you" (291). The somewhat chaotic patterns of the top panel with its mythic mermaids, armor-clad warriors, and hybrid figures seem to coalesce into the serpent that dominates the bottom panel—fairy tale morphs into nightmare. The serpent clutches and possesses an older and diminished Jean-Christophe, who is portrayed as barely conscious—his head is slumped to his chest; his one visible eye appears to be rolled back in its socket; his face is shadowed; and his hand is stiff and claw-like, resembling the serpent's own claws (291). In this graphic trope, becoming-epileptic leads to a metamorphosis into a more primitive being—epileptic here is becoming-serpent.

The caption that separates the two panels explains: "Now that I'm alone in Paris, I want to tell the whole story. My brother's epilepsy, the physicians, macrobiotics, spiritualism, the gurus, the communes" (291). At the center of the serpent's spiraling, kinetic body, next to Jean-Christophe's inert body, are the words, "But I don't know how to draw it." In the bottom right-hand corner of the panel and the page, David B. explains that knowing how to draw it—the fairy tales of his childhood along with the very real nightmare of his brother's becoming-epileptic—will take time: "And I don't yet realize that it'll take me another 20 years to get there" (291). This pair of panels provides a snapshot of the larger, longer project that the graphic memoir as a whole enacts, demonstrating David B.'s graphic heterotopic method of spatial and temporal juxtaposition and simultaneity, as well as the ethical burden of telling the whole story—his own and Jean-Christophe's.

That it takes him twenty years to draw "it" is a fascinating confession, in temporal, spatial, and graphic terms: the image of Jean-Christophe and the serpent stands as a kind of figurative resolution to the problem of not knowing how to draw it. Within the narrative structure of the text, David B. arrives at this graphic resolution by recalling his art school days in the mid-1970s, a period when he struggled to understand the effects of his brother's epilepsy on his own emergent self. At this earlier moment in his life, he puts all his energy into his writing and drawing as a bulwark against letting himself go. Despite the posture of self-protection, he admits to wanting to feel the relief that will accompany letting go, and he believes that "pretend[ing] to be an epileptic" (287) is a route to this feeling. David B., the art student in the 1970s, tells the reader, "I could imitate a seizure. I know how" (287), and David B., graphic memoirist, shows us, twenty years on.

In a series of five small panels over two pages, David B. makes good on his claim, at least graphically, by showing a younger David B. imitating a seizure, all in the hopes that being sick—or at least appearing to be sick—would lead to him being cared for and not having "to deal with day-to-day life" (288). His graphic process of becoming-epileptic is punctuated with a panel in which he leans over his brother, who after a seizure (a real seizure as opposed to David B.'s pseudoseizure, though, of course, both graphic-seizures are representations and not the seizure-thing itself) lies flat on his back on the ground with his legs in the air (Figure 15). The brothers' bodies appear imprisoned in the small panel, the top of the panel preventing David B. from standing upright. Their bodies create a box within the box of the panel, and in the middle of this double cell/panel is a speech balloon in which David B. says, "I see the state my brother's in and I don't really want to be like him" (288).

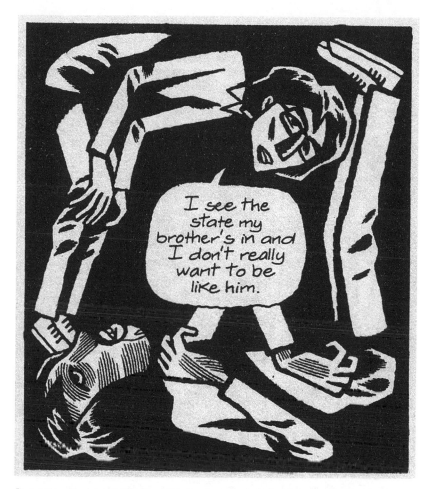

Figure 15. "I see the state my brother's in and I don't really want to be like him." David B., Epileptic, trans. Kim Thompson (New York: Pantheon, 2005), top middle panel, 288.

If David B. believes he can become—or not—epileptic, he feels less certain about his ability to control his own sanity, a graphic juxtaposition that suggests the enduring diagnostic and long historical association between epilepsy and madness discussed at the beginning of this chapter. We discover he doesn't really fear becoming-epileptic; by bragging about his ability to imitate a seizure, he indicates his certainty he will not in fact lose control in the way Jean-Christophe does. Yet he is less certain of his ability to control his sanity, and thus he fears becoming-insane, like the people he sees in the streets of Paris or on the Metro screaming and gesticulating. In this sequence, becoming-epileptic through imitation (a false convulsion) is juxtaposed with the possibility of being insane (another false convulsion). The categories of madness and epilepsy are linked through the spatial juxtaposition of David B.'s false convulsions confessional. We might even say that in this recollection of a moment from the 1970s, the ghost of hystero-epilepsy haunts the text, and imitation—the possibility of becoming-other—is understood as a form of power.

In coming to this revelation about his fears in relation to epilepsy and madness, David B. imagines and draws—imagines by drawing—his own desubjectification, as he feels the bones of his skull under the skin and the fat of his face. He imagines by drawing his own graphic suicide, in which he slices off his head with a knife, becoming a headless neck and shoulders with blood spewing out like an erupting volcano. This headless figure speaks the words, "My blood will speak for me," though the figure also realizes that the spewing/speaking cannot last long, because the "blood will dry off quickly" (290). The headless body then bends over to pick up its head, telling itself as it re-places its head on its shoulders, "Come on, admit it: You don't want to be sick, or crazy, or dead. It's just another way of telling stories. You can't help yourself. It's a way of conjuring unhappiness. It's magic" (290). And now, whole again, David B. says, "I've read many stories that have helped me. I want to touch people with my books in return." (290). In this sequence, becoming-epileptic and becoming-insane through drawing and writing are conjuring devices that David B. uses to touch others. They are also imitations—pseudoseizures, false convulsions, therapeutic *tableaux vivants,* graphic set pieces—and they provide an answer to the question, "So, what's it like, a seizure?" that won't disappoint.

Path 3: Of Other Spaces Not Yet Drawn

The moment when David B. admits to himself and his readers he doesn't want to be sick, crazy, or dead but wants, rather, to help others by telling stories, imitating seizures, and conjuring unhappiness is also a moment when his story diverges diametrically from his brother's. For Jean-Christophe there can be no dramatic scene in which he finally admits to himself that he doesn't want to be sick or crazy or dead—his creative possibilities are limited because he is, simply, sick. The question of choice is key to the chasm that opens up between David B. and his brother. While the capacity to get on or not with one's life is rarely, if ever, as clear-cut as being told to do so and doing it, the extent to which one is burdened and able to relieve that burden—through agency and self-representation—is highly variable. The figure of Jean-Christophe in *Epileptic* reveals this. I say "figure of Jean-Christophe" because, of course, I'm not really talking about Jean-Christophe himself, but the portrait of him drawn by David B. Jean-Christophe's experience is the foundation for David B's book, even as that experience remains murky, despite being starkly rendered in black and white. David B. notes poignantly, "He's drowning. He's my raft, I keep my head above water thanks to him" (214), and he captures these contrasting experiences with an image of Pierre-François straddling the back of a mostly submerged Jean-Christophe, whose translucent black skin merges with the translucent black water. In this image of one man surviving as or, perhaps, because another man drowns, an iconic image of a survivor's guilt that also haunts the experience and event of AIDS, the internal landscape of Jean-Christophe's body is externalized for all to see, his exposed organs appearing more botanical than anatomical. His body becoming-epileptic has come to resemble the thicket that the text of *Epileptic* attempts to traverse.

We are told frequently that as a young boy Jean-Christophe collaborated with his brother on creative projects.[29] We learn, for example, that together they wrote and illustrated the first eighteen pages of a novel called *The Great Convoy: An African Novel* (122). An eerie full-page portrait toward the end of the text captures the interconnectedness between the two brothers around the question of self-expression (Figure 16). In a series of nine interlocked panels on a page, David B. has drawn a face, which we recognize as Jean-Christophe's, blown up in the double sense of that term: both enlarged and exploded into pieces. The narrative captions explain that Jean-Christophe has returned from Paris to Olivet to live with his parents; the anger and rebellion at his situation has finally subsided, we are told, and he mostly stays in his room. "Even during the day the shutters are closed and the curtains drawn," the narrator explains (317). Filling the central panel on the page, David B. has drawn an outline of Jean-Christophe's nose, and within the contours of the enlarged, floating nose hovers a spooky, headless, black figure. This figure appears again in the bottom-right and left-corner panels, which contain smaller portraits, one of Jean-Christophe's face with distorted features, as if his face on the page is seizing, and one of David B's face, which is composed and without

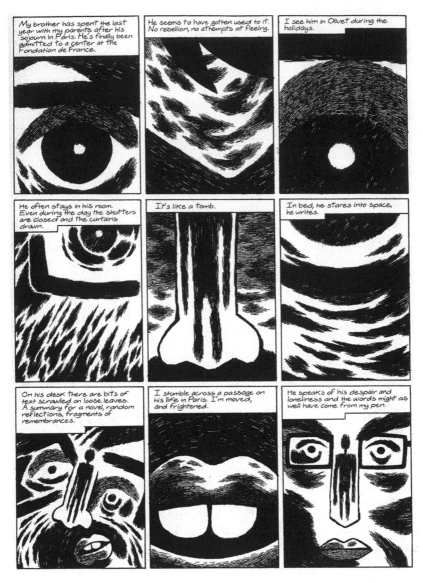

Figure 16. Jean-Christophe's face, blown up in the double sense of that term: both enlarged and exploded into pieces. David B., Epileptic, trans. Kim Thompson (New York: Pantheon, 2005), 317.

distortion from seizure or even, seemingly, emotion. The shadow figure hovers in the center of both faces, although Jean-Christophe's appears about to topple over, again as if the figure in the face is itself seizing, while David B.'s stands upright. In between these asymmetric faces is a blown-up image of Jean-Christophe's slightly opened mouth.

The question of self-expression signaled by the open mouth is also conveyed in the text above the three panels. In his bedroom, which David B. calls his "tomb," we learn that Jean-Christophe does two things: stares into space and writes. According to David B.'s account, "On his desk there are bits of text scrawled on loose leaves. A summary for a novel, random reflections, fragments of reminiscences. I stumble across a passage on his life in Paris. I'm moved, and frightened. He speaks of his despair and loneliness and the words might as well have come from my pen" (317). While David B. discovers words written by Jean-Christophe that he tells his reader might as well have come from his own pen, in *Epileptic,* of course, the words on the page are all his—quite literally, they are written and, even, inked by him. Put simply, we are not presented with any of Jean-Christophe's writings unmediated by David B., even though we are told that these writings exist and are moving and frightening.

When Jean-Christophe is away from Olivet, David B. scavenges for a key to Jean-Christophe's illness, searching through Jean-Christophe's stuff for clues to who he is and what he feels. Along with scraps of writing, he discovers that Jean-Christophe has appropriated an article in a literary magazine to tell his own story. We are presented with a drawing of David B. in Jean-Christophe's book-filled room reading the literary magazine that Jean-Christophe has doctored.[30] The caption describes Jean-Christophe's technique: "What he's done is recount his own life, crossing out proper names and replacing them with his own or with those of people from his world." And the figure of David B. in the panel explains further in three speech balloons: "Nietzsche becomes his doctor"; "Germany is the center for handicapped people where he is staying"; and "Nietzsche's madness was his epilepsy" (334). In the next panel, the reader is provided with a double interpretation of Jean-Christophe's writing practice, first in the caption, "He no longer has the strength to construct sentences to write," and then in a speech balloon spoken by the figure of David B., "Mom says he's reinvented the cut-up technique" (334). The reader (or this reader, at any rate) is tantalized by these two accounts from his brother and mother about Jean-Christophe's creative attempts to document his experience of illness, including by associating his own experience with Nietzsche's hystero-epilepsy—tantalized, in part, because the text of *Epileptic* only gestures to this work and does not attempt to reproduce it. Perhaps, this is another superficial gesture that makes a link between a past experience and a future event of illness. Certainly, it is a cautionary tale about the gap between the experience of illness and the stories of that experience, which is a central theme of this book.

In the last pages of *Epileptic*, David B. gestures again to what is left of Jean-Christophe's creativity after forty years of disease and at least a thousand little seizure deaths (358). In these last pages, Jean-Christophe appears as a rotund figure in an armchair with signs of his lifelong suffering, stigmata-like scars covering his face and a bald patch on the back of his head. From his armchair Jean-Christophe delivers what David B. calls his prophecies; according to David B. these prophecies are "a continuation of all his attempts at writing. It's his novel, his way of creating" (349). With David B. sitting attentively at his feet, Jean-Christophe haltingly delivers these divine revelations. Across two full pages, in scroll-like captions, we are presented with enigmatic aphorisms, including "Jesus speaks to me in my head" and "The water in my radiator has escaped to rejoin the 'mighty oceans'" (350). There is also an extended prophecy about a coming war between France and China and a description of attempts by Chinese soldiers to assassinate Jean-Christophe, who responds to the threat, as a good prophet might, with expressions of love not violence. The prophet figure suggests yet another diagnosis of the experience and event of Jean-Christophe's epilepsy, a diagnosis that is also a return to a premodern, pre-biomedical explanation of a falling sickness in which seizure is a divine gift—the ability to see into other worlds, including future worlds.

But as always, the real world of the present intrudes, even on Jean-Christophe's prophetic narrative: a disappointing Christmas with his family ends in a massive seizure. David B. and his sister are told to leave Olivet by their father, who is concerned that their presence upsets Jean-Christophe. The final panel in this scene shows a severe close-up of Jean-Christophe's scarred face, which echoes, on a smaller scale, the enlarged and cut-up image that appeared earlier. Also echoing the earlier full-page image, Jean-Christophe's mouth is slightly open but does not speak, and David B. gets the last word in a voice-over caption: "I feel like I've been chased off by his illness. I'm very bitter as I return to Paris" (353). What makes this panel so haunting is the juxtaposition and simultaneity of the silent, scarred face of Jean-Christophe overwritten by the words of David B. As in the earlier scene at the psychopedagogical institute in the late 1960s, drawing is contrasted with writing as interpretation. This time it is David B. himself who both draws and writes over Jean-Christophe's complex experience.

This is not the final image in the text, however. A two-page graphic reproduction of a dream of David B.'s from the night of September 26, 1999, is followed by an epilogue in which Jean-Christophe and David B. escape the family home on galloping white horses. The dream sequence seems to signify the range of emotions that David B., as dream figure, experiences in relation to the various members of his dream family: his mother accidentally hurts him when kissing him goodnight; his brother wants to do violence to him and, when he can't do so physically, does so emotionally through violent reproach; his sister sends him kisses, which manage to reach him across a great distance; and in the final panel, after he and his father are unable to express affection to each other, he becomes invisible to his father and the reader. This panel in which David B. disappears himself is in stark contrast to the hypervisible face of Jean-Christophe in the panel in the same position of the previous sequence. The implication seems to be that David B.'s own experience—his being itself—has disappeared into the dark shadows produced by Jean-Christophe's illness.

The epilogue as line of flight out of the shadows of illness returns the brothers to childhood and one of their childhood collaborations—the Martyr series—from before their creative lives diverged (359). Their creative divergence is signaled by a series of several panels leading up to the panel that re-creates an image from the Martyr series. In one panel the two young brothers ride the same white horse, an older Jean-Christophe, armed with a sword to kill the serpent/epilepsy that bites at the horse's heels, riding in front of the younger Pierre-François. In the next they are now adults riding a horse with two heads facing in opposite directions: a bloated and exhausted Jean-Christophe rides the horse to the left, and a thin David B. is to the right, echoing the earlier image of mother and father faced in opposite directions. The brothers openly discuss what connects and separates them: a shared passion for books and Jean-Christophe's wish to have written some, as his brother has. As a comforting response to his brother's admission to wanting to be like him, David B. tells his brother, "We're always afraid of falling short," and as his white horse flies off, while Jean-Christophe sits atop an open book, his motionless mount,

David B. compliments his brother on his prophetic stories, noting, "It's as if I'm hearing one of my own stories" (360). This leaves me with two final questions about other spaces of self-expression and illness: Are there stories Jean-Christophe tells that don't sound, look, and feel like David B.'s own? What might the fact of these other spaces of self-expression and illness-experience contribute to our understanding of the conjunction of illness-thought-activism in time? As David B. demonstrates in his graphic memoir about his brother's epilepsy, these are formal questions, but they are also political questions, even if the trajectory of the story he tells about his brother's epilepsy moves away from the political toward the personal. The question becomes even more complicated when the illness affects both an individual and, in the case of AIDS, an entire generation.

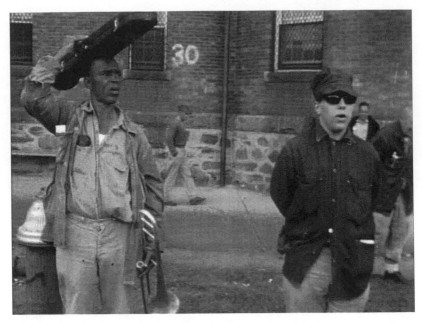

Figure 17. The political as internal to, not separate from, the experiences of patients at Bridgewater. Screen capture from Titicut Follies *(Frederick Wiseman, 1967).*

Disability Law Center's Investigation of Bridgewater State Hospital (2014) and Frederick Wiseman's *Titicut Follies* (1967)

In April 2014 the Disability Law Center (DLC) of Massachusetts began an investigation of the Bridgewater State Hospital (BSH) "based on . . . concern that individuals with mental illness were subject to abuse and neglect in the facility, including a deep concern about the excessive restraint and seclusion."[1] Under authority from the Protection and Advocacy for Individuals with Mental Illness (PAIMI) Act and the Developmental Disabilities Assistance and Bill of Rights (DD) Act, the DLC conducted numerous interviews (with patients at BSH, nonpatient inmates, corrections and mental health staff, and advocates for institutionalized persons) and reviewed the records of sixty-four patients and the relevant laws and policies. DLC's investigation found that "numerous conditions and practices at BSH violate the constitutional and federal statutory rights of its patients."[2]

The DLC report is terrifying in its unembellished presentation of Bridgewater as a place of harm and abuse rather than care and treatment for people with mental illness. The "fundamental problem," according to the report, is that "patients with serious mental illness are being held and 'treated' within a correctional facility, rather than within a mental health facility."[3] The report elaborates on this fundamental problem by describing in more detail how this arrangement contravenes therapeutic practices:

> Such a facility, with its correctional policies, practices and culture, is not an appropriate setting for men with significant psychiatric disabilities who need treatment and therapy, not just discipline and control. A significant number of patients, in addition to a psychiatric diagnosis, have trauma histories, including, but not limited to being victims of child sexual abuse. Some had problematic

behaviors tied to organic mental disorders, such as traumatic brain injury or AIDS dementia, which were unrelated to psychiatric disabilities. Yet their primary interactions were with DOC correctional officers, who have received minimal training in mental health treatment or trauma-informed care.[4]

The picture the DLC report paints is of a space that does exactly the opposite of what we might hope or expect of an institution for people who are mentally ill. The report argues that not surprisingly perhaps, considering their training, corrections officers are better at controlling and punishing, in particular through what the investigators found to be an excessive use of restraint and isolation as the main forms of treatment, than they are at calming, deescalating, and effectively treating with a variety of therapeutic practices.[5] Interactions between corrections officers and inmates operate in an emergency time that encourages restraint and isolation as always already inevitable responses to the problem of mental illness. Moreover, rather than exercising these forms of discipline and punish as short-term responses to crisis situations, the time of crisis is understood to be permanent, and thus, the violence of restraint and isolation is naturalized. What is demonstrated here is not only Bridgewater State Hospital as "total institution," in Goffman's sense, as "forcing houses for changing persons; each is a natural experiment on what can be done to the self,"[6] but also Bridgewater as permanent crisis institution: the extension of the time of crisis correlates directly to the compression of the spaces in which the patient can move freely or, even, at all. Emergency time shrinks space in the total institution.

Bridgewater State Hospital has been in the news before. Indeed, every decade or so, a pattern of mistreatment is exposed at Bridgewater, and changes are called for and promised. Most famously, or infamously, Bridgewater is the total institution profiled in Frederick Wiseman's *Titicut Follies* (1967), the first and arguably most controversial of Wiseman's many institutional documentaries, or "reality fictions," in the terminology he has used to describe his films.[7] For this snapshot I juxtapose the recent investigation at Bridgewater with an image from a scene cut into the middle of *Titicut Follies,* a scene shot in the liminal space of the hospital yard—at once outside and inside the institution—in which an inmate orates to a group of his fellow inmates against the war in Vietnam. I think it is important to note the event of oration and the figure of the orator at the center of this scene and the film itself because it distinguishes the scene from many of the other verbal and nonverbal exchanges we witness in the film. The inmate in the yard speaks at length to a fairly large crowd of his fellow inmates, seemingly gathered for the sole purpose of listening to his overtly political speech. Eventually, another inmate will interrupt his oration, and a political debate will ensue between the two. By pointing to the "mad" orator at the center of *Titicut Follies*, I want to draw a connection to Joan W. Scott's discussion of the female orator as one of her fantasies of feminist history. This fantasy figure "projects women into masculine public space, where they experience the pleasures and dangers of transgressing social and sexual boundaries."[8] For Scott one important aspect of fantasy is that it creates the setting not the object of desire. The "fantasies function as resources to be invoked": by attempting to see ourselves participating in a particular historical scene, we create links to a political past in order to craft a political present.[9] If the female orator is one of Scott's fantasies of feminist history, then the mad orator is one of my fantasies of illness history, in which the "mad" offer a trenchant critique of reason.

This scene isn't one of the more dramatic or commented on in the film, but in this snapshot I am interested in its function as a relay between two key scenes. In the first, one of the inmates, Vladimir, makes his case to the hospital psychiatrist, Dr. Ross, that he be "released" from Bridgewater and sent to a regular prison on the basis that the hospital and its drug treatments are making him sick. "I am here obviously well and healthy, and I am getting ruined," Vladimir explains. Vladimir's arguments, which appear for the most part more rational than Dr. Ross's often bizarre comments,[10] are made not only to Dr. Ross but to the filmmakers and for the cameras. It is clear from the way Vladimir occasionally turns to the camera instead of to Dr. Ross that his participation in Wiseman's film is an opportunity to make his case to the outside world.[11] I will take up a similar dynamic in my discussion in the next chapter of another documentary of a person with schizophrenia, who I argue uses the camera to become free.

Vladimir challenges not only his treatment at Bridgewater but also the manner in which he has been diagnosed as paranoid schizophrenic. In language anticipating Deleuze and Guattari's argument in *Anti-Oedipus* against the familial reductionism and "analytic imperialism" of the Oedipal complex and with similar humor about the domesticated and domesticating trap of the mommy-daddy-me triangle, Vladimir tells Dr. Ross and the camera: "You looked at me and you tell me I'm a schizophrenic paranoia. Just how do you know? Because I speak well? Because I, because I stand up for what I think?" When Dr. Ross responds that he knows Vladimir's diagnosis because Vladimir "got the psychological testings," Vladimir clearly enjoys ridiculing these tests, which ask questions about his toileting behavior, religious beliefs, and feelings for his mother and father. For Vladimir the tests are the source of amusement, but he also knows his capacity to defend himself is always already deauthorized within the space of the mental institution and in conversation with Dr. Ross (and later in conversation with Superintendent Gaughan and the review board). Quite powerfully and poignantly, Vladimir attempts to use the film to help him escape the phenomenon Goffman described as looping, whereby the inmate's statements are "discounted as mere symptoms" of his illness.[12]

The conversation between Vladimir and Dr. Ross takes place outside, the camera following them as the two men walk and talk in the hospital yard. The proximity and banter between the two also works to subvert the looping structure that would immediately capture Vladimir's speech as an aspect of his illness. The film then cuts from Vladimir making his case to an inmate wearing only white shorts exercising in the yard. On the soundtrack we hear the voice of another inmate, whom we have not encountered up to this point. Transcripts of the film designate this inmate as the "antiwar inmate."[13] The camera cuts to a close-up of the antiwar inmate's face at the moment his speech links the situation in present-day Vietnam to the situation in Europe before World War I. He then discusses the accusation that those who think and speak out as he does are "communists" ("We're for the community," he says) or "agitators" ("We're for the people," he says): "I'm a communist because I expound my views about the world conditions? It's the duty of every citizen to expound his views or her views of what goes on in the world." The antiwar inmate's position opposing U.S. intervention in Vietnam is challenged by a "prowar inmate," who asserts the people of North Vietnam are unfree and terrorized by the communist regime in North Vietnam. Eventually, the antiwar inmate's political speech devolves into a strange tale of America as a sex-crazed female in the "earth world," and the film cuts from this scene of speech to another inmate singing the patriotic song "Ballad of the Green Berets," which was popular at the time Wiseman and his crew were filming at Bridgewater and which lauds the Green Berets as "men who mean just what they say." What are we to make of this explicitly political speech and patriotic song in the middle of *Titicut Follies* and following Vladimir's questioning of his diagnosis, treatment, and oedipalization? Rather than use voice-over to tell us what to think, Wiseman's montage visually draws together debates over diagnosis and treatment with debates about politics. The effect of this technique is both to show the political as internal to, not separate from, the experiences of patients at Bridgewater and to extend our analyses of the political into the new domains of illness experiences and events, therapeutic thought and practices, and clinical and caring institutions and spaces. The film then cuts from the scenes outside the hospital to a harrowing scene inside of Dr. Ross tube-feeding an inmate, Malinowski, who like Vladimir is one of the main "characters" in the film. Both Vladimir and Malinowski practice an embodied politics of refusal—Vladimir refuses drugs, and Malinowski refuses food. Yet unlike Vladimir's protest, Malinowski's is completely silent, a passive form of resistance, a difference made more apparent placed next to the multiple forms of political speech that have immediately preceded the scene of force-feeding. Malinowski says three words in the film; when asked by Dr. Ross how he feels, he says, "Not too bad." During the force-feeding, Dr. Ross and the guards fill the silence of the soundtrack with banal speech, and when it is over, a guard says of Malinowski, in a kind of weird inversion of the line about "men who mean just what they say" from the "Ballad of the Green Beret," "Boy, this guy's a veteran, he's been tube-fed before, he's a veteran. Swallow, just swallow, swallow, swallow, that's-a-boy"—lyrics to a kind of "Ballad of the Tube-Fed Veteran."

The film's overall narrative arc (admission, institutional life, release) ends with Malinowski's death, which we are meant to understand is connected to his not eating, followed by the preparation of his body after death and his burial at a cemetery outside the grounds of the hospital. In Goffman's terminology Malinowski's death might be understood as a literal mortification, a final "curtailment of the self" that Malinowski had helped speed along by refusing to eat.[14] The grim reality fiction with which Wiseman leaves us is that Malinowski escapes Bridgewater before Vladimir. The DLC's investigation in 2014 updates the picture presented in *Titicut Follies.* What the DLC's report describes is not exactly a passage from institutionalization to deinstitutionalization of the mentally ill but of an institutionalized transfer of the "treatment" of mental illness from hospitals to correctional facilities—Vladimir's individual protest to be released to prison achieved writ large.

Witnessing Schizophrenia

In this chapter I continue to explore questions from chapter 5 regarding how best to document the physical, psychological, and social effects of illness on an individual and his or her family. I move from an ostensibly physical illness (epilepsy) to an ostensibly mental illness (schizophrenia) not to secure diagnostic categories but to reveal their constantly changing historical forms—or, we might say, to reveal the historical "ostensibility" of all illnesses. As in chapter 5, I analyze not only the experience of illness in a particular family during the 1960s and 1970s but also the event of illness in history in the period before the emergence of AIDS.

Susan Smiley's documentary film *Out of the Shadow* (2004)[1] opens with images of homeless people and these words narrated by Smiley herself: "We've all seen these people. Destitute. Delusional. Muttering to themselves. For the most part we just walk away and keep going. But every time I pass one of these people, I think: that could be my mother." The words and images with which *Out of the Shadow* opens frame what follows, which is both an account of Smiley's mother's struggle with mental illness and an investigation into various ways of seeing—practices of witnessing—mental illness. In chapter 3 I discussed doctoring as a practice of witnessing that enacts a particular medical experience at a particular time as described in Foucault's *Birth of the Clinic* and Berger and Mohr's *A Fortunate Man*. In this chapter, as in the previous, I shift my focus from the doctoring of doctors to the doctoring of patients and their families.

In her direct address to the viewer of *Out of the Shadow*, Smiley explains that the homeless person she sees on the street could be her mother, Mildred Smiley, because her mother suffers from schizophrenia, has been in and out of mental hospitals, and has endured a pharmacopeia of drug therapies. Although the exact date of the onset of her condition remains uncertain, the film shows that Mildred had what seems to have been a psychotic break after the birth of her first child in the early 1960s; that child is the filmmaker, who attempts to make sense of her mother's life in and through film. I read Susan Smiley's work with and against another account of the multiple effects of mental illness on the person who is ill and on her family: the memoir *Saving Millie: A Daughter's Story of Surviving Her Mother's Schizophrenia*, written by Susan's sister and Mildred's daughter, Tina Kotulski.[2] Mildred Smiley and her diagnosis of and treatment for schizophrenia are at the center of both daughters' treatments—filmic and narrative treatments—of mental illness, and in these texts all three become witnesses to the multiple experiences of mental illness and the multiple events of psychiatric power. Continuing themes raised in chapter 5 about other spaces of self-expression and disease expression, I argue these two texts are treatments of schizophrenia that both see *and* don't see Mildred Smiley's experience of mental illness. Through these texts we—viewer and reader—are asked to look again, or to look for the first time, at mental illness, and we are positioned as having the agency to look or look away. As we look and try to make sense of what we see (and don't see), we too participate in the production of mental illness as a category of analysis.

I extend the mother's and her two daughters' practices of witnessing by returning again and anew to Foucault's work on the historical category of madness by historicizing it as taking place in what I am calling the prehistory of AIDS. How Foucault thought about madness changed over time; in his breakthrough work *History of Madness* (1961), for example, he was already revising how he had thought madness in his very first publication, *Mental Illness and Psychology* (1954).[3] As touched on in chapter 5, madness would be one of the key objects through which Foucault delineated and transformed his historicoontological methods—methods that are explicitly described in his lecture series "The Government of the Self and Others" and in his essay "What Is Enlightenment?," in which he recommends a philosophical ethos that consists of "a critique of what we are saying, thinking, and doing, through a historical ontology of ourselves."[4] His archeological investigations into the discourses of madness would later be supplemented by his genealogical work on psychiatric power in his lectures at the Collège de France in 1973–74.[5] In each text Foucault returns to the object he studied earlier but approaches that object anew, in an overall arc that moves from a concern with the representations and iconic figures of madness that emerge at different points in history to an analysis of the multiple apparatuses of psychiatric power and the discourses of truth these apparatuses produce. In Foucault's later work, while representations are still utilized to provide historical images of the experiences of madness, he is now also concerned with how these representations are produced through particular discursive and nondiscursive practices of reason and unreason. By applying Foucault's methodology to Mildred Smiley's daughters' representations of her schizophrenia, we can begin to see how schizophrenia is enacted across multiple spaces, including the middle-class American home in the 1960s and 1970s, the hospital and mental institution, the group home, and, finally, Tina Kotulski's own home, into which Millie moves in 2003.

Throughout this book I have been interested in how illness is constituted directly and indirectly through different discourses, practices, and institutions—medical, political, conceptual, and aesthetic—in the period before the emergence of AIDS. Here, I will consider the ways we might discern the differences between what Foucault describes as the "truth of madness speaking in its own name" and the "truth of madness agreeing to first person recognition of itself in a particular administrative and medical reality constituted by asylum power."[6] In *Out of the Shadow* and *Saving Millie,* both truths of madness are enacted: we glimpse the truth of Millie's madness speaking in its own name, but we also witness the covering over of that truth with the potent truth of psychiatric power, expressed in the countless treatments Millie undergoes and in her daughters' treatments of those treatments. The film and memoir don't simply represent truths of madness but produce them through their particular ways of seeing (and not seeing) mental illness. One of Foucault's key interventions is to demonstrate how asylum power moves out into other domains and, indeed, into society at large. The image of homelessness with which *Out of the Shadow* opens haunts Susan Smiley's documentary treatment of schizophrenia, and it also haunts the text of *Saving Millie.* What Millie must be saved from is an existence that is homeless. The homeless and, in particular, the homeless who are mentally ill are, in Foucault's terminology, "the residue of all residues, the residue of all the disciplines, those who are inassimilable to all of a society's educational, military, and police disciplines."[7]

Smiley's awareness that "that could be my mother" signals her attempt to find a method to witness "the residue of all residues" not or not only in order to assimilate it through discipline but as a call to struggle against our impoverished response—conceptually, politically, practically, and aesthetically—to mental illness. Kotulski also issues a call to struggle, but her way of seeing mental illness and the struggle that way of seeing produces is different from her sister's, emphasizing a privatized rather than a structural perspective. And yet despite their differences, both *Out of the Shadow* and *Saving Millie* suggest a teleological narrative trajectory that moves from a state of homelessness to the happy resolution of finding a home for Millie. In *Out of the Shadow,* the resolution finds Mildred Smiley settled in a group home, holding down her first job in some thirty years, and reveling in the "normal" she feels at long last.[8] Although *Out of Shadow* ends with hope, even triumph,[9] *Saving Millie* reveals the failure of this earlier resolution (the group home, Mildred's job, the "normal") and replaces it with another, supposedly even better, resolution. In Tina's updated version of Mildred's story, Mildred goes to live with Tina and her family and is "saved" again, this time by a different normal, here signified by her role as grandmother in a loving family. The desire to create stories that help others motivates both Susan Smiley and Tina Kotulski, as it did David B. Yet as these stories also demonstrate, this creative desire exists alongside the everyday exhaustion of and from illness that dissipates creativity and desire. What we see again is the difficulty of creating what I described in chapter 2, citing Guattari's writing on and work at La Borde, as alternative spaces for a "therapeutic social life."[10]

Despite the seemingly happy resolutions in the narratives presented in *Out of the Shadow* and *Saving Millie,* uncertainty regarding Mildred's situation remains, if most obviously when we consider the texts together. Foucault's formulation of the concept of the social residue, an unwanted trace that remains despite our attempts to eliminate it, evokes another, related concept for framing my analysis of Susan Smiley's documentary film, Tina Kotulski's memoir, and Mildred Smiley's experience of schizophrenia. That concept is the shadow or, perhaps I should say, *shadows,* in the plural, because there are at least three shadows I delineate here.[11] The first shadow refers to the social structures of shame and stigma that often keep mental illness out of view in the hopes of preempting or avoiding the gaze of society, a normalizing gaze that David B. draws as a landscape of eyes. As her film's title suggests, Susan Smiley attempts to bring the experience of mental illness out of the shadows that shame and stigma cast in order to not only make the experience of mental illness visible but also expose the structures of power that exclude whole categories of experience from public domains and discourses. The second shadow, which is less central in Smiley's documentary but is the focus of Kotulski's memoir, is the shadow that Mildred Smiley's mental illness casts over the experiences of others—in particular, the experiences of her two daughters' emergent selves as children and young adults. If the first refers to the ways structures of power cast shadows by making visible the experiences of some and invisible the experiences of others, then the second refers to the way individual subjectivity always emerges in relation to the subjectivity of others. We come into being in the shadow of others; our subjectivity is overshadowed, often quite literally and in a double sense—to overshadow can mean to protect and shelter or, paradoxically, to obscure or overwhelm.

The final shadow I want to address is an ethical one and relates to those shadows Smiley's film and Kotulski's memoir cast over Mildred Smiley's experience of schizophrenia. In an echo of the turn in the final section of the previous chapter, as well as in relation to the function of the snapshots in the overall structure of this book, I want to examine how the practice of witnessing creates its own shadows. In order to explore how this happens, we must understand witnessing in temporal as well as spatial terms, which is one of the central tasks of my approach to the experience of illness and health activism in the period before AIDS. As I understand it, witnessing is not something that happens in a single place or moment in time. To witness we must always anticipate other witnesses in other places and times. One obvious way we can grasp the temporal and spatial aspects of witnessing is by reading Smiley's and Kotulski's texts together. When we do this, we discover a tension between the two texts with regards to how best to treat schizophrenia, and taking the two texts together helps to illuminate the way shadows can be cast by both social structures and individuals. But what still remains oblique is what schizophrenia is for Mildred Smiley, unmediated by her daughters' desire to understand their mother's story and render it for others to witness. Witnessing is a practice of illumination, and illumination changes the substance of that which is illuminated. Simply put, shadows disappear when we illuminate them. How, then, do we apprehend them? Or in Foucault's terms, how do we see the shadows of unreason in the glare of reason?

Using Foucault's concept of the "truth-thunderbolt," I conclude this chapter by presenting what I take to be several flashes of Mildred Smiley's experience of schizophrenia in the stories Susan Smiley and Tina Kotulski tell about their mother. I do not claim to be the final arbiter on Mildred Smiley's experience of schizophrenia; rather, my hope is to extend the practices of witnessing she and her daughters have already enjoined us to participate in. In that spirit this conclusion is open-ended, suggesting pos-sibilities rather than resolutions out of respect for the complexity of mental illness and its traumatic effects. By placing a story of schizophrenia in the context of the prehistory of AIDS, I also want to draw links—direct and indirect—between illness experiences, practices of health activism, and historical shifts in medical diagnoses and treatments.

Before I turn to the various shadows cast over the experience and event of schizophrenia, a brief note on terminology seems called for and will help to locate Mildred Smiley's and her daughters' experiences of schizo-phrenia within the prehistory of AIDS. Thus far I have used three terms interchangeably: *unreason, madness,* and *mental illness.* Although I don't have the space here to trace a genealogy of the use of these terms, I want to make clear that the term both Smiley and Kotulski use for their moth-er's condition is *mental illness* and to briefly acknowledge the historical shift this term demonstrates. That this term is now used almost univer-sally demonstrates the medicalization or scientization of madness and the hegemonic view, in contemporary Western culture at least, that the pri-mary etiology of most mental disorders is biological. This new perception of psychological disorders emerged in the 1970s with new brain-imaging technologies that aided diagnosis and new-and-improved pharmacologi-cal treatments for formerly intractable conditions like schizophrenia. In his foreword to Kotulski's memoir, Marvin Swartz, head of the Division of Community Psychiatry at Duke University Medical Center, indicates this hegemonic view when he writes: "Fortunately, the scientific revolu-tion in psychiatry has dramatically increased our understanding of the etiology of schizophrenia. While stressful social environments do seem to play some role in the development of the disease, genetics and neuro-biology appear to be much more significant—indeed, usually decisive—factors."[12] What the "scientific revolution in psychiatry" replaced was a regime of diagnoses and treatments influenced by psychoanalysis.[13] As we consider Mildred Smiley's experience of schizophrenia as it is produced in her daughters' texts, I want us to keep in mind Swartz's confidence in the dramatic progress that has been made in diagnosing and treating schizo-phrenia. From his comments and from the fact they are used to introduce Kotulski's memoir about her mother, we might gather that Mildred Smiley has somehow benefited from the scientific revolution in psychiatry. Yet the texts themselves, as well as Mildred's position as articulated in them, at the very least complicate this narrative of scientific progress.

Structures/Shadows

"We know the images," Foucault states at the beginning of the penultimate chapter of *History of Madness,* entitled "The Birth of the Asylum."[14] Those well-known images from the history of psychiatry to which Foucault refers are of the liberation of the mad from their confinement, that ostentatious removal of their chains by reformers in the "philanthropic" impulse that led to the birth of the asylum at the beginning of the nineteenth century. Over 150 years later, at the same time as Foucault is diagnosing the earlier birth of the asylum, the mad, who are no longer "mad" but now "mentally ill," are liberated again, as we saw in my earlier snapshot of a snapshot and echo of an echo—Isaac Julien's "Frantz Fanon" liberating patients from shackles at Blida-Joinville Hospital during the Algerian war of liberation from France. This later "liberation" will become, paradoxically, the death of the asylum, a casualty of the massive deinstitutionalization of the mentally ill in the United States beginning in the 1950s.[15] This historical moment is also when the first signs of Mildred Smiley's schizophrenia appear, although, tellingly, she will not be diagnosed with and treated for schizophrenia until 1985.[16]

Against the supposedly well-known images of the mad being "liberated" as the asylum comes into being, Smiley begins *Out of the Shadow* with other well-known images, of homelessness, and a comment on our abiding historical and contemporary desire to look away from mental illness. The opening shots of homeless people, some muttering to themselves, all absolutely alone yet surrounded by their possessions, which signify both their struggle to survive and the burden of that survival, are familiar scenes from the urban United States in the late twentieth and early twenty-first century. After these all-too-familiar scenes, the film cuts to footage from a grainy home movie, probably from the early 1960s. This is our first image of Mildred Smiley, and we see a striking young, blonde woman wearing a pink top and white shorts in what appears to be a suburban backyard during the summer. A large, black dog on a leash pulls her toward the person who holds the camera and toward us, the viewers. She is smiling slightly as she closes in on the person with the camera and the viewers of Smiley's film. The young woman in the 1960s appears to be pulled from the past into the viewer's present; the film links the ghostly past depicted in this home movie with the possibility of future witnesses. The colors in the home movie fade to black and white, and the shot freezes when the woman arrives directly before the camera, filling the screen, smiling, yet slightly out of focus, as the film's title appears (Figure 18). This image of a person being brought into our field of vision so that we may get a closer look sets the scene for the film's practice of witnessing mental illness. It also suggests that we must look back at the ghostly evidence from the past, including home movies and family photographs, in order to discern when and why Mildred Smiley became mentally ill. Some of the same family photographs Smiley incorporates into her film will appear again in the pages of Kotulski's memoir. The person behind the camera is not identified in either documentary film or memoir, and how these remnants of family history have endured in spite of the many upheavals in Millie's and her daughters' lives is never explained, though I will speculate further about their survival.

Smiley's film stages an examination into the experience and event of mental illness. The filmmaker adopts a clinical gaze—one that looks intently but almost always from a distance, sometimes literally in terms of the position of Smiley's camera, and most often at a slight emotional remove, expressed especially in Smiley's prominent voice-over, which provides an organizing perspective for the film as a whole.[17] Although Susan states that one of the "most confounding aspects" of her mother's illness is that "she has no insight about it, no awareness that she has it," Millie does have an explanatory model for her condition. Early in the film Mildred describes what was happening in her brain when years earlier she "slit [her] throat and wrists," explaining matter-of-factly that it was a kind of "noise pollution, . . . like 10 billion years of hell slamming through my head. The noise pollution temporarily set something off in my head." According to Millie's explanatory model of illness, at times some of the circuitry in her brain doesn't connect properly, causing her brain to misfire. Hers might be said to be a biosocial model of illness (brain circuitry interacting with noise pollution); the discourse of psychoanalysis or even of psychology more generally is apparently not useful to her in describing her experience of schizophrenia. Interestingly, while Millie's explanatory model may be antipsychological, if not quite antipsychiatric, in this moment at least it can hardly be said to be without insight or awareness.

Susan follows her mother's assessment of the misfiring in her brain with a statement about why she wants to make this film: "Her mind intrigues me. I find being curious helps keep at bay all that I feel." Later in the film, Susan describes an earlier instance of using this same approach,

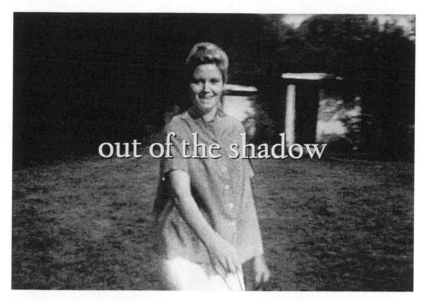

out of the shadow

Figure 18. The image of a person being brought into our field of vision so that we may get a closer look sets the scene for the film's practice of witnessing mental illness. Screen capture from Out of the Shadow (Susan Smiley, 2004).

what I call her clinical practice of witnessing. When her mother is finally diagnosed with paranoid schizophrenia when Susan is in her early twenties, Susan researches the illness and learns that children of schizophrenics have a 10 percent chance of becoming mentally ill like their parent. Fearful of the possibility of inheriting schizophrenia from her mother, Susan tells her viewers, "[I] started to analyze my mind and scrutinize my behavior," suggesting a certain faith that by examining her mind and behavior she might protect herself from the same fate as her mother. For Smiley filmmaking becomes an extension of this earlier, nascent clinical examination into schizophrenia and its biological and social effects. Film becomes an instrument that helps her to analyze the experience of schizophrenia, but it is also a means to control the story by keeping emotion at bay. Indeed, for Smiley filmmaking is one indirect effect of the trauma of living with a person with schizophrenia and of violence; with her camera she attempts to analyze an experience that is always beyond—or prior to— her awareness of it. Smiley's filmmaking as practice, as much as the content of the film itself, reveals schizophrenia as something traumatic that happened to her but that she cannot fully comprehend.[18] Like David B.'s drawing, Smiley's filmmaking becomes a line of flight out of the trap of illness. Smiley's documentary film and David B.'s graphic narrative are the creative offspring of their genetic predispositions—in Smiley's case, to schizophrenia, and in David B.'s, to epilepsy.

We can see how Smiley's clinical gaze structures our perception of schizophrenia in particular in two scenes of illness presented in the film. The first is footage from what appears to be a single incident, though Smiley has split this footage and incorporated it into two different sections of the film. In Smiley's direct address, we learn this sequence is, chronologically, the beginning of Smiley's filming of her mother's experience of mental illness. She explains that Mildred had been living in her "mother's empty house" and that she was "withdrawn, isolated, and hadn't taken her medication in weeks." Susan returns to check on her mother (where she returns from, we aren't told), and for the first time she brings her camera, as her voice-over explains. We first see the "empty" house from the outside and then accompany the handheld camera down a corridor toward a room, and there, we see Mildred, at first from a distance. The film then cuts to a mundane shot of Mildred in the kitchen getting something out of the refrigerator before quickly cutting again, this time to a close-up of Mildred back in the room where we had seen her before.

Smiley captures an angry and paranoid outburst from Millie, an outburst clearly meant to show the viewer a psychotic episode. Millie rants at Susan, accusing her of talking to strangers and of "dragging me into it too." Millie sits alone on a chair in the small room in her mother's house, which we can see isn't precisely empty (and isn't Mildred living there, after all?), although it is clearly in some disarray. The camera stays tight on Mildred's face as she hurls accusations at Susan, who we can hear softly asking her mother to explain why she is so angry. Although Susan zooms in on her mother's face, the impression is that Smiley shoots the scene through the door to the room from the threshold, not unlike some shots in *Titicut Follies* of patients in their cells at Bridgewater. It is as if Susan fears getting too close to her mother's anger and wants to keep enough distance to ensure a means of escape. During her diatribe Millie does not look directly at the camera; her eyes dart toward Susan and the camera but don't make contact as she gets more and more enraged. As Mildred finishes her paranoid outburst, the camera zooms in close, and Susan's voice-over explains, "As usual she was furious with me for meddling in her affairs. When mom's illness takes over, I become the enemy." This early scene of psychosis ends

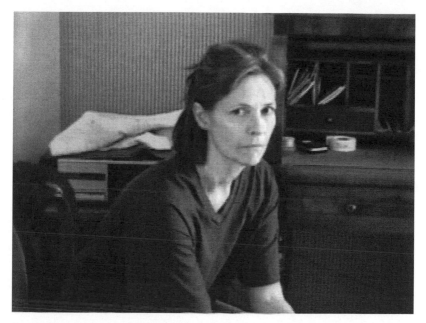

Figure 19. The visual and narrative trope of Millie's eyes—what they see and don't see, what they reveal and don't reveal—recurs throughout the film. Screen capture from Out of the Shadow (Susan Smiley, 2004).

as the shot zooms out again and Millie turns to face the camera, Susan, and the film's spectators. In this moment the film freezes, and we are confronted with Mildred Smiley's dark eyes looking directly at us (Figure 19).

As with Berger and Mohr's *A Fortunate Man* and David B.'s *Epileptic*, eyes figure prominently in *Out of the Shadow*, suggesting again Foucault's point in *Birth of the Clinic* that particular arts of seeing enact particular experiences of illness. The visual and narrative trope of Millie's eyes—what they see and don't see, what they reveal and don't reveal—recurs throughout the film. Tina's husband, Jeff, describes Millie's eyes as "steely" and says that when he first met Millie, her eyes "weren't looking at me; they were looking through me." Later, in a scene in the car after a shopping trip, with Susan driving and Millie sitting in the back while a third person with the camera films them both from the passenger seat, Millie says plainly, "I have an unhappy face, don't I?" Looking at her mother in the car's rearview mirror, Susan replies without pause, "You have sad eyes." Millie considers this and then suggests a way to solve the problem of her sad eyes: "I'll have to make them up again. Get the right medication; put make up on."

This is one of the few times Millie herself brings up the potential benefits of medication; it's as if, for a fleeting moment, she sees herself as others see her—clinically. Yet this statement also tells us something about what Millie thinks medication does: here it is linked with a cosmetic covering over of the problem of sadness. Both medication and makeup can mask feeling sad.

After the scene of psychosis and the searing shot of Mildred's black eyes, the film cuts to black. The next scene introduces Mildred's ex-husband and Susan's father, Alan Smiley, who in an interview with Susan tells the story of Mildred's breakdown after the birth of their first child. We first see Alan working on the yard of his rather palatial suburban home, and then the film cuts to Susan interviewing her father as he sits comfortably in a leather armchair in what looks to be a fairly elegant upper-middle-class living room. Alan's home, shown several times in the film, stands in stark contrast to Mildred's mostly depressing and ever-changing accommodations. In response to Susan's query, "When did you first know something was wrong, Dad?" Alan describes being blindsided by his wife's breakdown after the birth of their first child: "She cut her wrists. I said, 'My god, what am I dealing with here?' This is an unusual circumstance. She's not rational. I think she's nuts. I said, 'What did I do?'" Alan's narrative is accompanied by home movies of Mildred with Susan as an infant and toddler; the juxtaposition of words and images is apparently meant to illustrate Mildred's dramatic emotional highs and lows that Alan describes, although without his narrative it would be difficult to discern from the movie clips themselves that they are evidence something is seriously wrong with Mildred. The clips at this juncture in the film's narrative, accompanied by Alan's voice-over, indicate he is most likely the person behind the camera in the moving and still images of Mildred from the 1960s incorporated into Susan Smiley's documentary. It also seems likely Alan's house has served as the repository for the collection of images of Mildred Smiley and family that serve as visual evidence in the documentary of all her mother has lost.

In a continuation of the interview, Alan anticipates possible criticisms of his subsequent actions as selfish and even presents a case of sorts against his eventual decision to leave the house, saying with visible discomfort, "How could any human being, a father, leave children that are one and a half and three years old? . . . How can a man leave like that?" By speaking in the third person about "any human being," "a father," "a man," Alan

Smiley's grammar shields him from personal responsibility. Only when he defends his actions does he speak in the first person: "I had to survive." As the film makes clear, he has survived, even thrived, without the burden of a wife who was "not rational," "nuts." Although Kotulski is far more critical of her father for leaving than Susan is, neither film nor memoir explores the way gender norms contributed to the response to Mildred Smiley's breakdown within her immediate and larger family and within society. By placing the cut of Mildred's scene of psychosis right before we first meet Alan and hear his story of desperation and survival, Susan, unconsciously perhaps, offers a visual and narrative justification for his escape.

We witness more of the scene of psychosis later in the film. Although Smiley doesn't indicate this is an extension of that earlier scene, it appears to be, as Millie is in the same clothes and position as before. While the earlier use of footage from this incident helps to illustrate Susan's precarious position, as daughter and witness, in relation to her mother's anger, this later cut provides an explanation of sorts for one of Millie's breakdowns, as well as a structural critique of the public health system. That this story can now be told this way seems to me to be the result of mental health activism that began in the late 1960s and early 1970s, although unlike David B's *Epileptic* the text itself delves only into personal histories, not into what I describe earlier as queer clinical histories. The film demands we view Mildred's psychosis by both zooming in to get a closer, if still safely removed, look at Mildred's individual experience and zooming out to get a wider view of the experience of schizophrenia within the structures of the family and the public health system.

We see Millie visiting her own dying mother in a nursing home. As she and Susan leave the home, Millie is clearly disturbed by what she has seen. She describes the people in the home as nothing more than "carcasses in clothes" and admits, "I feel like I'm locked up in a nursing home too. I'm on my death bed too." Of her own mother's situation, Millie notes, "I feel so sorry for her. I could just lay down and die." This visit appears to be a contributing factor to the psychotic episode captured by Susan on film. Amid the accusations directed at various individuals, whom she apparently encountered at the nursing home, and at Susan, who is accused of standing "there listening to that fucking bullshit," we glimpse something else behind the anger: the terror of becoming a "carcass in clothes" or, in Foucault's phrase, "the residue of all residues." Millie states emphatically, drawing a disturbing parallel between the treatment of the elderly in nursing homes and homosexuals, "I'm not going to wind up being treated like some kind of faggot, like she is." In her paranoia Mildred discerns what I have been describing in this book as the interconnectedness between the experiences and events of illness and sexuality.

Considering the film documents Mildred Smiley's often harrowing journey through an at best "fractured" public health system, on many levels her fears of such treatment are entirely rational. What she sees in the nursing home is not simply the possibility of an unwanted future of involuntary institutionalization at the end of her life, which is a common fear among the elderly in the West, but a permanent shadow of institutionalization that has and continues to mark her life. This permanent shadow of the terrors of institutionalization is illustrated by the film's narrative structure. After Millie's angry and fearful response to witnessing her own mother's experience of institutionalization, we next see Millie in a hospital gown in a psychiatric ward. She is psychotic and refusing to take antipsychotic medication. When Susan explains that if she doesn't take her meds, she will lose her place in her apartment, Millie corrects Susan's characterization of where she is living at that time: "It's not an apartment. It's not even a prison."

We then become witnesses to what might be described as a scene of *mis*informed consent as Tina lies to her mother to get her to sign a form that consents to the administration of the antipsychotic drug Prolixin. Tina explains to Millie that the form is for placement in a group home, and her mother signs, saying, "I can't wait to get out of here. There are better things to do." Outside the hospital the two daughters discuss the ethics of what has just occurred and disagree over whether lying was justified in this situation. Tina insists, "She has to be medicated to get her brain straight," and she regards "lying to her [as] a sweet thing to do," whereas Susan is concerned about the consequences of the lie once their mother realizes she won't in fact be going to the much desired group home. This particular ethical conflict between the sisters signifies a difference between their practices of witnessing and their treatments of and for schizophrenia. In this instance Tina becomes a relay for the administration of psychiatric power, utilizing Mildred's desire for freedom to justify an, arguably, temporary usurpation of her autonomy. In Tina's understanding, freedom for Millie can come only through submission to psychiatric power, first in the form of Millie admitting she is ill and then by submitting to the pharmacological treatments that might help her. Tina's attitude regarding the benefits of Mildred's medications changes somewhat by the end of *Saving Millie*. Tina takes Mildred into her home after Mildred nearly dies from an adverse reaction to the combination of medications she is taking, noting "her body's decreasing ability to metabolize them, [and] . . . compromised . . . kidney function, which led to a low blood sodium level" (205). Tina and her husband, Jeff, an osteopathic family doctor, put Mildred on a new regime: orthomolecular medicine, which Tina says in the postscript "aims to restore the optimum environment of the body by correcting imbalances or deficiencies based on individual biochemistry using substances natural to the body, such as vitamins, minerals, amino acids, trace elements, and essential fatty acids" (218). One of the goals behind the publication of *Saving Millie* appears to be promoting orthomolecular treatment for schizophrenia, which although an alternative to conventional biopsychiatry is nonetheless an individual, not structural, response to illness.

The daughters' ethical debate over the function of the lie illustrates the difficulty of both successfully treating schizophrenia and witnessing as a form of treatment. The film stages this as a central question of ethics: How can they convince or force their mother to take antipsychotic medications when she resists these drugs because they themselves make her feel bad, not some abstract disease entity with the name *paranoid schizophrenia*? For Tina this can be accomplished only by deceiving her mother, who in Tina's assessment already deceives herself, unwittingly or not, about her illness. Although she questions the deception, Susan is also complicit with it. By filming the moment of deception and the debate between the daughters that follows, Susan demonstrates the way this decision must be seen in relation to Millie's long history of failed treatment and her, always precarious, freedom. The centrality of this sequence in the overall structure of the film's narrative, as well as the relative length of the scene and the fact it is one of the few sequences where a musical track is added to the soundtrack, suggests Smiley has self-consciously produced an ethical set piece for the film. I think, however, this set piece also covers over another ethical question, which is not about the particular lie the daughters tell their mother to get her to, unwittingly, agree to drugs she does not want but the possibility the film itself might—indeed must—also lie about Mildred Smiley's experience of mental illness.[19] I will return to this ethical question in the final section of the chapter.

Although both *Out of the Shadow* and *Saving Millie* show the problem of the fractured U.S. public health system, with its "long line of nameless, faceless doctors to offer a panacea for [Millie's] condition," Susan appears more sympathetic than her sister to her mother's resistance to the plethora of medications she has been prescribed for most of her life. It is Kotulski's memoir, however, that reveals the extent of Mildred Smiley's highly medicated past. Doctors began prescribing drugs for Millie long before she was diagnosed with schizophrenia. In her teens, after the death of her stepfather, Millie's mother, concerned about Millie's frequent outbursts combined with a general lethargy, took her to a doctor, who diagnosed hypothyroidism and prescribed Synthroid, which Kotulski describes as "a hormone-replacement medication that had just come on the market" (23). During her sophomore year of high school, Millie was sent to a strict boarding school. When she began to put on weight and started smoking, Millie's mother again took her to a doctor, who this time prescribed Dexedrine. Kotulski notes that Millie became addicted to Dexedrine and speculates that "Millie could have experienced toxicity from overuse of the drug. Side effects of Dexedrine overdose can include restlessness, insomnia, and even a psychosis clinically indistinguishable from schizophrenia" (24–25). Kotulski admits that "much of Millie's medical history, especially from the sixties and seventies, is no longer available" but says there is "evidence" she was also prescribed Stelazine, a tranquilizer and antipsychotic; Fiorinal, a barbiturate; and Darvon, a painkiller. I will return to the effects of the historicoclinico imperative "drugs into bodies" in my conclusion, but for now it suffices to say that as in the case of Jean-Christophe's treatments for epilepsy, it is often difficult to separate the negative physical effects of an individual's illness from the also negative physical effects of her or his treatments. We are still learning about the long-term effects of taking the protease inhibitors introduced to treat HIV/AIDS in 1995.

Toward the end of the film, Millie shows us the various medications she is taking and describes what she knows about each. She then states matter-of-factly to Susan and to us: "They all have side effects and they all interact—not very well." But Millie doesn't simply tell us about the drugs' side effects; she embodies these effects for us. Throughout most of the film but especially in this scene where she describes her drug regimen and its side effects, Millie's movements are stiff, and her speech is halting. She does not move through the world with ease, and the film wants us to see that her struggle is with both her illness *and* its treatments. Susan asserts Mildred is a victim of both her illness and an ineffective mental health system. Smiley argues it is impossible to understand her mother's illness outside these structures that at best have failed to help her and at worst have done violence to her.[20]

Selves/Shadows

Susan wants us to see her mother as a victim, and she documents Mildred's long history of being trapped in a fractured public health system. Smiley's focus on these larger structures, the various and sundry drug regimens and institutions her mother has wandered through and lost herself in, helps to keep Susan herself—and her emotions—out of the picture. Tina, however, disrupts Susan's attempt to maintain her clinical gaze, first within the text of the film and then by supplementing Smiley's account with her own in *Saving Millie*. In Smiley's film the present is interrupted by a past to which Susan both does and does not want to return. The trope of the interruption is used in David B.'s narrative, too, but it is his mother in the present who interrupts the narrative of the past David B. is trying to tell when she pleads, "No, David, I don't want you to tell that story," about her mother's alcoholism, which she worries might be perceived by some as a genetic explanation for Jean-Christophe's epilepsy—that is, as her fault. In both texts the interruptions indicate, paradoxically, a haunting family heritage.

If Susan presents the shadow of structural violence that looms over Millie's life, then Tina testifies to another shadow of violence that looms over Millie's daughters. We learn from Tina that Millie was sometimes violent to her daughters when they were growing up. When their father leaves, the two young girls became isolated with their increasingly paranoid mother in their middle-class suburban home as relatives and neighbors refused to see—or allow themselves to register—what was going on. In the film Tina recalls, in tears, it was Susan in particular who was the focus of their mother's violence: "She beat you horribly. That was my first memory of her: being terribly horrid to us." As we hear this and witness Tina's emotion in telling it, we are confronted with the limit of Susan's clinical gaze and with another piece of this story, which is the story Susan doesn't want to tell. In a voice-over she admits, "I did not want Tina to bring this up. That was not part of the movie I wanted to make." In this moment we witness the story as evasion of another story; even Tina, in insisting Millie's violence must be chronicled, uses rather evasive, almost quaint, language to encapsulate that violence.[21]

Susan's desire not to focus on Millie's abuse of her and Tina as children reveals her desire to present not simply the shadow of her mother's illness but also the "sweet soul hidden deep within her," as she says in a voice-over. Indeed, the film ends with Millie proclaiming to Susan what Susan seems to want the film to illustrate: "I'm still your mother." Millie, however, immediately undercuts this assertion, seeming to realize how precarious this subject position is for her, when she adds, hedging, "I'm supposed to be the mother." Unlike Susan, Tina seems to have less interest in witnessing Millie's ability to mother her—in the past, but especially in the present and future. Throughout both film and memoir, she never calls Mildred "mother" or "mom" but always refers to her by her first name. As we learn in the film and memoir, Susan escaped to live at her father and stepmother's house when she was twelve. Why Susan was able to escape while Tina stayed behind is never made entirely clear in either the film or the memoir. Tina seems to accept that because Susan bore the brunt of Mildred's abuse, this arrangement made sense at the time. Susan explains that she thought her leaving would make things easier for Tina and her mother because Tina had a knack for ingratiating herself with their mother. Susan says in a voice-over, "I was sure when I left [Tina would] be all right. I was wrong."

In *Saving Millie*, Tina describes how she and Susan as young children "became inhabitants of [their mother's world]—a terrifying and unpredictable place to live" (9), but she also emphasizes that the two of them had different relationships to this world and to their mother. While Susan was constantly escaping the terror and unpredictability by riding off on her bicycle or spending time at her grandmother's, father's, or friends' houses, Tina "tried to follow her [mother] into that strange world" of psychosis (71). In a statement that reveals the extent to which her own sense of self developed in an intimate relation to her mother's own precarious self, Kotulski states: "I became her shadow, her understudy—not realizing I was emulating a woman who didn't understand her own role. For years, I analyzed Millie" (71). In a desire to protect her mother, she became the shadow of a shadow, and her memoir is an attempt to give a kind of narrative substance to this impossible subject position. Unlike Susan, who tried to keep her distance, both physically and emotionally, and seems to have succeeded, at least to some extent, Tina got as close to her mother as possible, thinking that proximity rather than distance allowed her to better understand, and control, her mother's moods. "Until I was about nine or ten," Kotulski writes, "I actually slept in the same bed with my mother, fearing abandonment; I also believed my constant proximity would ensure that I wouldn't 'miss' anything. Even when I wasn't in the same room with her, I was forever aware of where she was, how she was seated and what mood she was in. The strings that tied us together were strong and many" (72).

Tina admits she also believed her tactics protected her from her mother's unpredictable anger, whereas "Susan did not develop the acute observational skills required to 'handle' Millie when she was at the breaking point. Often, because of her relative innocence, lack of strategy, and visible fear of Millie, Susan became our mother's 'hostile' target" (73). In Kotulski's assessment Susan's desire to keep her distance signified a potential weakness in handling her mother, and this criticism extends to Susan's filmic practice of witnessing, which Tina seems to suggest fails to confront the depths of Mildred's illness because Susan fears looking too closely. Rather than argue that one form of witnessing is better than the other, I juxtapose them as two different ways of seeing and attempting to control mental illness—from up close and at a distance.

When Susan moved out of their mother's terrifying world, Tina's world grew even smaller. Susan's "innocence" and escapes had functioned, if only obliquely, to bring the wider world back into the enclosed, paranoid world in which they lived with Millie. Tina's skills at handling Millie no longer served the purpose of protecting Susan, and she began to feel it would be better for her mother if she (Tina) were dead. In 1979, when she was fourteen years old, Tina attempted suicide by taking an overdose of her mother's Fiorinal pills, which Tina's medical records note, "her mother used for tension headaches" (115). When admitted to Hinsdale Hospital after the suicide attempt, she is described as "in a catatonic, withdrawn state" and unable to "relate to those around her" (115). Later, she was admitted to Old Orchard Hospital for an extended stay, and her speech at the time of her admission is described as "fragmented," contributing to "the social worker's assessment that [she] was suffering from a 'psychotic condition'" (115). While the psychologists and social workers were able to see Tina's illness, Millie's own illness and the effects of that illness on her daughter, remarkably, remained hidden from them. This seeing and not seeing is repeated in Saving Millie, as Tina's experience of mental illness and institutionalization in the late 1970s is presented, whereas Millie's experience, at this same time, can remain only a shadow in the text.

The only way that Tina could witness her mother's illness was to get so close to her that she almost became her by becoming ill. She succeeded in this all too well, diagnosed by psychiatrists and social workers as "psychotic" after her suicide attempt. She continued to "protect" her mother, in this case by helping to keep her mother's illness out of view from the agents of psychiatric power, who, as young Tina recognized, terrified her mother. Yet in the psychiatric hospital, she began to establish some distance between herself and her mother; the physical distance from her mother's world allowed her to begin to see alternative ways of living. Looking back on her time in the hospital, she realizes that she "lacked the words and perspective to describe what it was like living on Vine Street" (120). A major aspect of her treatment included being encouraged by the staff to voice her own needs and "to step out of the shadow [she'd] been hiding in for years" (122). *Saving Millie* is a continuation of that treatment, the finding of words to describe her own experience in the shadow of her mother's paranoid schizophrenia.

Film and memoir reveal that as children the daughters were unwitting witnesses—they were made to witness what they could not fully understand—and part of that witnessing was the recognition that others didn't want to see what was happening to them. Their later attempts to put words and images to what they witnessed as children demonstrates the temporal aspects of witnessing. Through documentary film and memoir, the daughters return to their past, a past they couldn't fully comprehend as they were living it. The tension within and between the texts comes from a double desire: to see their mother's illness and its effects on them and, having seen, to now be able to look away. Through the artifice of their texts, they are able to create the conditions of possibility for a kind of controlled looking.

The ends of both film and memoir reveal this attempt to witness and contain, or put another way, they reveal witnessing as containment. *Out of the Shadow* ends with Mildred upbeat about her future, having lived in the same group home for two years and feeling content with her job as a dishwasher at a sandwich shop. *Saving Millie* updates us on Mildred's situation since the film was finished and reminds us again of the difficulty of treating schizophrenia. Despite or, perhaps, because of the relative stability of this particular period of her life, while on a trip to California to see Susan, who is living in Los Angeles, Millie yet again stops taking her medications. Tina, who is living in Minnesota, is called by the group home after Millie's return to Illinois because she is "threatening to kill herself along with everyone around her" (197). Tina's impression from childhood

that Susan lacks the acute observational skills to handle Millie in such moments is reinforced by this instance of Millie's treatment going awry. Susan
fails to check that Millie has actually swallowed the pills she watched her
take in Los Angeles rather than "cheeking" them, as she is wont to do if
not monitored properly. Neither text makes much of the fact that both
daughters are living far from their mother and seem to have been doing so
for quite some time when this incident occurs. I mention this not to call
into question their commitment to their mother's care but to acknowledge
their ambivalence at having to be responsible for her.

Out of the Shadow witnesses to the many ways that the public health
system has failed to properly treat Mildred Smiley, but it also demonstrates
the possibility of creating a better system. Indeed, as witness to both failure
and possibility, Smiley and her film help produce the conditions of possibility for new treatments for mental illness. In the film the group home
becomes a symbol of a more effective—and humane—form of treatment,
a kind of domesticated clinical milieu. Kotulski's memoir even suggests
that community mental health workers, who had seen parts of Smiley's
documentary before it was completed, might have facilitated Millie's placement in the group home. Saving Millie, as its title suggests, offers a critique
and solution that is less structural and more privatized. By taking Millie
into her own home at the end of her memoir, Kotulski once again seeks
to save Millie by keeping her close. Although she wonders in the film if
she has the "fortitude" to look after Millie, she now believes she is ready,
both because she knows—has always known—how to handle Millie and
also because unlike her mother before her, she now understands her own
role, having successfully raised children of her own. The possibility that
the limits of the role itself might have contributed to Mildred's condition
is never considered. From inadequate state institutions to group homes to
the private home of a daughter with a family of her own, Mildred Smiley's
journey offers a microcosm of the neoliberalization of health care beginning in the prehistory of AIDS and continuing in the present.

Paranoid Schizophrenic/Mildred Smiley

We see through the daughters' practices of witnessing what it means to
grow up in the shadow of schizophrenia in a world where mental illness
itself remains in the shadows cast by the structural violence of a broken
health system and by shame and stigma. What we see less clearly is what it

means to be schizophrenic, to be the shadow, to be Mildred Smiley. There are flashes of insight, or what I want to think about as negative flashes, flashes of darkness rather than flashes of light. In his lectures on psychiatric power, Foucault discusses a "standpoint of truth in our civilization" that challenges a "philosophico-scientific standpoint of truth."[22] For Foucault this "will be the standpoint of a dispersed, discontinuous, interrupted truth which will only speak or appear from time to time, where it wishes to, in certain places."[23] Foucault calls this other, "discontinuous truth the truth-thunderbolt, as opposed to the truth-sky that is universally present behind the clouds."[24] To conclude this chapter, I examine, briefly, three of these negative flashes, these "truth-thunderbolts" that appear against the truth-sky of psychiatric power in *Out of the Shadow* and *Saving Millie*: one is an image of Mildred Smiley; the second is a statement from Mildred about psychiatry; and the third concerns Mildred's performance in front of the video camera.

The first image is used in both film and memoir, though neither text comments on it explicitly. It is a family snapshot of Millie in the backyard of what Tina calls "the house on Vine Street" (141). This is the house that Alan and Mildred Smiley bought when they were first married, where the Smiley family lived together as an apparently average, middle-class American family in the early 1960s: a father, a mother, and two children. This is also the house that provides the backdrop for the home movies incorporated into *Out of the Shadow*. By the time this photograph was taken in 1980, according to its caption in *Saving Millie*, Millie was the only one who remained in the house on Vine Street. All of its other residents had left, one by one: first father, then older daughter, and, still later, younger daughter. They had all left to save themselves. The photo is reprinted in *Saving Millie* in black and white, but we can tell the day is bright: the trees on the right side of the photograph and Millie at the center cast shadows. Millie is a pale, spectral figure. She is not smiling; her eyes are dark shadows, and her mouth seems to grimace. Her posture is awkward; she cowers slightly, almost as though she has been cornered, and her right arm is behind her back, as if she is keeping something from view (Figure 20). Although she appears to be pictured in the same backyard, she is no longer the robust young woman pulled toward camera and viewer in the sequence at the beginning of the film.

In *Saving Millie* this picture faces the opening of a chapter entitled "Last Days on Vine Street," which begins with these words:

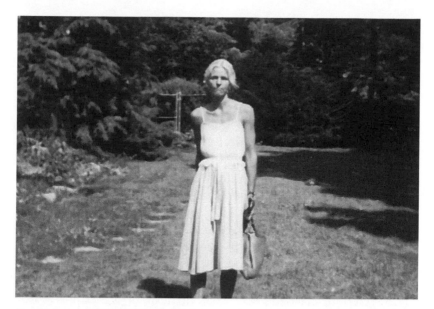

Figure 20. Image as truth-thunderbolt. Although she appears to be pictured in the same backyard, she is no longer the robust young woman pulled toward camera and viewer in the sequence at the beginning of the film. Screen capture from Out of the Shadow *(Susan Smiley, 2004).*

In the summer of 1983, Millie made a serious attempt to kill herself. At home by herself one night, she slashed her throat and wrists and ingested large amounts of Librium, diuretics, and rubbing alcohol. At some point, she called the police, and they brought her to Hinsdale Hospital, where I'd been taken after my suicide attempt. A few days later, Kathryn [Millie's mother] went back to the house and dutifully cleaned the blood off the walls and floors. She would never be able to rid her mind of the gruesome scene she found there. (141)[25]

There are three years between the photograph and the suicide attempt, three years of which we have no record, though looking back at the photo from 1980 surely we see—and feel—the darkness of this time in Millie's life. In the film Smiley also shows us this snapshot: she cuts to it from a home movie image of a teenage Susan on a merry-go-round. Smiley's direct address creates continuity between the moving merry-go-round image of the daughter and the still photo of the mother in the backyard of the house on Vine Street: "By my mid-twenties," Smiley explains, "I knew I had escaped Mom's fate. And, frankly, I wanted to escape her." Visually redoubling the voice-over narrative of her own escape and her mother's inability to escape, the shot slowly zooms in to give us a closer look at her mother's face (Figure 21) as Susan's voice-over continues: "For many years I did. It was hard knowing Mom was becoming more and more disabled. She became increasingly withdrawn and despondent. She sold her house and lost all her money. She attempted suicide and was then sucked into the public health system." Getting a closer look at Millie's shadowed eyes in the photograph doesn't help us to see them or her more clearly, but drawing nearer to, though never arriving at, those shadowed eyes does give us a feeling of the darkness of which they are a sign. The truth-thunderbolt is that feeling of darkness, which exceeds not only the comforting resolutions of the group home in *Out of the Shadow* and Tina Kotulski's home in *Saving Millie* but also, more generally, the consolation of the daughters' filmic and narrative treatments.

The second truth-thunderbolt takes the form of Millie's own words, which offer a counternarrative to psychiatric power but also, perhaps, a counternarrative to the counternarrative that her daughters' texts present. Millie speaks these words, in slightly different form, in both *Out of the Shadow* and *Saving Millie*. In the film she articulates them after her psychiatric interviews to determine whether she can handle the environment of the group home. Worried about the impression she has made, she tells Susan: "They don't treat any other mentally ill people successfully. They just get worse all the time. They don't know what they're doing with the drugs or anything. They don't know if it's chemical. There's no way of testing someone's brain. They don't even know what they're doing." A version of this same account is repeated in *Saving Millie* at the end of the book, after Millie has almost died from the toxic interaction of the many drugs she has been prescribed, which is the incident that finally leads to Tina's decision to take Millie into her own home.[26] Millie's statement, with its repetition of the two words "they don't," is a sign of both her paranoia and her refusal of the reality imposed on her by psychiatric power. Under the diagnostic terms already established in both texts, Mildred's statement is a sign of her illness, her lack of insight, which both daughters confess is one of the great difficulties of dealing with their mother, but it is also a sign of what her illness has allowed her to see quite clearly: the failure of psychiatric power to know and treat mental illness. The truth-sky is that as

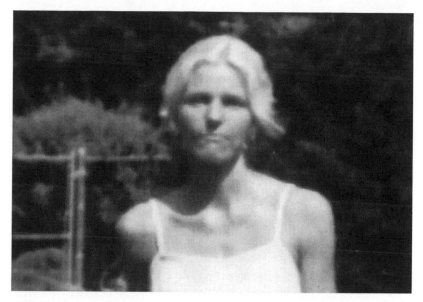

Figure 21. Getting a closer look at Millie's shadowed eyes in the photograph doesn't help us to see them or her more clearly, but drawing nearer to, though never arriving at, those shadowed eyes does give us a feeling of the darkness of which they are a sign. Screen capture from Out of the Shadow *(Susan Smiley, 2004).*

a paranoid schizophrenic she has no insight into her illness, which makes her adherence to proper treatments unlikely, while the truth-thunderbolt that she also articulates is that her doctors have no insight either, calling into question the rationality of their treatments.

The final truth-thunderbolt relates to Mildred Smiley's relationship to the camera. We learn from both daughters' texts that one sign of Mildred's paranoia over the years has been her belief that she is surrounded by tiny cameras, watching her every move. It is somewhat surprising then to see her take such apparent pleasure in the camera that films her for Smiley's documentary. The first time in the film she comes into the camera's field of vision is when she is discharged from Elgin Mental Health Center, a place, Susan's voice-over explains, "my mother hates; it makes her feel like she's in jail, and she can't figure out what she did to get here." Yet as Mildred hugs Susan, she looks over her shoulder at the camera, aware of its presence, watching it watch her with what looks like a slight smile of anticipation. Although Susan never asks Mildred about being filmed and we never get a sense of a negotiation between the two about what can and cannot be filmed,[27] we do on several occasions see Mildred show an awareness of the camera and how it functions; once, for example, she asks if the sound is on, and when Susan says it isn't working well, Mildred asks, "So, my lips are just moving?" We also get a sense from their conversations of Millie's acute interest in film and film stars. Mildred's quirky sense of humor comes out in some of these discussions: she's disappointed when she learns Richard Chamberlain is gay and unimpressed by whatever it is that Al Pacino has done to his mouth. Although Kotulski criticizes her sister in *Saving Millie* for sometimes appearing to be more concerned with filming Millie's suffering than with alleviating it, there is no sign, in the film at least, that Mildred is ever troubled by the presence of the camera.[28] Indeed, quite the opposite. Whereas for Vladimir in *Titicut Follies* being filmed is an opportunity for him to make a case for his freedom, for Mildred Smiley in *Out of the Shadow* film is a medium through which she can imagine another world for herself. She relates her own situation of frequent confinement to the horrific story the film *Midnight Express* tells of an American in a Turkish prison for a drug violation. Like the protagonist at the end of that film, Millie dreams of jumping in the air, clicking her heels, saying, "I'm free," and becoming free. Perhaps, she believes starring in her own film is a route to this mode of becoming free. And perhaps, the camera becomes witness to her performance of becoming free.

ACT UP's "Drugs into Bodies," the Near Present

Indirection as method means there can be no dramatic flourishes at the end or tidy resolutions and statements of certainty in conclusion. In keeping with *Indirect Action*'s open and indirect trajectories—into remembered, unremembered, and disremembered pasts and toward uncertain futures—as well as my emphasis throughout on multiple and divergent ways of seeing and doing illness, thought, and politics, I will not so much offer a conclusion as leave readers with an afterimage of health activism that I take to be operating in the present moment. After tracing back from the emergence of AIDS and AIDS activism to earlier experiences and events of illness and politics before AIDS, I want to return explicitly to the history of AIDS and AIDS activism and to the memories and forgettings constitutive of the conjunction illness-thought-activism in the present moment.

I deploy the concept of the afterimage as yet another method-image to help explore how illness-thought-activism operates in the present. An afterimage is, according to the *OED*, "a visual sensation which remains after the stimulus that gave rise to it ceases," and it is used to suggest literal or, perhaps we should say, physiological images that remain in the field of vision, as well as figurative or mental images that recur or linger. Despite the emphasis on the visual in the phrase itself, afterimages "may also be experienced in the case of smells, tastes, tones, and impressions of contact."[1] For me the concept of the afterimage suggests how our experiences of events in the past continue into the present and the future—literally and figuratively, materially and immaterially, physiologically and psychologically. Such a method-image is useful for considering the multiple and complex effects of particular practices of health activism as impressions of contact across scales, linking individual bodies and biologies with larger medico-political structures, as well as impressions of contact across time, linking the prehistory of AIDS with the present.[2] What I hope readers will take from this book is not only the specific experiences and events of illness-thought-activism documented here but also the importance of a multifocal and multiscalar approach for exploring the conjunction illness-thought-activism in history.

The afterimage I consider here is ACT UP's phrase and campaign "Drugs into Bodies," a slogan and cause that transformed the experience and event of AIDS in very concrete, material ways and is usually taken as an image of political success. I explore the phrase as a clinical and political performative in order to open up questions for the future that relate back to other possibilities that might yet emerge out of health activism. My analysis of "Drugs into Bodies" as clinical and political performative seeks to undermine the seduction of scientific, political, and conceptual reductionism by exploring the ongoing repercussions not only of treatment failures but also of so-called treatment successes. I take this phrase to express an ontology of the late-capitalist present, a condensation of the complexities of the interaction of medicine, politics, and the multiple and conflicting demands of different temporalities: the emergency time of immediate action and the tentative time of reaching for new forms and phrases to articulate what is and is not yet coming into being, directly and indirectly. Suggesting, among other things, the overreliance on pharmaceuticals in contemporary, especially U.S., medicine, the enduring hope for surefire cures and quick fixes, and the pleasures and dangers of recreational drug use as a form of self-care for various biosocial groupings, "Drugs into Bodies" is an almost magical phrase that encapsulates the messy experiences and events of illness into the always already present tense of late capitalism.[3]

I discuss this magical phrase and its clinical and political performative effects in relation to two recent films: David France's documentary *How to Survive a Plague* (2012) and Jean-Marc Vallée's feature film *Dallas Buyers Club* (2013), which taken together would seem to signal a desire in the present moment to return to the early days of AIDS and AIDS activism in U.S. popular culture. Yet despite historical work like Jennifer Brier's *Infectious Ideas* and Deborah Gould's *Moving Politics* and cultural memory work like Martin Duberman's *Hold Tight Gently* and Sarah Schulman's *Gentrification of the Mind* produced around the same time as the films, in these popular accounts we nonetheless see the continuing dominance of one particular story of AIDS and AIDS activism, as I discussed in the introduction and chapter 1. That hegemonic story suggests that once there were drugs to put into bodies we had won the battle against AIDS. In this concluding afterimage, then, I take up again the question of how we do politics, thought, and illness as well as how that doing of politics, thought, and illness is remembered in the near present as demonstrated in these films about treatment activism. In both *How to Survive a Plague* and *Dallas Buyers Club,* time is short, and direct action is presented as a necessary strategy to stem the tide of deaths, both the many, as depicted in the running body count in *How to Survive a Plague,* and the singular, as captured in the "inspired by true events" story of the two main characters—one straight, one transgender, one "real," one "imagined"—of *Dallas Buyers Club.*

I am far from the first to use the phrase "Drugs into Bodies" as part or all of a chapter title in a book about health activism, and the phrase's ubiquity in analyses of health activism post-AIDS and the performative effects of its repetition and circulation in different disciplinary contexts also interest me.[4] In her important political history of AIDS and AIDS activism, Brier's final chapter, "Drugs into Bodies, Bodies into Health Care: The AIDS Coalition to Unleash Power and the Struggle over How Best to Fight AIDS," invokes this magical phrase but also places it in relation to larger questions about access to health care and best practices of health activism, a differend I highlight here.[5] The brief pause grammatically signaled by the comma between "Drugs into Bodies" and "Bodies into Health Care" marks a scaling up but also belies the intensity of the rift she describes between activists concerned with the availability of treatments, narrowly understood as pharmaceutical treatments, and activists concerned more broadly with structural questions, including how race, class, gender, and sexuality intersect with illness and disability, or with, following Guattari, ways of creating a "therapeutic social life."[6]

As Brier notes, some activists expanded the concept and practices of "treatment" in order to make the argument that "the only way to get drugs into bodies was to deal with structural inequalities that made it difficult for certain people to access health care more generally."[7] Yet this structural—or ecological and indirect—approach contrasted sharply with a targeted approach that focused single-mindedly on making new drugs available to treat AIDS. This relates to Lewis Thomas's concern, discussed in chapter 4, about the increased emphasis on "direct, frontal approach[es]" to scientific research at the expense of less direct, more open-ended blue-sky approaches, a shift Thomas locates in what we now diagnose as the neoliberalizing 1970s. In this later moment, Brier mentions, for example, Mark Harrington's system of drug buddies, whereby members of ACT UP's Treatment and Data Committee would closely monitor the progress of a particular drug through direct contact with the scientists researching the drug. Although Brier doesn't note the contrast herself, "drug buddies" encapsulates a relationship quite different from the relationship evoked by another buddy figure of AIDS activism: the buddy for persons with AIDS (PWAs). In the first figure, the relationship is to a scientist searching for a drug cure for AIDS or, even more intriguingly, to the drug itself as object of special and personal concern, and in the second the relationship is to a person with AIDS in need of care and assistance. Drug buddies become invested in the production of new drugs they can consume in order to survive, whereas PWA buddies help PWAs maintain their normal lives in their own homes for as long as possible. Thus, the first figure instantiates a capitalist logic of choice (more drugs to choose from = better health care),[8] whereas the second instantiates a different logic, of care, which gets co-opted by capitalism in the form of surplus value but nonetheless remains a decidedly queer logic in the emergency time of neoliberalism. In thinking about what these different figures of treatment activism do, I use "encapsulate" to suggest something about the capacity of drugs to enact a rather paradoxical idea of desire (for cure, for health) as both containment and escape.[9]

Echoing but also personalizing Brier's historical discussion, Duberman's memoir about writer/activists Michael Callen and Essex Hemphill and their involvement in early AIDS activism also includes a chapter entitled "Drugs into Bodies." In his double memoir—or we might even call it his memoir of a generation, since he refers to many other, mostly unsung activists as well as his own involvement in the early "battlefield of AIDS"—Duberman is interested, like me, in correcting the origin story that says AIDS activism began with ACT UP. Neither Callen nor Hemphill were members of ACT UP, and Callen in particular challenged the "Drugs into Bodies" mantra that drove a rush to approve experimental drugs and encouraged people with AIDS to start taking approved drugs like AZT early, even prophylactically.[10]

Following the advice of his doctor, Joseph Sonnabend, Callen did not take AZT or other experimental conventional and alternative therapies that were tried and almost universally failed during the late 1980s and early 1990s. Duberman writes of Sonnabend and Callen's skepticism about, for example, Martin Delaney's Project Inform, which encouraged "early intervention" with substances that had not been shown to be helpful or even safe: "The result was that some PWAs, given the lack of alternatives, were still 'injecting, ingesting and imbibing' any new substance that came down the pike."[11] Callen was impressed by Sonnabend's idiosyncratic and ecological—or multifactorial—theory of AIDS causation, and he agreed with him that one must not lose sight of the fact that the effect of drugs on bodies is complex, a point demonstrated in my discussions of the often negative effects of drug treatments for complex diseases like epilepsy and schizophrenia. Mildred Smiley and Jean-Christophe Beauchard suffer not simply from their illnesses but also from their ever-changing drug treatments and overtreatments. Recall Smiley's observation about the drugs she takes: "They all have side effects and they all interact—not very well."

In Duberman's discussion of Callen's oppositional stance to the biologic of early drug intervention, he notes that Callen

attributed his survival to having followed Sonnabend's advice *not* to experiment with whatever drug was currently being touted. In this regard, Mike rejected the widespread assumption that a drug either worked or it didn't work. He insisted on a third alternative: taking a given drug could actually *harm* you, could hasten your death. Mike believed that he and other long-term survivors had rightly taken "a wait-and-see attitude about experimental drugs."[12]

Sonnabend did not deny the relationship between HIV and AIDS, but he also did not think "HIV causes AIDS" adequately captured the complexity of causation and treatment of illness in general and AIDS in particular, even in the emergency time of the 1980s and early 1990s.[13] I read Duberman's return to the ecological alternative that Callen and Sonnabend offered in the early days of AIDS as reminding us of the importance of thinking about things together and more slowly, even, or especially, in a time of crisis. In this concluding afterimage, then, I want to supplement the imperative "Drugs into Bodies" by posing the questions: What do drugs in bodies do over time and in relation? What are the biological, social, and political side effects of drugs into bodies? What are the pleasures and dangers (and pleasure in danger) of drugs into bodies?

Screening Treatment Activism 1: *How to Survive a Plague*

In order to consider "Drugs into Bodies" as both imperative and question, I turn now to two recent examples of what I am calling "screening treatment activism" in order to suggest both the ways treatment activism is depicted on screen as well as what these representations screen from our view. The documentary *How to Survive a Plague* begins not at the "official" beginning of AIDS in the United States, around 1981, but, as the opening subtitle indicates, in "Year 6"—that is, 1987, the year ACT UP was formed. The opening titles also tell us that the events we are witnessing are happening in Greenwich Village, identified as the "Epicenter of AIDS." Already, then, in this opening scene the event of AIDS has been compressed for us, temporally and spatially. Rather than seeking to understand how AIDS and the response to AIDS emerged historically, the film begins by sedimenting the origin story of AIDS activism I have been working to counteract in both the content and the form of this book. Recall the powerful method-image that Wojnarowicz gives us in his work of "history . . . reached through the compression of time," discussed in snapshot 2.[14] In contrast to the expansive historicizing effects created in Wojnarowicz's art, writing, and activism, I argue that history in *How to Survive a Plague* works, paradoxically, to dehistoricize AIDS activism.

In the film's foreshortened historical narrative, then, health activism happened between 1987 and 1995, beginning with the founding of ACT UP and ending with the discovery of the protease inhibitors. The first six years of the epidemic are apparently not worth recounting, and by this omission we are led to believe there was no response to AIDS until year six, reiterating the passivity-to-activism narrative arc I describe as characterizing discussions of AIDS since its emergence. Through a series of subtle inclusions and exclusions, the film builds a fascinating picture of this response-beginning-in-year-six. The first person to speak in the film is a woman activist; she is one of two facilitators at an ACT UP meeting. She is not identified, the first of many unidentified women activists who make appearances in the film. We are introduced by a caption to the next activist to speak, David Barr, who will become one of several mostly white gay male "stars" of the film. This pattern of identifying some participants and not others at ACT UP events is repeated throughout the film, with the effect of authorizing some speakers and their statements and deauthorizing others.[15] As a result viewers know who Larry Kramer is when he screams, "Plague!! We are in the middle of a fucking plague, and you behave like this! ACT UP is taken over by a lunatic fringe?" but the lunatic fringe he rails against remains safely on the margins of the history presented in *How to Survive a Plague,* unnamed and thus unremembered, becoming some of the many who won't survive this *Plague.*

Publicity for the film notes it presents the "story of two coalitions—ACT UP and the Treatment Action Group (TAG)—whose activism and innovation turned AIDS from a death sentence to a manageable condition,"[16] and while the film certainly shows tensions between these groups, by failing to articulate clearly both the links and the rifts—the "dis/continuities"[17]— between them, this statement manages to forget the intersections and shared histories of the two groups. While the film makes good use of archival video footage shot by members of ACT UP's video collectives and media activists, it is less adept at reflecting on the contested politics of representation at work in AIDS activism in particular and all activism in general. By presenting the activist video footage as a document of what really happened beginning in 1987, the film is not very interested in taking experience itself (of AIDS and AIDS activism) as a category of analysis. What we get, then, is an attempt by the filmmakers to make visible a history hidden from view rather than, or as well as, a meditation on the evidence of experience itself.[18] The film effectively makes us feel as if a forgotten history is being recovered and that this in itself is a good thing. What it does less well is problematize the sprawl and mess of historical events and nonevents and of historical events becoming nonevents. As in my snapshot linking Samuel Delany's memory of his experience attending Allan Kaprow's happening with Joan Scott's historicizing of the evidence of "experience" in her reading of Delany's memoir in the late 1980s, I have been attempting to articulate throughout *Indirect Action* a method of documenting illness and politics that does not take representations of the experience of either illness or politics as always already self evident but rather seeks to show how illness events—diagnoses, treatments, health activisms—constitute new subjects, objects, forms of expression, and worlds.

In an early sequence, the film cuts from footage of then-mayor Ed Koch describing ACT UP's tactics as "fascist" to the film's first image of activism—a not-very-fascist-looking group of protesters singing and dancing—to shots of the Twin Towers and city hall to a crowd shot that includes Keith Haring to a meeting of what appears to be the same support group described in Bordowitz's "Boat Trip," discussed in my first snapshot. Peter Staley, identified in the archival footage as a bond trader, is the first person to be interviewed in the near present, and he will be the film's main protagonist. When we first meet him, he discusses looking around in desperation for treatments in the early days of the epidemic, explaining the brutal reality of a personal moment of crisis in which "everything [he] read said [he] had about two years to live." Staley's personal experience of illness leads directly to his politicization; he understands his survival may depend on his ability, personally, to politicize illness. As I've shown throughout, such an understanding and analysis of health and illness as political was not new in 1987, but the urgency of an emerging epidemic created both a crisis and an opportunity for the politicization of the experience of illness, which I have argued would then become *the* image of doing health activism, covering over a much longer and more diffuse history of illness and/ as thought and politics.

Moving from archival footage to interviews with survivors in the present, the film somewhat didactically presents its viewers with strategies for survival. The lessons the film teaches might be boiled down to three main ones: (1) work to become scientists, (2) work to speed up the drug approval process, and (3) work with the drug companies to make more drugs. One hero of the film then is Iris Long, a chemist who though "not gay" agreed to teach members of the Treatment and Data (T&D) Committee the science they needed to know about AIDS and its treatments. After we hear about Long's importance, several members of the T&D Committee are introduced, including Jim Eigo, who tells us he sought out Long after she spoke at a meeting about the science of AIDS; Garance Franke-Ruta, who describes the T&D Committee as a "science club"; and other key T&D members Spencer Cox and Mark Harrington.

The film then cuts from this discussion of activists becoming scientists to an ACT UP meeting where an unnamed activist speaks about a PWA who is being evicted from his home. From this scene the film cuts to footage of ACT UP member Bob Rafsky and his family. Rafsky features prominently in the film as a key figure in ACT UP who is not a member of the T&D Committee. His story and approach is meant to offer a contrast to Staley's; these individual stories come to stand in for the stories of the two coalitions that the film's promotional material describes as important to the film's narrative structure. The film portrays Rafsky as an immensely appealing and effective activist, as well as a loving husband and father, who came out at forty: "It's bad to come out in an epidemic," he tells us. Yet I contend Rafsky's is a minority voice in the film, outnumbered as he is by the T&D (later, TAG) boys. He is also the one key protagonist who will die and be eulogized in the film. Tacitly, then, the stories of those fighting for something other than drugs into bodies are associated with failure and death.

When illness appears in the film, it is usually presented as separate—

temporally and spatially—from the politics that is the film's focus (Figure 22). Images of people in hospitals sick with AIDS, sometimes on their own, sometimes being cared for, usually by loved ones not professional health practitioners, are used to link and separate scenes of politics in action. Accompanied by music on the film's soundtrack, these scenes are elegiac set pieces of illness and care not so much in action but rather as inaction. Bodies at rest—ill and dying—are contrasted with bodies in protest: the suffering of the sick structurally interrupts the scenes of activism. One obvious lesson in the differend between these cuts is that the film cannot present the voices and lives of most of the people who have died of AIDS; it cannot speak for the dead, despite the fact that as the closed captioning in Figure 22 shows, Jim Eigo's voice speaks over an image of an unknown person with AIDS, presumably now dead. Thus, a subtler lesson is also at work in the film's temporal and spatial structures, and that other lesson seems to be that those who survived survived for a reason. The clearest explanation the film gives is that a single-minded focus on drugs—both personally and politically—is the right (read: rational) approach to surviving a plague. Why spend time on housing issues for PWAs or, more generally, creating alternative spaces for a therapeutic social life when one could be working on getting drugs into bodies as quickly as possible? By the end of the film, we see the positive effects of this specific "drugs into bodies" work in the simple fact of the survival of several of the key activists that the film tracks from 1987 to the present.

In footage from an episode of the CNN program *Crossfire* entitled "Against All Odds," Peter Staley sits between commentators on the right and the left, with whom he discusses speeding up the drug approval process. Dressed in a *Silence = Death* T-shirt, Staley's youthful boy-next-door looks, calm demeanor, and obvious intelligence make him an effective and compelling spokesperson for people with AIDS desperately seeking drug treatments. Staley tells his fellow panelists—regulars Tom Braden and Pat Buchanan—that the current approval process often takes seven to ten years, and he adds, "I don't have that long. AZT is the only drug approved. I can't take it. It's far too toxic." Braden, articulating the left position, offers rather tepid sympathy to Staley personally but worries it might be dangerous to rush the approval process. Buchanan, commenting from the right, clearly disapproves of Staley's homosexuality but tells him, "You'll be surprised to know that I agree with you. You should be allowed to take these drugs, even if they haven't been approved."

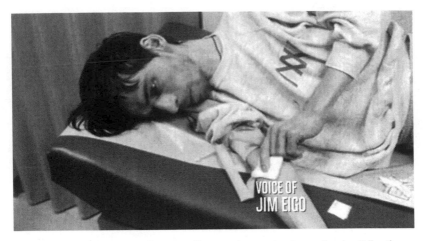

Figure 22. When illness appears in the film, it is usually presented as separate—temporally and spatially—from the politics that is the film's focus. Screen capture from How to Survive a Plague *(David France, 2012).*

The dichotomous left/right conception of politics presented here, between those who favor government regulation of new drugs and those who don't, is instructive in considering the long-term effects of policies that came into being as a result of the AIDS crisis and AIDS activism. Buchanan's sense that because of their different sexual orientations, he and Staley would normally be opposed to each other politically oversimplifies the complex network of interests at work in the fight against AIDS, as well as the strange alliances that emerge from illness. Buchanan's comments also fail to account for the multiple temporalities of illness and politics, or what I have been calling the temporopolitics of illness. What happens when the emergency time of the late 1980s for people with AIDS becomes the chronic time of the late 1990s? How were, and are, both temporalities operating at once? Attending to continuities and discontinuities between acute and chronic conditions is important not only in relation to experiences and events of illness but also in relation to experiences and events of thought and politics. As the many cases in this book show, both acute and chronic temporopolitics of illness are at work in particular historical moments. We are never operating in one temporality at once— illness, politics, and thought all teach us this.

Cut between the footage of the *Crossfire* episode and footage of AIDS activists heckling Dr. Ellen Cooper, an FDA regulator, about the foot-dragging of the FDA to approve a drug for cytomegalovirus (CMV), an opportunistic infection that often causes blindness in PWAs, we see an image of a person giving himself the drug ganciclovir (DHBG) through a drip in his chest to treat CMV (Figure 23). Like the portraits of the sick and dying cut between scenes of public protest, this short vignette of self-treatment is intimate to the point of being claustrophobic. The viewer is made to feel like a voyeur as she watches at very close proximity the bare-chested man insert the drip into a line right above his left nipple. The lighting of the shot creates a feeling that something illicit and, perhaps even, erotic is happening in a seedy place, and the impression is that we are witnessing something we shouldn't. The man's gloved hands holding the needle give off an eerie yellow glow, appearing detached from his body and otherworldly. The shot draws on a visual rhetoric often deployed in depictions of people shooting up in public bathrooms, and although I don't think the filmmakers intended this link, in this scene of therapy a visual association is created between the pleasures of drug taking for recreational use and the taking of experimental drugs for treatment. That is, an image of experimenting with drugs for personal enhancement or transformation is itself transformed through the scientization and privatization of experimental drug practices.

This short scene of what we might call self-medication as privatized treatment activism is followed by shots of public treatment activism and an interview with Mark Harrington, one of the leaders of T&D and TAG, who describes the FDA as "like the Wizard of Oz" and expresses amazement at how activists managed to write a treatment agenda, on the bus back from the ACT UP protest at the FDA, that would then influence the practice of clinical trials and the process of drug approval in the United States. We then see footage from the 1989 International AIDS Conference in Montreal, which is notable in the history of international AIDS conferences as "when the activists took over." Staley is prominent in these scenes, too. He is the activist who addresses the conference delegates, and as with his appearance on *Crossfire*, he hits the right note of defiance and inclusivity, showing a savvy know-how of both political and clinical best practices.

Yet the film shows the activists didn't so much take over in Montreal as become part of the AIDS science and research communities—that is, become ingested into a larger pharmaceuticalizing agenda. The film shows this both by discussing the importance of the T&D Committee's National AIDS Treatment Research Agenda and by interviewing a pair of research

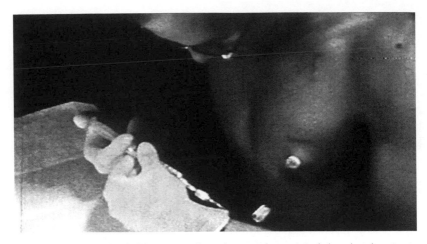

Figure 23. The viewer is made to feel like a voyeur as she watches at very close proximity the bare-chested man insert the drip into a line right above his left nipple. Screen capture from How to Survive a Plague *(David France, 2012).*

scientists who worked for Merck at the time. These men describe how they came to discover the function of protease in HIV, and the film seems to want to suggest a direct link between the inclusion of activists in the research process and the later development by drug companies of the protease inhibitors, which turned AIDS from a death sentence into a manageable chronic condition. By pointing this out, I am less interested in questioning the important influence of activists on the research process, which is clearly a significant result of AIDS activism, than in noting the film's overall trajectory toward getting activists on the inside, as signaled in the film by the appearance of Merck scientists speaking in the present as on the same side as the treatment activists or even as treatment activists themselves. While the film does highlight some of the tensions between those in ACT UP who saw success as a seat at the tables of power and those who worried, as Ann Northrop notes in an interview in the film, "that we were getting too close to people in power," the film's rhetorical arc and its own forms of inclusion and exclusion suggest that getting in (getting drugs into bodies, activists into research, and bodies into drug trials) = how to survive a plague.

This is most clearly articulated in a scene toward the end that opens with David Barr in the near present saying that 1993 to 1995 were the worst years, before stating with a look of disbelief, "And then we got lucky." The camera shows current headshots of the "we" who got lucky, a group of seven white male activists still alive at the time of the making of the film: Barr, Harrington, Derek Link, Gregg Gonsalves, Cox, Bordowitz, and Staley.[19] In case we don't recognize a particular activist twenty years on, each is named again. These, then, are the men who survived a plague. What is powerful about this scene is that these seven men have rather divergent views on what it means to have survived. In keeping with the single-minded and heroic image of him the film presents, Staley marvels, "It wasn't until we started putting the drugs into our bodies that we realized what we'd done. Viral load disappears within months. The dying was stopping." This comment is followed by images of empty hospital beds, as if to say the AIDS crisis was under control immediately upon discovery of the protease cocktail treatment. In this moment in the film's narrative, the ill and dying magically disappear from view. And while Bordowitz and Barr admit to the many difficulties that survival brings, especially after experiencing the deaths of so many comrades and loved ones and feeling sure one would soon die too, Kramer gets the last word in *How to Survive a Plague*: "Every single drug that is out there is because of ACT UP. Proudest achievement that gay people have given the world." It isn't clear from Kramer's statement whether the proudest achievement that gay people have given the world is the activist group ACT UP and its response to AIDS or drugs. And finally, it isn't clear what to make of the gnomic statement, "The number of companies making effective protease inhibitors is 7," appended at the end of the film, presumably to bring us up to date on the positive effects of treatment activism. With this statement the filmmakers seem to suggest the importance of drugs over politics or, even more insidiously, that the desirable outcome of politics is more companies making more drugs.

Screening Treatment Activism 2: *Dallas Buyers Club*

A year after the release of *How to Survive a Plague*, another film about treatment activism was released in North America—the feature film *Dallas Buyers Club*. Directed by Jean-Marc Vallée and starring Matthew McConaughey, *Dallas Buyers Club* tells the story of Ron Woodroof, a straight rodeo cowboy[20] who is diagnosed with AIDS in 1985 and given just thirty days to live, long odds he will beat for seven years. By telling a story of treatment activism that takes place before the events chronicled in *How to Survive a Plague*, *Dallas Buyers Club* reminds us that there was AIDS activism before

ACT UP emerged in 1987 and also that AIDS and AIDS activism were happening not only in the gay meccas of New York City and San Francisco but all across the United States, including places like Dallas. Yet the picture we get from *Dallas Buyers Club* of the early days of AIDS and AIDS activism in the United States is a curious one, and reading the film with and against *How to Survive a Plague* helps us to think about how AIDS activism is being remembered now. Who are the figures at the center of these recent stories of AIDS activism? How is health activism portrayed, and what are its goals? How are links made to other forms of activism, or not?

Unlike the collectivist, two-coalitions ideology and structure of *How to Survive a Plague, Dallas Buyers Club,* in keeping with mainstream Hollywood cinema, gives an impression of treatment activism as a kind of rugged individualism. Ron Woodroof must take the law into his own hands—rodeo cowboy must become outlaw, or in the sequence of identity terms used to describe Woodroof's personal transformation in the film's trailer, he must become Cowboy, Gambler, Hellraiser, Hustler, Savior—in order to have a chance at surviving the desperate circumstances he finds himself in. As in many classic cowboy films, Ron pairs up with a sidekick who somehow manages to see the decency hidden behind Ron's cold exterior, allowing the film's spectators to see that underlying decency, too. In *Dallas Buyers Club*'s blending of film genres, then, the Lone Ranger meets the Odd Couple as Ron Woodroof teams up with Rayon,[21] the loquacious, campy transwoman with a heart of gold who like Ron is HIV+. The buyers club the two create attempts to circumvent federal laws regulating the importation of drugs from overseas and the sale of drugs not yet approved by the FDA. In *Dallas Buyers Club,* the treatment activist is a savvy entrepreneur who goes on buying trips abroad and sets up a pop-up shop, or pop-up club, for drugs that have shown some potential in treating AIDS on the black market and outside the United States. By focusing on the phenomenon of buyers clubs and, in particular, on the Dallas Buyers Club, the film commodifies AIDS activism by reifying a particular picture of activism for our consumption in the late-capitalist present. By noting this, I am not arguing we should dismiss *Dallas Buyers Club* because it gives a false picture of AIDS activism, but rather, I am asking us to consider how it functions to both contain and expand our understandings of how we do illness and politics. I argue that the film creates its own buyers club, facilitating the distribution of a capsule history of AIDS activism with many side effects.

In a brief exchange between Ron Woodroof and Dr. Eve Saks, treatment activism is presented as a late-capitalist form of self-help. Dr. Saks, usually identified as simply Eve in the film script, is a young doctor who is shown to genuinely care for her patients and to be concerned about the lack of treatments she has to offer them. In scenes with other doctors, she is the only woman and significantly younger than her colleagues, which is perhaps the film's small gesture to the feminist challenge to the age-old hierarchies of organized medicine, a challenge that was prominent in the years immediately before AIDS arrived, as I have shown. Promotional materials on the film's official website describe Eve as the "heart at the center of the film." She and Rayon are old friends, which accounts for the close relationship between this straight woman doctor and her transgender patient with AIDS. In one particularly intimate scene between the two, Rayon pulls Eve close, linking her fingers behind Eve's neck, and looks deeply into her eyes, the way a lover might. Perhaps not surprisingly, considering the somewhat cloying sentimentality of their relationship, Eve and Rayon are not based on any one person in the "real" Ron Woodroof's life (even their names hammer this point home—Eve as natural and Rayon as artificial woman). Rather, they are composite characters invented for dramatic purposes who seem to have been sent from an idealized present to the past to heroicize and humanize—to make us feel good in the present about who we (read: the general public) were in this past. More than any other character, the film wants and needs us to identify with Eve, since her good doctoring will continue after both Rayon and Ron have died, perhaps even into the present moment in which we watch the film. She is the tolerant and empathic doctor celebrated here as a historical side effect of AIDS.

In a scene where Eve confronts Ron about the treatments he is providing for her patients—including, in Ron's down-home medicalese, "Vitamins, Peptide T, DDC. Anything but that poison you're hawkin'"—Eve responds in a manner not unlike the medical establishment's response to women's health activists in the early 1970s, with a professional concern about the problem of someone offering medical treatments without a license as well as a personal concern about giving false hopes, responses discussed in my earlier chapter on health feminism's practices of self-help and the medical establishment's reaction to and appropriation of these practices. In order to protect himself from the accusation of treating without a license, Ron says the patients are "treating themselves"; self-help here is a tried-and-true way around the system, although none of this longer history of self-help is shown or even alluded to in the film. Moreover, the collective endeavor of most self-help projects is elided in the film. Ron teams up with Rayon mainly to give him access to gay buyers, and Rayon uses this fact to negotiate a better cut of the profits.

The collaborative ethic of the network of buyers clubs, most of which emerged out of gay communities in cities across the United States, is also not accounted for in the film. The official website for the film includes the section "AIDS Activism in the Time of Dallas Buyers Club," which, it explains, serves to provide "additional context . . . to give a larger sense of the fight."[22] We might call this Web material a gay and collective supplement to the film's straight male cowboy individualism. Interestingly, this section reveals that the Dallas Buyers Club was one of the few buyers clubs that was not explicitly nonprofit but had "money-making in mind" and that it never subscribed to the Ft. Lauderdale Principles, which established a code of ethics for buyers clubs that included the requirement to provide services at the lowest possible cost.[23] Despite this extratextual information provided on the website for the film, the film itself presents a picture of a kind of accidental activism emerging in the unlikely personage of Woodroof. As with Staley's story in *How to Survive a Plague,* Woodroof's activism emerges as a result of his own experience of diagnosis and his shock at the lack of treatments available for him. Whereas Staley's class background infuses him with confidence and financial resources in the face of homophobia and hopelessness, Woodroof draws on a different class background and a fount of cussedness, which the film suggests is a resource as valuable as money in fighting to survive a deadly disease.

Ron's cussedness, his will to survive, is combined with signs of an ability to reign in the bad habits the film posits as the reason he contracted HIV/AIDS in the first place. The film opens with a scene that moves between the rodeo ring and a cowboy riding a bull to Ron having wild sex with two different women and snorting cocaine in between partners. The cowboy is thrown from the bull and trampled on and has to be carried from the ring by the rodeo clowns at the same time as Ron's drug- and sex-induced high climaxes. All through this opening scene, what the film script describes as a "strange ringing" can be heard on the soundtrack, an ominous tolling foreshadowing doom to come. Later, after Ron is diagnosed with AIDS, he participates in another dream-like scene of sex and drug taking, though this time his illness keeps him at a remove from the hedonistic events taking place around him. We are clearly meant to feel relief that he restrains himself from having sex with the women. In the new reality of Ron's life, pleasure has become danger, yet individual will can protect us from ourselves and others. The hallucinatory quality of this scene, however, seems to work against such a narrative of containment. Pleasure still lures and escapes our attempts to contain it. There is a fine line or short drop between drugs into bodies to fight AIDS and drugs into bodies to heighten the experience of sex.

In these popular filmic accounts, personal character becomes the key to fighting the hopelessness, stigma, and discrimination that people with AIDS faced in the 1980s. Such representations stand in for and cover over a more complicated and longer history of the interconnectedness of illness, thought, and politics in late capitalism. Although the politics of direct action in general and the goal of drugs into bodies in particular presented in both *How to Survive a Plague* and *Dallas Buyers Club* were critical in the emergency time of the early days of AIDS in the United States, we are still living the effects of such politics in the present. Considering that the use of pharmaceuticals has become virtually the only means by which we treat illness today, it seems clear the emergency time of the early 1980s has not ended, and we must ask, therefore, Who has benefited and continues to benefit from the extension of a temporality of crisis?

The phrase "drugs into bodies" becomes the distillation of one story that covers over other stories, literally and physiologically. Delivered in capsules that hide the bitter taste, our treatments—of illness and of our stories of illness—have become scientized and commodified, and we have little choice but to take these capsules as directed. By looking back to the prehistory of AIDS, I am interested in counteracting this very specific clinical and political imperative by demonstrating other therapeutic and political practices, those varieties of politico-therapeutic experience less easily encapsulated and operating less directly in and on the present moment. Thinking illness, thought, and activism together and across multiple spaces and temporalities suggests treatments and treatment activisms beyond drugs into bodies. This is the challenge in and to the emergency time of neoliberalism: to remember and bring into being other temporal registers—living with chronicity, the social habits of endurance, and the politics of indirect action.

Acknowledgments

Many people and places, (inter)disciplinary spaces and institutional structures influenced this project in direct and indirect ways. Wonderful colleagues at Stony Brook University have made my time there intellectually stimulating and convivial. Nancy Tomes is not only a brilliant scholar but also a mentor who goes above and beyond time and time again. I have been inspired by a group of amazing scholars and teachers in the Program and now Department of Women's, Gender, and Sexuality Studies at Stony Brook: Kadji Amin, Mary Jo Bona, Ritch Calvin, Francoise Cromer, Robyn DeLuca, Melissa Forbis, Nancy Hiemstra, E. Ann Kaplan, Liz Montegary, and Teri Tiso. The emergence and growth of disability studies at Stony Brook, under the tireless leadership of Pamela Block, has been a source of inspiration for my work. I am grateful to the provost's office and the FAHSS Committee for grants to support archival research for this project.

A big thank you goes to my comrades, mentors, and friends: John Bailyn, Nerissa Balce, Michael Beck, Mark Bowen, Lena Burgos-Lafuente, Ed Casey, Lou Charnon-Deutsch, Matthew Christensen, Fidelito Cortes, Joanne Davila, Patty Dunn, Daniela Flesler, Michele Friedner, Lauren Hale, Dijana Jelaca, Tiffany Joseph, Michael Kimmel, Eva Kittay, Shirley Lim, Sara Lipton, Ira Livingston, Kristina Lucenko, Iona Man-Cheong, Peter Manning, Gary Marker, Celia Marshik, Ryan Minor, Adrienne Munich, Anne O'Byrne, Adrián Pérez-Melgosa, Brian Phillips, Joseph Pierce, Mary Rawlinson, Joel Rosenthal, Naomi Rosenthal, Jeffrey Santa-Ana, Sabina Sawhney, Susan Scheckel, Carrie Shandra, John Shandra, Katherine Sugg, Kathleen Vernon, Tracey Walters, and Kathleen Wilson.

I am continuously enriched by the opportunity to teach and work with fabulous undergraduate and graduate students at Stony Brook University. The classroom provides material and emotional sustenance for my research.

I appreciate the opportunity to present my work at various sites, and I thank those who extended invitations and hospitality, including Margrit

Shildrick and Azrini Wahidin for the Retheorising Women's Health Seminar at Queens University Belfast; Hendrik Hartog for the American Studies Workshop at Princeton; Victoria Pitts-Taylor for the Gender and Sexuality Seminar at City University of New York; Sayantani DasGupta and Marsha Hurst for the Narrative, Health, and Social Justice Seminar at Columbia and the opportunity to present with the amazing Alondra Nelson; Franziska Gygax and Miriam Locher for the Narrative Matters in Literature, Linguistics, and Medical Humanities Symposium at the University of Basel; and Jane Thrailkill and the Literature, Medicine, and Culture Research group in the Department of English at the University of North Carolina at Chapel Hill. Others near and far have helped me think anew about illness-thought-activism, critical pedagogy, and institutional analysis, including Rita Charon, Therese Jones, Ranjana Khanna, Allison Kimmich, Bradley Lewis, Vivian May, Annemarie Mol, Kelly Oliver, Cindy Patton, Susan Squier, Benigno Trigo, and Robyn Wiegman.

Danielle Kasprzak, my editor at the University of Minnesota Press, has been an enthusiastic supporter of my work and calming influence on me throughout the process of bringing this work to fruition. Her assistant, Anne Carter, has responded helpfully to all my queries while chasing permissions and preparing the final manuscript. Copy editor Mike Hanson kept my voice while cutting commas. I thank the Press's anonymous readers of my manuscript, one of whom revealed herself to be Catherine Belling. I am grateful to both readers for reading my work so closely and well. Their readings were both generous and incisive, pinpointing my key interventions in regards to illness, thought, and politics in the period before the emergence of HIV/AIDS, as well as making helpful and specific suggestions for revision that strengthened my arguments about method, history, and health activism. I thank Jennifer Brier, who read an early, partial version of the manuscript and offered constructive comments on AIDS and its (pre)histories.

Thanks go to Gregg Bordowitz, John Berger, and Jean Mohr, who readily granted permission to use copyrighted images of their work in my book. The use of their images is one gift, and the generosity in allowing them to be used freely, another. I thank staff at the P.P.O.W. Gallery in New York City, the Getty Research Institute in Los Angeles, the Iowa Women's Archives, and the Linda Lear Center for Special Collections and Archives at Connecticut College for helping me with permissions as well as staff at the Schlesinger Library at Radcliffe and the Beinecke Library at Yale for assistance on my visits to the Boston Women's Health Book Collective and Rachel Carson archives. Thanks go to Patrice Scanlon at Stony Brook Library and Paul St. Denis in the media lab, who helped me produce high-quality reproductions of several images.

I am grateful as always for the long-standing and unconditional love and support of my mother, Fran Diedrich, my father, Richard Diedrich, and my sisters, Dawn Diedrich and Andrea Kumar. It's been thrilling to see my nephews, Nikhil Kumar and Jack Boyette, and niece, Sona Kumar, exploring the world and figuring out, not too quickly, what to do with their lives.

Victoria Hesford suggested the title and helped me stay the course.

Notes

Introduction

1. The event was at the Center for Lesbian and Gay Studies (CLAGS) at the Graduate Center of the City University of New York. CLAGS board director Daniel Hurewitz moderated a roundtable discussion between Sarah Schulman, Douglas Crimp, and Nathan Lee.

2. ACT UP's earliest mission statement confirms Schulman's point about the single-issue politics of ACT UP: "ACT UP is a diverse, nonpartisan group of individuals united in anger and committed to direct action to end the AIDS crisis" (actupny.org). Interestingly, ACT UP London has recently ratified a more elaborate and more broad-based mission statement. It begins with this revision of the original ACT UP New York statement: "ACT UP London is a diverse, nonpartisan group of individuals united in anger and committed to direct action to end the HIV pandemic, along with the broader inequalities and injustices that perpetuate it." ACT UP: London website, http://actuplondon.wordpress.com.

3. Tadiar, *Things Fall Away.* In her last chapter Tadiar begins by wondering if the time of revolution has passed and asks whether interest in the 1960s and 1970s is simply nostalgia for a revolutionary moment.

4. Carson, *Silent Spring,* 188.

5. My concept *indirect action* draws on recent work in the humanities and social sciences that seeks to challenge a hegemonic temporopolitical logic of crisis for understanding current sociopolitical events, including Rob Nixon's work on slow violence, *Slow Violence and the Environmentalism of the Poor,* and Lauren Berlant's work on slow death, "Slow Death (Sovereignty, Obesity, Lateral Agency)." For recent work on ecological thought styles, see, for example, Chen, "Racialized Toxins and Sovereign Fantasies" and *Animacies,* and Morton, *The Ecological Thought.*

6. This historicizes my earlier analysis of illness as a queer performative in *Treatments.* Lynne Huffer's brilliant work *Mad for Foucault,* on madness and queer theory, makes a similar point, if only in relation to madness not illness more generally.

7. Foucault, *The Government of the Self and Others,* 20–21.

8. I am using the term *deeventalization* in order to suggest a historicoontological effect rather than a psychological effect of an individual or collective trauma. To be sure, the experience of AIDS was and is traumatizing, and trauma theory

provides many useful concepts for understanding not only the immense losses experienced by a generation of gay men and others but also the biopsychosocial difficulties for those who were certain they would die shortly after diagnosis but have survived. For a fascinating account of the relationship between the trauma of AIDS and queer theory, see Castiglia and Reed, *If Memory Serves*. They argue that "well-received versions of queer theory in the 1990s often signaled their novelty in ways that participated in post-AIDS unremembering and, at the same time, registered the traumatic aftereffects of their own unremembering" (5).

9. For some examples of the practices of reparative reading and weak theory, see Sedgwick, *Touching Feeling*; Cvetkovich, *Depression*; Freeman, *Time Binds*; Berlant, *Cruel Optimism*; Povinelli, *Events of Abandonment*; and Stewart, *Ordinary Affects*.

10. I thank the anonymous reader of my manuscript who encouraged me to think more about the historical relationship between weak theory and AIDS.

11. See, for example, Love, "Truth and Consequences." Love cautions against a reading of Sedgwick as having sought to replace paranoid reading with reparative reading, noting that in "Paranoid Reading and Reparative Reading, or, You're So Paranoid, You Probably Think This Essay Is About You," "the paranoid aspect of the essay is evident not only in the subtitle but throughout the essay, and Sedgwick says so all but directly" (238). Love's "all but directly" is an intriguing and oblique turn of phrase that suggests the importance of both direct and indirect modes of reading for Sedgwick.

12. Wiegman, "The Times We're In," 12.

13. Schulman, *The Gentrification of the Mind*, 11–12.

14. Here, I am drawing on Viego, *Dead Subjects*. For other recent work that usefully deploys queer as method not as identity, see Freccero, *Queer/Early/Modern*; Muñoz, *Cruising Utopia*.

15. Diedrich, *Treatments*.

16. In his introduction to Deleuze's *Essays Critical and Clinical*, Daniel W. Smith explains that Deleuze first links the critical with the clinical in his 1967 essay on Sacher-Masoch, "Introduction: 'A Life of Pure Immanence,'" in Deleuze, *Essays Critical and Clinical*, xi. See also Deleuze, "Coldness and Cruelty," in *Masochism*, 14.

17. Peter Cohen, for example, argues there was little continuity between ACT UP and earlier social movements. According to Cohen, "In the history of social and political movements in the United States, ACT UP is something of a standout, an anomaly during a decade in which the vibrant activism of the 1960s and early 1970s (second-wave feminism, black civil rights, the New Left) had largely been abandoned. At the same time, ACT UP must also be understood as . . . something of a paradox—a movement for social change that was created in large part by individuals with a significant investment in the status quo." *Love and Anger*, 17. Although I think Cohen makes some very useful points about the gender and class

politics of ACT UP, I also think he contributes to a misreading of activism around AIDS as dominated by white middle-class men.
18. Patton, *Sex and Germs* and "AIDS Industry." She made this point quite explicitly to me when she directed my dissertation in the late 1990s and early 2000s.
19. Brier, "Locating Lesbian and Feminist Responses to AIDS, 1982–1984" and *Infectious Ideas*; Gould, *Moving Politics*.
20. See the portraits taken by Bill Bystura of key players in ACT UP "who survived—to live their lives, and to recall the extraordinary days in the trenches." France, "Pictures from a Battlefield."
21. A review of the New York Historical Society's exhibition on the early years of AIDS in New York by Hugh Ryan, the founding director of the Pop-Up Museum of Queer History, highlights some of the ways this covering over, or, as the headline suggests, "whitewashing," happens. Ryan writes that the show "takes a black mark in New York City's history—its homophobic, apathetic response to the early days of AIDS in the early 1980s—and transforms it into a moment of civic pride, when New Yorkers of all stripes came together to fight the disease. It's a lovely story, if only it were true." Ryan, "How to Whitewash a Plague." I would argue that this whitewashing follows a trajectory that Sara Ahmed describes in "Shame before Others," in *The Culture Politics of Emotion*, in which nations or, in this case, cities pass quickly from shame to pride in recalling a shameful past.
22. Kramer, *The American People*. Prepublication publicity called *The American People* the "long-awaited magnum opus of America's master playwright and activist" and noted it has been "forty years in the making," which makes the text almost as old as AIDS. As I have been completing this project, Kramer has been in the news not only in anticipation of the publication of his novel but also because of HBO's adaptation of his play *The Normal Heart*, first produced at the Public Theater in New York City in 1985. Patrick Healy's positive review of the film and gushing profile of Kramer in the *New York Times* emphasizes Kramer's frail health and the amazing fact of his having lived to see his play produced for television. "A Lion Still Roars, with Gratitude." The response to HBO's *The Normal Heart* was generally positive among mainstream critics, although several queer critics objected strongly to its "sanitized, fictional 1980s New York." Lalonde, "I Hate *The Normal Heart*." In her fascinating reading of the film and its representation of the early days of the AIDS epidemic in New York, Lalonde notes that "the entire film explicitly supports the thesis that gay men, through promiscuity and infidelity, brought an epidemic upon themselves."
23. Mass, "Interview with a Writer," 333.
24. Ibid.
25. Ibid.
26. Spivak, *Outside in the Teaching Machine*, 67. Tani Barlow develops Spivak's literary concept into a historical one in *The Question of Women in Chinese Feminism*.

27. Mass, "Interview with a Writer," 334.

28. I take the term *nonevent* from Michel-Rolph Trouillot, who uses it to signal the way that some historical events, such as the Haitian Revolution in Trouillot's case study, are unthinkable as they are happening. *Silencing the Past,* 73.

29. Barad, "Shifting Sands of Time."

30. Nelson, *Body and Soul.* Nelson discusses the concept of biological citizenship in relation to the Black Panther Party's social health work but worries about the "transaction costs" when citizenship is reduced to "damaged biology or presumed biological pathology or disproportionate illness rates or disease identity" (185). *Biological citizenship* is a term that emerges in the period I explore here, and others have studied the varieties of practices of biological citizenship in different global contexts. Adriana Petryna first coined the term in *A Life Exposed,* her ethnographic study of the myriad responses—political, scientific, medical, social—to the explosion at the Chernobyl nuclear reactor in the Ukraine in the former Soviet Union in 1986. In Petryna's formulation health and illness become the means through which vulnerable people make claims for citizenship and human rights on the basis of their damaged biological condition. Others have used the term to think through the ways new developments in genetics and medical technology have transformed the rights and responsibilities of citizenship in the late twentieth and early twenty-first centuries. See, for example, Rose, *The Politics of Life Itself.*

31. I am inspired in this task of pursuing linkages between illness experiences and events across time and space by the work of anthropologist and science studies scholar Kim Fortun on the industrial disaster in Bhopal, India, in 1984. In its approach *Advocacy after Bhopal* considers how the disaster in Bhopal in 1984 reverberates beyond that particular moment and place, into the past and future. Organizations like the Bhopal Group for Information and Action and the Bhopal Gas Affected Working Women's Union, middle-class advocates, including Fortun herself, and also the text of *Advocacy after Bhopal* all struggle to respond to a disaster. That disaster is not over and done with once the gas has stopped leaking but continues in small things like mutated genes and damaged bodies and in large things like ethnic and religious conflict and grassroots challenges to corporate malfeasance. We can only respond, Fortun believes, "tentatively. Reaching for something that can't yet be named. Pursuing new linkages, as a way around available—and obsolete—idioms and social forms" (194).

32. In his now classic work of science studies *Impure Science,* Steven Epstein offers an exhaustive analysis of the relationship between AIDS activism and science, especially with regards to debates and controversies surrounding AIDS causation and treatment. I trace back from the period Epstein covers—1981 to 1995—to explore the political and scientific (and politicoscientific) landscapes into which

AIDS would later emerge. In his introduction Epstein argues that "analysts of science have paid little attention to the extensive theoretical and empirical literature on 'new social movements'—works describing the ecology movement, the women's movement, the antinuclear movement, racial and ethnic movements, the gay and lesbian movement, and so on—a literature with obvious relevance to the study of the AIDS movement" (20). Epstein's own analysis, focused as it is on activism around AIDS, doesn't go much beyond suggesting that some of these links, especially with the women's health movement, might be considered. I am interested more explicitly in what does and does not get brought into AIDS activism from these "new"—yet earlier—social movements.

33. Riley, *Am I That Name?*, 97.

34. Guattari, *The Machinic Unconscious*, 10.

35. Ross, *May '68 and Its Afterlives*.

36. Ibid., 149.

37. Thanks go to Catherine Belling, one of the readers of the manuscript, for providing this evocative term for the formal work I am trying to do in *Indirect Action*. As I was completing *Indirect Action*, I had been reading, teaching, and writing about what has come to be called graphic medicine—comics and other graphic forms on the experience and event of illness and health care. In an essay on Alison Bechdel, I had used the term *graphic analysis* to describe the long and difficult therapeutic and creative process of doing and undoing the self in words and images that Bechdel practices. Diedrich, "Graphic Analysis."

38. For a discussion of the "politics of absorption" in relation to the social movements of the 1960s and 1970s, see Omi and Winant, *Racial Formations in the United States*. For a recent use of this term in relation to the interdisciplinary experiments, especially ethnic studies and women's, gender, and sexuality studies programs that emerged as a result of social and political transformations of the university in the 1960s and 1970s, see Ferguson, *The Reorder of Things*.

39. Berger and Mohr, *A Fortunate Man*.

40. Thomas's columns were later anthologized in two collections, *The Lives of the Cell*, published in 1974, and *The Medusa and the Snail*, published in 1979.

41. Fanon, *The Wretched of the Earth*.

42. Smiley, *Out of the Shadows*; Kotulski, *Saving Millie*.

43. Guattari uses this phrase in the essay "Mary Barnes's 'Trip,'" in *Chaosophy*, 135, in which he discusses the experimental clinic, Kingsley Hall, created by R. D. Laing in London in 1965, and one of Laing's most famous—or infamous—patients, Mary Barnes. See also Barnes's autobiographical account of her time at Kingsley Hall, written with one of her doctors, Joseph H. Berke, *Two Accounts of a Journey Through Madness*.

44. Deleuze and Guattari, *Anti-Oedipus*.

1. Doing Queer Love, circa 1985

1. Kamau, "Feminists Asleep in AIDS Fight."

2. The call to "wake up!" is of course a fairly common rhetorical strategy. Such rhetoric was used to great effect by Larry Kramer in his now legendary diatribe "1,112 and Counting" published in the *New York Native* in 1983, which exhorted gay men to stop sleeping—and sleeping around—when they were dying in such large numbers. In his essay "Not-about-AIDS," David Román discusses a later article by Michelangelo Signorile entitled "641,086 and Counting" published in the gay magazine *Out* in 1998 that echoes Kramer's earlier wake-up call in an effort to "counter apathy and denial" now made even more monstrous by the exponentially larger number in the headline.

3. Kamau, "Feminists Asleep in AIDS Fight."

4. Ibid.

5. Ibid.

6. Ibid.

7. Spivak's own phrase is "white men saving brown women from brown men." Spivak, "Can the Subaltern Speak?" Thanks go to Victoria Hesford for suggesting this reading to me.

8. Barbara R. Bergmann, letter to the editor, *Denver Post*.

9. Rotello, *Sexual Ecology*.

10. Some of the works Lorber mentions include Alonso and Koreck, "Silences"; Campbell, "Male Gender Roles and Sexuality"; Hammonds, "Missing Persons"; Osmond et al., "The Multiple Jeopardy of Race, Class, and Gender for AIDS Risk among Women"; Patton, *Last Served?*; and Schneider and Stoller, eds., *Women Resisting AIDS*.

11. For a related analysis of how one figure may cover over the complexities of a social movement, see Victoria Hesford's discussion of the feminist-as-lesbian figure in the second-wave women's movement in *Feeling Women's Liberation*. For an analysis of competing cultural memories of AIDS activism, see Castiglia, "Sex Panics, Sex Publics, Sex Memories."

12. Foucault, *Discipline and Punish*, 271.

13. Ibid., 290.

14. Ibid., 292.

15. Scott, "Fantasy Echo," 287. Scott further develops the concept of the echo for feminism in "Feminist Reverberations." She argues that "reverberations is a good way to think about this global circulation of feminist strategies, of feminism itself, and also of the analytic term gender" (12). Both of these essays are collected in Scott's recent collection *The Fantasy of Feminist History*.

16. Scott, "Fantasy Echo," 286.

17. Ibid., 287.

18. Ibid., 290–91.

19. Ibid., 291.

20. For more thinking on doing illness, see Annemarie Mol's praxiographic approach in *The Body Multiple*. Mol investigates not how we know a particular disease but how doctors, patients, nurses, caregivers, technicians, etc., do it in practice.

21. In the inaugural volume of *TSQ: Transgender Studies Quarterly*, partially devoted to keywords of the field of transgender studies, Heather Love discusses the uses of "queer" in relation to "transgender" in ways that I find helpful in thinking queer and illness together. She notes that "while *queer* at its most capacious is understood to indicate a wide range of differences and social exclusions, it has often been critiqued for functioning more narrowly in practice." "Queer," 174. She then cites Cathy J. Cohen's article "Punks, Bulldaggers, and Welfare Queens" as an indictment against "*queer* as a false universal, one that claims to address the situation of all marginal subjects but in fact is focused on the concerns of gays and lesbians" (174).

22. Foucault, "The Subject and Power," in *Power*, 326. This essay was first published as an appendix in Dreyfus and Rabinow, *Michel Foucault*.

23. Foucault, "The Subject and Power," 327.

24. Ibid., 335.

25. Ibid.

26. Ibid., 336.

27. The interview with Foucault was published just a few months before the *New York Times* published the article "Rare Cancer Seen in 41 Homosexuals," written by Lawrence K. Altman in 1981.

28. Foucault, "Friendship as a Way of Life," in *Ethics*, 135.

29. Ibid.

30. Ibid., 136.

31. Foucault, "Friendship as a Way of Life," 136. This perhaps explains why the prospect of gay marriage is such a threat to many conservatives, who like to characterize the "gay lifestyle" as hedonistic and irresponsible and, thus, purportedly so radically unlike their own.

32. Foucault, "Friendship as a Way of Life," 137.

33. Foucault, "Friendship as a Way of Life," 138–39. Lillian Faderman, *Surpassing the Love of Men*.

34. Foucault, "Friendship as a Way of Life," 139.

35. Virginia Woolf's portrait of homosociality and homoeroticism among men in the professions in *Three Guineas* is revealing in this context. She describes the professional world from a woman's perspective, which is also the perspective of the outsider, as one that "seen from this angle undoubtedly looks queer" (18).

36. Foucault, "Friendship as a Way of Life," 139–40.

37. *Around 1981*, by feminist literary scholar Jane Gallop, explores the changing terrain of feminist literary theory by moving backward and forward from 1981.

38. Schulman, *My American History*, 11.

39. Patton, *Globalizing AIDS*, 4.

40. Brier, "Locating Lesbian and Feminist Responses to AIDS, " 234–35. This article forms the basis for chapter 1 of Brier's *Infectious Ideas*.

41. Brier, *Infectious Ideas*, 203n15. Brier also mentions David Román's work as attempting to counter the myth that AIDS activism didn't exist before ACT UP. See, for example, *Acts of Intervention*.

42. Gould, *Moving Politics*, 42–43.

43. Ibid.

44. Martin Duberman's recent memoir *Hold Tight Gently*, about Essex Hemphill and Michael Callen, reminds us of the political conservatism of most of the men who founded and ran Gay Men's Health Crisis.

45. Schulman, *My American History*, 1. For histories of 1970s feminism in the United States that have sought to complicate this story, see Echols, *Daring to Be Bad*; Hesford, *Feeling Women's Liberation*; and Rosen, *The World Split Open*. For an oral history of this period, see DuPlessis and Snitow, eds., *The Feminist Memoir Project*.

46. Schulman, *My American History*, 1.

47. Ibid.

48. Ibid., 5.

49. Hollibaugh, *My Dangerous Desires*, 248.

50. Hollibaugh, *My Dangerous Desires*, 248. For more on the Barnard Conference, see Vance, ed., *Pleasure and Danger*, as well as the archival material from the conference recently published in "The *GLQ* Archive" and introduced by Heather Love, "Diary of a Conference on Sexuality, 1982," in the special issue on "Rethinking Sex" in *GLQ*.

51. Wolfe, "The Mother of Us All," 282.

52. Schulman, *My American History*, 11.

53. Schulman, *My American History*, 120. Note that by publishing in the *New York Native*, Schulman already serves as a kind of relay between the two communities Wolfe delineates in the earlier quotation.

54. Schulman, *My American History*, 120.

55. Ibid.

56. Ibid., 122.

57. Ibid., 123.

58. Ibid.

59. Ibid.

60. Sedgwick, *Touching Feeling* and *Tendencies*. Elsewhere, I have argued that Sedgwick utilizes shame and what she calls "the queer performative" as a means to politicize the experience and event of patienthood. Diedrich, *Treatments*.

61. Schulman, *My American History,* 123.
62. Schulman, *My American History,* 124. The notion that those on the margins are better able to understand how power works is one of the key tenets of feminist standpoint epistemology. See, for example, Hartsock, "The Feminist Standpoint."
63. Schulman, *My American History,* 124.
64. For an important critique of community as a usually unexamined concept, see Joseph, *Against the Romance of Community.*
65. "The term 'community' has political valency in the United States," Patton argues in *Inventing AIDS,* "but fails as an analytic concept; for it cannot illuminate the shifting personal or network of allegiances lived by individuals in face-to-face relations" (7).
66. Schulman, *People in Trouble,* 159.
67. Gregg Bordowitz, interview, ACT UP Oral History Project, A Program of MIX: The New York Lesbian and Gay Experimental Film Festival, December 17, 2002, http://www.actuporalhistory.org.
68. Dreifus, *Seizing Our Bodies.* Other important texts from this period include Lorde, *The Cancer Journals;* Ehrenreich and English, *For Her Own Good;* Kushner, *Why Me?* (originally titled *Breast Cancer: A Personal History and Investigative Report*); Boston Women's Health Collective, *Our Bodies, Ourselves;* and Frankfurt, *Vaginal Politics.* All attempt to provide the knowledge necessary for making the patient her own health expert. See also chap. 2, note 29, of this book.
69. Dreifus, *Seizing Our Bodies,* xxiv–xxv.
70. Ibid., xxviii.
71. Ibid., xxix.
72. Coburn, "Off the Pill," 136.
73. Bordowitz, interview.
74. Ibid.
75. Ibid.
76. Sarah Schulman, statement, ACT UP Oral History Project, A Program of MIX: The New York Lesbian and Gay Experimental Film Festival, May 12, 2003, http://www.actuporalhistory.org.
77. Ibid.
78. Schulman, *The Gentrification of the Mind,* 4.
79. Howard, *Men Like That,* 12–13.
80. Cvetkovich, *An Archive of Feelings,* 158.
81. Cvetkovich interviewed Schulman for her project but, interestingly, does not quote from that interview in *An Archive of Feelings.*
82. Schulman, *The Gentrification of the Mind,* 2.
83. See her recent genre-defying *Depression,* which describes the collective work of public feelings. See also Staiger, Cvetkovich, and Reynolds, eds., *Political Emotions.*

84. Cvetkovich, *An Archive of Feelings*, 166, 167.

85. Ibid., 194.

86. Ibid.

87. It might be interesting to think about being preoccupied in relation to the political activism that has become the Occupy movement. Being preoccupied seems to suggest less direct forms of action than occupying.

88. Scott, "Fantasy Echo," 291.

89. Bordowitz, *The AIDS Crisis Is Ridiculous*, 25.

90. Ibid., 38.

91. Ibid., 39.

92. Bordowitz, *The AIDS Crisis Is Ridiculous*, 270. For a reading of *Habit* as a "genre of the present," see Berlant, *Cruel Optimism*, 60.

93. Bordowitz, *The AIDS Crisis Is Ridiculous*, 273.

94. Ibid.

95. Ibid., 274.

96. Ibid.

97. Ibid., 275.

98. Ibid.

Snapshot 1

1. Bordowitz, *The AIDS Crisis Is Ridiculous*, 245.

2. Ibid.

3. This essay was first published in Gever, Greyson, and Parmar, eds., *Queer Looks*.

4. Bordowitz, *The AIDS Crisis Is Ridiculous*, 44.

5. Ibid., 46.

6. Ibid., 48.

7. Ibid., 49.

8. Ibid., 50.

9. Ibid., 51.

10. Williams is the author of the influential cultural studies text *Keywords*.

11. Williams discusses the concept in *Marxism and Literature*, which is a text that opens with a discussion of four basic concepts: culture, language, literature, and ideology. The short chapter "Structures of Feeling" is situated between the chapters "Dominant, Residual, and Emergent" and "The Sociology of Culture" in the book's middle section, "Cultural Theory." I mention how Williams situates this key concept because he is quite explicit in the linkages he makes between concepts; one concept gets him so far, and then he must move on to another. Here is how he ends "Dominant, Residual, and Emergent": "Again and again what we have to observe is in effect a *pre-emergence*, active and pressing but not yet fully

articulated, rather than the evident emergence which could be more confidently named. It is to understand more closely this condition of pre-emergence, as well as the more evident forms of the emergent, the residual, and the dominant, that we need to explore the concept of structures of feeling" (126–27). For a demonstration of how he utilizes the concept in relation to literature, see Williams, *Culture and Society*, esp. "The Industrial Novels." I would argue that his own use of the concept in this earlier work (first published in 1958) came before his full articulation of it.

12. Williams, *Marxism and Literature*, 128.
13. Bordowitz, *The AIDS Crisis Is Ridiculous*, 49.
14. Williams, *Marxism and Literature*, 129.
15. Ibid., 132.
16. Two recent films, *United in Anger: A History of ACT UP*, directed by Jim Hubbard, and *How to Survive a Plague*, directed by David France, make use of this early AIDS activist video footage.
17. Bordowitz, *The AIDS Crisis Is Ridiculous*, 96.
18. Ibid., 106.
19. Ibid.
20. Ibid., 98.
21. Ibid., 99.
22. Ibid., 96.
23. Bernstein, "Surviving AIDS, but Not the Life That Followed."
24. Voelcker, "The Death of Activist Spencer Cox."

2. Que(e)rying the Clinic, circa 1970

1 Wachter, "AIDS, Activism, and the Politics of Health," 128.
2. Ibid.
3. Ibid.
4. In his influential analysis of stigma first published in 1963, Erving Goffman discusses "action groups" as offering a protopolitical critique of stigmatization as a form of normalization. These action groups challenge stigmatization via the publication of counternarratives "that give voice to shared feelings" and help to "consolidate belief in the stigma as a basis for self-conception." *Stigma*, 27.
5. Wachter, "AIDS, Activism, and the Politics of Health," 128.
6. Ibid.
7. Patton, *Inventing AIDS*, 13. A version of a chapter in *Inventing AIDS* was first published in 1989 as "AIDS Industry: Construction of 'Victims,' 'Volunteers' and 'Experts,'" in Erica Carter and Simon Watney's *Taking Liberties*.
8. *Personal Politics* is the title of Sara Evans's important history of the emergence of the women's liberation movement in the United States out of the civil rights and new left movements of the 1960s. For a discussion of the phrase "the

personal is political" as, first, "powerfully enigmatic statement" and, then, "empty phrase," see Hesford, *Feeling Women's Liberation*, 96.

9. See, for example, Preston and Swann, *Safe Sex*.

10. In his effective and affective history of May 1968, Bourg discusses the transformation from the "revolutionary-political modes of social experience" that characterized the uprisings of May 1968 and after to an "ethics of liberation." *From Revolution to Ethics*, 8. As Bourg notes, "During the 1970s, the ethics of liberation occasionally fizzled out in dead ends. Aspects of the 1960s never made it to the 1980s" (10).

11. Patton, "Introduction: Foucault after Neoliberalism; or, The Clinic Here and Now," in *Rebirth of the Clinic*, xvii.

12. Contra Sontag, I am intentionally metaphorizing the experience of AIDS to help think about the relationship between a 1990s queer theory—read as full-blown—and earlier theoretical and political formations—read as not-yet queer. For Sontag's position, see *Illness as Metaphor* and *AIDS and Its Metaphors*.

13. Wachter, "AIDS, Activism, and the Politics of Health," 131.

14. Keyword searches in the *New England Journal of Medicine* online database show the following: "women's liberation" is mentioned in fifteen articles between 1960 and 1979, seven articles between 1980 and 1999, and once between 2000 and 2010; "women's lib" is mentioned in three articles between 1960 and 1979; "women's health movement" is mentioned twice between 1960 and 1979, once from 1980 to 1999, and twice from 2000 to 2010; "feminist" is used in nineteen articles between 1960 and 1979, seventy articles between 1980 and 1999, and seventeen articles between 2000 and 2010. Search conducted at www.nejm.org on January 13, 2011.

15. Howell, "What Medical Schools Teach about Women"; and Spiro, "Myths and Mirths: Women in Medicine."

16. Ingelfinger, "Doctor Women," 304.

17. Ibid., 303.

18. Ibid., 304.

19. Ibid.

20. Ibid.

21. Howell, "What Medical Schools Teach about Women," 304.

22. Ibid., 305.

23. Ibid., 306.

24. Ibid., 307.

25. Spiro, "Myths and Mirths," 354.

26. Ibid., 355.

27. Ibid., 356.

28. Ibid.

29. Dreifus, *Seizing Our Bodies*. For other accounts of the women's health

movement published at the time of or just after the height of the movement, see, for example, Boston Women's Health Collective, *Our Bodies, Ourselves*; Ruzek, *The Women's Health Movement*; Frankfort, *Vaginal Politics*; and Seaman, *The Doctors' Case against the Pill*. For a selection of original literature from the women's liberation movement, including a section on bodies with a subsection on health, see Baxandall and Gordon, *Dear Sisters*. For more recent histories of the women's health movement, see, for example, Davis *Moving the Mountain*; Davis, *The Making of "Our Bodies, Ourselves"*; Dresser, "What Bioethics Can Learn from the Women's Health Movement"; Morgen, *Into Our Own Hands*; Murphy, "Immodest Witnessing" and *Seizing the Means of Reproduction*; and Wells, *"Our Bodies, Ourselves" and the Work of Writing*.

30. Murphy, *Seizing the Means of Reproduction*, 26. Murphy describes self-help as kind of a protocol, defined as "a procedural script that strategically assembles technologies, exchange, epistemologies, subjects, and so on" (25).

31. Boston Women's Health Book Collective, *Our Bodies, Ourselves*. The collective initially had a series of pieces developed for consciousness raising sessions on women's health published by the small radical press the New England Free Press. Later, when the Free Press was unable to keep up with demand for the book, the collective made the difficult decision to go with a mainstream press. "History: Decision to Go with Simon and Schuster (1973 edition)," file, Boston Women's Health Book Collective Records, 1972–1997 (no. 102.4), Schlesinger Library, Radcliffe Institute, Harvard University, Cambridge, Massachusetts.

32. Boston Women's Health Book Collective Records, 1972–1997 (no. 102.2), Schlesinger Library, Radcliffe Institute, Harvard University, Cambridge, Massachusetts.

33. I use the term "medical sovereignty" here to suggest the ways medicine participates in both modes of power—sovereign and disciplinary—that Foucault delineates in his work beginning in the 1970s. Although Foucault has often been read as arguing that disciplinary power replaces sovereign power in the nineteenth century, I think it is more accurate to understand these two modes of power in relation to each other and to consider how that relation functions. Elaborating on Foucault's concepts, Agamben makes the important observation that biopower is often exercised in support of a sovereign power. Gorgio Agamben, *Homo Sacer*. I discuss medical sovereignty in two mediatized medical events from 2005—the legal and medical case of Terri Schiavo and Hurricane Katrina and its aftermath—in "Speeding Up Slow Deaths."

34. "Physicians and Feminist Patients: Conflict Grows," *Medical Tribune*, November 7, 1973, 15, Boston Women's Health Book Collective Records, 1972–1997 (no. 102.3), Schlesinger Library, Radcliffe Institute, Harvard University, Cambridge, Massachusetts.

35. Ibid.

36. Ibid.

37. *How to Do a Pelvic Examination, 1976,* Boston Women's Health Book Collective Records, 1972–1997 (no. 102.1), Schlesinger Library, Radcliffe Institute, Harvard University, Cambridge, Massachusetts.

38. "Transmission of affect" is feminist philosopher Teresa Brennan's term from her book of the same title. For an influential analysis of the affective in relation to feminism, see Ahmed, *The Cultural Politics of Emotion.* In the chapter "Feminist Attachments," Ahmed discusses how many women, including herself, come to feminism through positive affective experiences like wonder as much as through negative affective experiences like anger.

39. Foucault, *The History of Sexuality,* vol. 1, 57. In diagnosing the relationship between *ars erotica* and *scientia sexualis* in Western culture, Foucault writes, "*Scientia sexualis* versus *ars erotica* no doubt. But it should be noted that the *ars erotica* did not disappear altogether from Western civilization; nor has it always been absent from the movement by which one sought to produce a science of sexuality" (70).

40. Price, *The Self Help Clinic,* reprinted from *Women's World* 1, no. 4 (March–May 1972), Boston Women's Health Book Collective Records, 1972–1997 (no. 102.3), Schlesinger Library, Radcliffe Institute, Harvard University, Cambridge, Massachusetts.

41. *How to Do a Pelvic Examination, 1976.*

42. In his fascinating discussion of the clinic and/as tea room, "Clinic and the Tea Room," Geoffrey Rees describes the inchoate queer ethical potential of the clinical encounter. For Rees the clinic itself is an intimate public space, and comparing how intimacy happens in the clinic with other intimate public spaces allows bioethics to draw on an elaborate discourse and practice of queer sexual ethics.

43. Price, *The Self Help Clinic.* See also Downer, "Covert Sex Discrimination against Women as Medical Patients," address to the American Psychological Association meeting in Hawaii, September 5, 1972, Boston Women's Health Book Collective Records, 1972–1997 (no. 102.3), Schlesinger Library, Radcliffe Institute, Harvard University, Cambridge, Massachusetts.

44. Davis, *The Making of "Our Bodies, Ourselves,"* 43. In her discussion of the *OBOS's* transnational travels, Davis describes the aspects of the project's theories and practices that are emphasized, downplayed, or deleted in various locations. For example, she notes that the "editors of the Latin American adaptation were critical of the U.S. *OBOS,* which they regarded as individualistic, consumer oriented, and insufficiently political. In their view, the U.S. text over-emphasized the power of the individual woman to take care of herself as epitomized by the 'completely Anglo' notion of self-help" (180).

45. Wachter, "AIDS, Activism, and the Politics of Health," 132.

46. Mol, *The Logic of Care*, x.

47. Ibid., 11.

48. Mol argues that care is a strange process: "It is difficult to act strangely; difficult to do something that does not fit with the company you keep. Yet this is exactly what the logic of care wants you to do. In order to take care of yourself, you may need to deviate." *The Logic of Care*, 60.

49. Deleuze and Guattari, *Anti-Oedipus* and *A Thousand Plateaus*. Deleuze and Guattari also collaborated on two other books, *Kafka* and *What Is Philosophy?*

50. A recent biography of the two together goes a long way to restoring Guattari's primary not secondary influence on the thought of the pair. See Dosse, *Gilles Deleuze and Félix Guattari*. Nonetheless, the frequency with which in published—and thus peer-reviewed and edited—articles and books Deleuze alone is discussed as the author of *Anti-Oedipus* and *A Thousand Plateaus* is nothing short of astounding, to this reader at least.

51. According to Bourg, the "term Institutional Psychotherapy was first used in print in 1952 by the French psychiatrists Georges Daumézon and Philippe Koechlin." *From Revolution to Ethics*, 125.

52. Bourg, *From Revolution to Ethics*, 126.

53. Interestingly, in *May '68 and Its Afterlives*, Kristin Ross notes, in one of her few explicit references to Guattari, that he, along with Henri Curiel, Francis Jeanson, the cartoonist Siné, among others, acted as relays, or "*porteurs de valise,*" for the Front de Libération Nationale, "moving cash, not arms, across the city, and over national borders" (51).

54. Genosko, "The Life and Work of Félix Guattari," 47. As Genosko notes, Guattari's essay "Transversalité" was first written in 1964 and published in French in 1977.

55. See Félix Guattari's interview with Arno Munster, "The Best Capitalist Drug," in Guattari, *Chaosophy*, 147.

56. Ibid.

57. *Oxford English Dictionary Online*, s.v. "transversal," accessed October 5, 2010, dictionary.oed.com.

58. For an interesting account of how they came to work together, see Catherine Backès-Clément interview with Deleuze and Guattari on *Anti-Oedipus* first published in *L'Arc* 49 in 1972, in Deleuze, *Negotiations*, 13–15.

59. Deleuze, *Negotiations*, 15.

60. Ibid., 17.

61. Guattari, *Chaosophy*, 181–82.

62. Deleuze, *The Fold*, 33.

63. Ibid., 3.

64. Ibid., 56.

65. Bourg, *From Revolution to Ethics*, 126.

66. Guattari, "La Borde: A Clinic Unlike Any Other," 178.
67. Ibid, 180.
68. See Brian Massumi's "Translator's Forward: Pleasures of Philosophy" in Deleuze and Guattari, *A Thousand Plateaus*, x.
69. The clinic as a kind of laboratory for social change was one of the tenets of the community health movement. For an insightful comparative analysis of two community health centers—the Delta Health Center in rural Mound Bayou, Mississippi, and the Watts Health Center in Los Angeles—established in the 1960s as part of Johnson's War on Poverty program, see Loyd, "Where Is Community Health?" and *Health Rights Are Civil Rights*.
70. Cooper, *Psychiatry and Anti-psychiatry*, 37.
71. Genosko, "The Life and Work of Félix Guattari," 53.
72. Sedgwick, *Touching Feeling*, 123.
73. Ibid., 124.
74. Ibid., 126.
75. Ibid., 146.
76. Guattari, "La Borde: A Clinic Unlike Any Other," 189.

Snapshot 2

1. Lotringer is another relay between Guattari and Scemama and Wojnarowicz.
2. Lontringer and Ambrosino, eds., *David Wojnarowicz*, 131.
3. Wojnarowicz, *In the Shadow of the American Dream*, 176.
4. Agamben, *Means without Ends*, 57.
5. Lotringer and Ambrosino, eds., *David Wojnarowicz*, 118.
6. Guattari, "David Wojnarowicz."
7. Ibid.
8. Ibid.
9. Rizk, "Looking at 'Animals in Pants,'" 151.
10. Lotringer and Ambrosino, eds., *David Wojnarowicz*, 136.

3. Enacting Clinical Experience, circa 1963

1. Foucault, *The Birth of the Clinic*, 54.
2. Foucault, *The Birth of the Clinic*, x. Later in the text, he describes the years 1760–1800 as "forty years that witnessed the formation of the clinical method" (126).
3. Foucault, *The Birth of the Clinic*, 57.
4. Ibid., xv.
5. Ibid.
6. Ibid., xviii.

7. Berger and Mohr, *A Fortunate Man*. Subsequent references are cited parenthetically in the text.

8. Barlow, *The Question of Women in Chinese Feminism*.

9. See Diedrich, *Treatments,* esp. chap. 5; Diedrich, "Complexity and Cancer," about Richard Powers's novel *Gain*; and Diedrich, "Gathering Evidence of Ghosts," about W. G. Sebald's practices of witnessing. What I think connects writers like Sebald and Powers and my own analysis of their works is a desire to delineate the complex structures that allow or prevent the practices of witnessing, practices that are crucial for bringing about social change.

10. My choice of *doctoring* is inspired by Annemarie Mol's *The Logic of Care*, in which she describes doctoring as a kind of tinkering that involves many persons, objects, and technologies. In her formulation patients doctor as much as doctors themselves do.

11. Although there is not a lot of critical work on *A Fortunate Man,* some of the little work there is ignores Mohr's important contribution to the text. For example, Fred L. Griffin's essay "The Fortunate Physician" mentions at the outset and in passing Mohr's contribution but then refers only to Berger's written account, never discussing the photographs and the aesthetic and cultural work they do. This elision of Mohr's participation in the enactment of the story that *A Fortunate Man* tells is strange because Mohr's name is equally prominent on the book's cover as one of the authors. Berger and Mohr have collaborated on two other works, *Another Way of Telling* and *A Seventh Man*. For an essay that does acknowledge Mohr's contribution and that reads the photographs and narrative together but that nonetheless focuses on Berger's work more generally, see Martyn Hudson, "The Clerk of the Foresters Records." Yet even in the section of his essay headed "The Pictures," Hudson's analysis of the use of photographs in *A Fortunate Man* remains rather abstract, rarely looking very closely at particular photographs. This style of reading fits with Hudson's primary concern with Marxist history writing.

12. Berger, *Ways of Seeing*.

13. This is how Griffin reads *A Fortunate Man* in "The Fortunate Physician."

14. Foucault, "Foreword to the English Edition," in *The Order of Things*.

15. Foucault, *The Birth of the Clinic,* 198.

16. For Foucault's encouragement to others to use and transform his gadgets, see the interview "Questions on Geography," in *Power/Knowledge,* 65. In his biography of Foucault, David Macey describes a conversation the feminist philosopher Jana Sawicki had with Foucault when she met him at a seminar in Vermont in 1982. As she explains to Macey, she told Foucault, "I had just finished writing a dissertation on his critique of humanism. Not surprisingly," Sawicki continues, "he responded with some embarrassment and much seriousness. He suggested that I do not spend energy talking about him and, instead, do what he was doing, namely, write genealogies." Macey, *The Lives of Michel Foucault,* 450. I am motivated by

Foucault's methods to incorporate Foucault's own work as part of a genealogy of the changing experience of medicine in the 1960s.

17. Macherey, *The Object of Literature*, 211. For another text that explicitly takes up Foucault's work with and as literature, see During, *Foucault and Literature*. For a collection of some of Foucault's own writings on "language and the birth of 'literature,'" see part 1 of *Language, Counter-memory, Practice*.

18. Foucault, *Death and the Labyrinth*.

19. Macherey, *The Object of Literature*, 218.

20. Ibid., 211.

21. Macherey, *The Object of Literature*, 219. In *The Age of the World Target*, Rey Chow argues that, early in his career, Foucault "seemed invested in none other than a repressive hypothesis of literature, whereby literature, rather than being the vehicle and effect of power (as he would teach us about sexuality), is conceived of, romantically, as power's victim and opposition" (8). While I agree with Chow's assessment that literature or the literary sometimes figures romantically in Foucault's early work, I also think that by drawing attention to those literary methods that reveal the sickness of language itself, Foucault manages to skirt around the accusation of a latent or not so latent romanticism.

22. *Oxford English Dictionary Online*, s.v. "clinical," http://dictionary.oed.com.

23. Ibid.

24. In "The Disappearance of the Sick Man from Medical Cosmology, 1770–1870," a classic text in medical sociology published in 1976, Nicholas Jewson describes three "medical cosmologies"—bedside medicine, hospital medicine, and laboratory medicine—and the historical shift between the dominance of one to the other. Other medical sociologists have since extended Jewson's cosmologies into the contemporary period by discussing various other cosmologies, including "surveillance medicine" and "e-scaped medicine." See Armstrong, "The Rise of Surveillance Medicine"; and Nettleton, "The Emergence of E-Scaped Medicine?" All of this work on shifts in medical practices and thought, including Foucault's, is indebted to the historicophilosophical work of Georges Canguilhem. Canguilhem diagnoses the shifts between several "points of view" or forms of medical perception: the physiological point of view, the statistical point of view, and the applied or public health point of view. As Canguilhem himself understood, such shifts are not simply epistemological but also ontological. See Canguilhem, *A Vital Rationalist*.

25. Collings, "General Practice in England Today."

26. Petchey, "Collings Report on General Practice in England in 1950." Petchey also rightly makes much of the massiveness of the article, which at thirty double-columned pages was an anomaly in scientific publishing, even at a time of less standardization of the scientific article form.

27. Petchey, "Collings Report on General Practice in England in 1950."
28. Collings, "General Practice in England Today," 555.
29. Ibid.
30. Ibid., 559.
31. Ibid., 560.
32. Ibid, 579.
33. Here, Collings's recommendations foreshadow the family practice movement that would begin in the 1960s as a response to years of decline in general practice in the United States. As Nicholas J. Pisacano, the first executive director of the American Board of Family Practice, has written, "The American Board of Family Practice was born many years before it was officially recognized in February, 1969 as the 20th primary medical specialty." "History of the Specialty." Pisacano and others have described family practice as a "revolutionary movement" that sought to overturn the increased specialization of medicine with, paradoxically, a new specialization in general medicine. For a fascinating account of the early years of the family practice revolution in the United States, see McPhee, "Heirs of General Practice." McPhee describes the reaction to the overspecialization in the U.S. health care system in the mid-1960s and says this "reaction became known as the family-practice movement. Its aim was to shift some of the emphasis in medicine, to give refreshed importance to generalism; and it arose . . . at a time when many people had come to distrust the pervasion of technology in every field from high-energy physics to superfast foods, and to look upon the dehumanization of medicine (a phrase much in vogue) as just one of a great number of unfortunate results" (110).
34. Collings, "General Practice in England Today," 566.
35. Armstrong calls this new medical thought style "biographical medicine," and he cites Michael Balint's *The Doctor, His Patient, and the Illness* as an important text exemplifying this thought style. *A Fortunate Man* could also be categorized as demonstrating biographical medicine by emphasizing the patient's biography and environment. See Armstrong, "The Emancipation of Biographical Medicine," 5. J. S. Huntley explains that Balint's work had a profound influence on Berger's conception of *A Fortunate Man*. "In search of *A Fortunate Man*," 547.
36. Later, Foucault will begin *Discipline and Punish* with another shocking image of a body and its treatments. That shocking image is of the public execution on March 2, 1757, of Damiens, the regicide, who is described as having "molten lead, boiling oil, burning resin, wax and sulphur" poured on his torn flesh before his body is "drawn and quartered by four horses and his limbs and body consumed by fire, reduced to ashes and his ashes thrown to the winds" (3). Interestingly, Foucault quotes from an article in the *Gazette d'Amsterdam*, in which the regicide is described as "the patient."

37. The patient does need to answer the question "Where does it hurt?" but of course, she might remain silent in response, answering the question by pointing. Foucault's point, however, is that the question signals an effacement of the patient's experience. The patient is reduced in this exchange to a collection of body parts, some of which might hurt. The quality of the hurt—its feeling for the patient—is less important than its location and visibility to the doctor. If the hurt cannot be seen by the doctor, the patient's report is not likely to give the hurt substance, at least not physiological or organic substance.

38. Recalling my opening snapshot juxtaposing Bordowitz's diagram *The Order of Image Production* and his concept "queer structures of feeling," Berger and Mohr's text might also be read in relation to a British cultural studies tradition beginning with Raymond Williams that combines a Marxist analysis of social structures with an investigation into less formal, more practical elements of consciousness that are "not yet recognized as social but taken to be private, idiosyncratic, and even isolating," what Williams calls "structures of feeling." *Marxism and Literature*, 132. For a Marxist reading of *A Fortunate Man*, see Hudson, "The Clerk of the Foresters Records." Hudson's reading of Sassall as an intellectual among the peasants has the unfortunate effect of heroicizing Sassall and objectifying his patients/the foresters. Another classic British cultural studies text that resonates with *A Fortunate Man* in interesting ways both theoretically and methodologically is Steedman, *Landscape for a Good Woman*. One reader of an earlier draft of this chapter noted that *A Fortunate Man* might be read as a nostalgic rendering of a disappearing form of doctoring exemplified in the figure of the country doctor. I think this is indeed the way the text is often read, and I appreciate my reader's astute assessment of the potentially conservative effects of nostalgia. Griffin's essay "The Fortunate Physician," for example, discusses the text as a tool utilized in a contemporary medical humanities workshop context to encourage doctors to talk about their feelings and explore the ways that contemporary medicine is dehumanizing for doctors as well as patients. Yet Berger, Mohr, and even Sassall himself work against this nostalgic view of the figure of the country doctor by challenging the simplistic idea of the rural idyll isolated from the time and place of postmodernity.

39. I gesture here to Althusser's "Ideology and Ideological State Apparatuses," in *Lenin and Philosophy and Other Essays*, partly to suggest his theories of subjectification as a link between Berger and Mohr's Marxist-inflected text and Foucault's protopoststructuralist text.

40. Armstrong, "Space and Time in British General Practice," 208.

41. Ibid., 213.

42. Ibid., 214.

43. As in my analysis of figures and forms of health activism in history in chapters 1 and 2, Scott's formulation of the echo is a key method-image for my analysis

of the clinic as event in history. See Scott, "Feminist Reverberations"; and "Fantasy Echo."

44. In her reading of Foucault's lectures on race and biopower, Ann Laura Stoler provides a brilliant summary of Foucault's method, which I am attempting to apply to his own *Birth of the Clinic* and *A Fortunate Man*. Stoler argues that in Foucault's analysis "the changing force of racial discourse is not understandable in terms of clean semantic breaks. Again, what occupies Foucault are the processes of recuperation, of the distillation of earlier discursive imprints, remodeled in new forms." *Race and the Education of Desire*, 68.

45. Diedrich, "Complexity and Cancer." I take the term "emergency of the long term" from Bindé, "Toward an Ethics of the Future."

46. Foucault, *The Birth of the Clinic*, 97.

47. Ibid., 101.

48. Ibid., 97.

49. Ibid., 108.

50. Ibid., 109.

51. Ibid.

52. Ibid., 114–15.

53. See Balint, *The Doctor, His Patient, and the Illness*.

54. For a genealogical discussion of this particular moment in the history of psychiatry, see Metzl, *Prozac on the Couch*. As his title suggests, Metzl argues that a psychoanalytic thought style still influences this new evidence-based era in psychiatry.

55. Foucault, *The Birth of the Clinic*, 198.

56. Ibid.

57. Ibid., 199.

58. I take the term "structural violence" from Paul Farmer, who defines this concept as "historically given (and often economically driven) processes and forces [that] conspire to constrain individual agency." *Infections and Inequalities*, 79.

59. Berger calls Sassall an "objective witness" to his patients' lives but thinks a humbler term is more fitting: "the clerk of their records" (109). In an essay on Berger's work, Robin Lippincott says that "witnessing" is one of Berger's favorite terms. "One Big Canvas," 134.

60. The real John Sassall would eventually commit suicide. In his fascinating article for the Literature and Medicine section of the *Lancet* entitled "In Search of *A Fortunate Man*," Huntley grapples with what he sees as the "apparent paradox" of Sassall's suicide. He concludes that the text itself bears witness to Sassall's place and life (549). I mention his death in the final note to this chapter to make a slightly different, if more banal, point, which is that who John Sassall really was, conclusively, is precisely what *A Fortunate Man* cannot give us. And it seems to

me that the title, as a kind of cliché, might be understood ironically as working to discourage such conclusive readings. Sassall's death by suicide is outside the story *A Fortunate Man* tells, but like Spencer Cox's death discussed earlier, it is another image of future (mental) illness that belies any easy interpretation of the temporal and spatial contours of a crisis.

Snapshot 3

1. The first edition of Delany's memoir was published by Arbor House, an imprint of William Morrow, in 1988. The original edition was subtitled *Sex and Science Fiction Writing in the East Village, 1957–1965*. When the University of Minnesota Press reprinted the book in 1993 and again in 2004, the dates were cut from the subtitle. Delany did not significantly revise the text, although the numbers (some with decimal points) Delany used to organize the text were reduced, creating longer "chapters" and less numerical cuts in the narrative. Subsequent references are to the 2004 edition and are cited parenthetically in the text.

2. See especially José Esteban Muñoz's elegant reading of the centrality of Delany's experience of Kaprow's happening to the form and content of *The Motion of Light in Water* in *Cruising Utopia*, 50–52.

3. Scott, "The Evidence of Experience." Scott's essay cites the 1988 edition of *Motion of Light in Water: Sex and Science Fiction Writing in the East Village, 1957–1965* (New York: Arbor House, 1988).

4. Or in Foucault's oft-cited words: "The nineteenth-century homosexual became a personage, a past, a case history, and a childhood, in addition to being a type of life, a life form, and a morphology, with an indiscreet anatomy and possibly a mysterious physiology." *The History of Sexuality*, vol. 1, 43.

5. For more on the frequent readings and misreadings of Scott's essay, see Hesford and Diedrich, "Experience, Echo, Event"; and "On 'The Evidence of Experience' and Its Reverberations."

6. Scott, "The Evidence of Experience," 774, quoting Delany, *Motion of Light in Water* (1988), 173.

7. Ibid.

8. The person whose recollections most frequently triangulate Delany's own is Marilyn Hacker. Hacker's recollections are presented in both prose and poetic form, as *The Motion of Light in Water* includes poems Hacker wrote during the period they lived together on the Lower East Side.

9. Scott, "The Evidence of Experience," 775.

10. In her fascinating work historicizing the emergence of the happening out of the coupling of theater and action painting, Judith Rodenbeck argues that desubjectification was at work in happenings: "These works figured participants—*and*

attention *and* senses—as objects, collage elements, exchangeable tokens." "Madness and Method," 60.

11. Foucault, "Nietzsche, Genealogy, History," in *Language, Counter-memory, Practice*, 153.

4. Thinking Ecologically, circa 1962 and 1971

1. In my attempt to bring together the ecological and the conceptual, I am indebted to both Morton, *The Ecological Thought*, and Code, *Ecological Thinking*. Morton brilliantly elucidates what "ecological thought," as object, might be, and by materializing both sides of the human/nature binary, he elegantly challenges romantic notions of humans, nature, and the ecological. Nonetheless, I find my tongue tripping on the definite article and noun phrase of "the ecological thought," as asserted in the opening statement of the book: "The ecological crisis we face is so obvious that it becomes easy—for some, strangely or frighteningly easy—to join the dots and see that everything is interconnected. This is *the ecological thought*. And the more we consider it, the more our world opens up" (1). Although I prefer Code's phrase "ecological thinking" to Morton's "the ecological thought," by inverting "ecological thinking" into "thinking ecologically," I turn a noun phrase into a verb phrase, emphasizing process over product.

2. Thomas, *The Lives of the Cell*; and *The Medusa and the Snail*. Further references will be cited parenthetically in text.

3. For the significance of *Silent Spring* at fifty, see, for example, Nixon, "Rachel Carson's Prescience." Sandra Steingraber, who like Carson is a biologist and cancer survivor, offers an example of how contemporary scientists and thinkers draw on Carson's legacy, in this case to make an argument against the twenty-first-century practice of fracking. "The Fracking of Rachel Carson."

4. Code cites Linda Lear's biography of Carson, which traces a genealogy of ecological thinking in Carson's work as far back as the 1940s, even though this approach was not common to wildlife science at the time. *Ecological Thinking*, 25–26. See Lear, *Rachel Carson*, 132. Code also cites Sharon Kingsland's history of ecology, *Modeling Nature*, and Raymond Williams's engagement with the history of the term *ecology* in *Keywords*, as well as Deleuze's uses of the related concept of ethology in *Spinoza*. Interestingly, although Code appreciatively reads the work of Deleuze and Guattari on the formation of concepts in her introduction, when she discusses ecological aspects of their work, Guattari no longer figures, thus repeating a recurring habit in philosophy of disappearing Guattari from the work of Deleuze and Guattari, which I think functions in general to recapture Deleuze for philosophy with an effect of depoliticizing his (and Guattari's) work. This is especially surprising because Guattari explicitly takes up the ecological and what he

called "ecosophy" in his later work without Deleuze, *Three Ecologies*. My thinking on philosophy's capture of Deleuze (minus Guattari) has benefited from conversations with Briana Martino. For a fascinating account of the "ecological consciousness" of thinkers associated with the mass protests of 1968, including Guattari, see Conley, *Ecopolitics*.

    5. Code, *Ecological Thinking*, 14.

    6. Ibid., 15.

    7. Friedan, *The Feminine Mystique*. Friedan's essay opens, "The problem lay buried, unspoken, for many years in the minds of American women" (15).

    8. For a fascinating review of the reviews of *Silent Spring*, see Smith, "'Silence, Miss Carson!'" Smith notes that "the most sexist, most unbalanced review of *Silent Spring* appeared in *Chemical and Engineering News* in October 1962, shortly after the publication of the book. William Darby of the Vanderbilt University School of Medicine attacked Carson from the first paragraph of his review, entitled 'Silence, Miss Carson!' The title itself (which the journal later admitted was its own creation, not Darby's) expresses the prevailing attitude among many of Carson's critics that she was an uninformed woman who was speaking of that which she knew not. Worse, she was speaking in a man's world, the inner sanctum of masculine science in which, like the sanctuary of a strict Calvinist sect, female silence was expected" (172).

    9. For an excellent online discussion of the reception of *Silent Spring*, see Mark Stoll's virtual exhibition entitled *Rachel Carson's "Silent Spring," a Book That Changed the World*. Spinsters figure in both positive and negative reviews of *Silent Spring*. In her biography of Carson, Lear describes in detail the attacks on Carson, including from former agriculture secretary Ezra Taft Benson, who wondered "why a spinster was so worried about genetics." *Rachel Carson*, 429. A positive review in the *American Institute of Biological Science Bulletin* ends with the rather bizarre story of a "spinster in Los Angeles" who "indignantly called the Air Pollution Control office, asking why they did not stop the smog, for her poor canary was dying herself. Heroically she added that she herself was dying, too, but that did not matter." Went, "Review of *Silent Spring*," 42. Went calls upon us "not to emulate the attitude of the spinster" and her canary, which is especially ironic if we think of Carson as spinster as dying canary.

    10. Ferguson, "Review of *Silent Spring* by Rachel Carson," 208.

    11. Egler, "Pesticides—In Our Ecosystem," 116.

    12. The term "normal science," of course, comes from Thomas Kuhn's *The Structure of Scientific Revolutions*, which, like Carson's *Silent Spring*, was first published in 1962. Although it isn't clear that Egler and Kuhn were familiar with each other's work, they were both early proponents of taking science, scientific practices, and scientists and their communities as objects of study.

13. Frank Egler to Rachel Carson, June 6, 1962, box 84, folder 1461, Rachel Carson Papers, Beinecke Library, Yale University.

14. Ibid.

15. Ibid.

16. Ibid (emphases in original).

17. In his Findings column for the *New York Times,* conservative writer John Tierney argues that the *Bulletin*'s and Baldwin's review of *Silent Spring* offered real science, whereas Carson presented a "hodgepodge of science and junk science." "Fateful Voice of a Generation Still Drowns Out Real Science." Tierney portrays Baldwin as a heroic leader of a group of scientists studying the impact of pesticides on wildlife. In keeping with his overall tone of "everything was fine until that silly woman butted in," Tierney offers this nugget of revisionist history (contained so neatly and assuredly in a brief parenthetical): "(Yes, scientists were worried about pesticides long before *Silent Spring.*)"

18. Frank Egler to the Letters Department at *Science,* October 3, 1962, box 84, folder 1462, Rachel Carson Papers, Beinecke Library, Yale University.

19. Frank E. Egler, "The N.A.S.-N.R.C. in Defense of the Pesticide Industry," manuscript, box 84, folder 1462, Rachel Carson Papers, Beinecke Library, Yale University.

20. Frank Egler to Rachel Carson, April 4, 1963, box 84, folder 1465, Rachel Carson Papers, Beinecke Library, Yale University. For a more detailed description of Carson's triumph on *CBS Reports,* see Lear's account in *Rachel Carson,* 449–50. According to Lear, "It would have been a masterful performance even if there had been no one else to compare her to, but in juxtaposition to the wild-eyed, loud-voiced Dr. Robert White-Stevens in white lab coat, Carson appeared anything but the hysterical alarmist that her critics contended" (449).

21. Nixon, *Slow Violence and the Environmentalism of the Poor,* ix.

22. In Nixon's wonderfully succinct terms, Carson is an "insurrectionary generalist" and a "renegade synthesizer." *Slow Violence and the Environmentalism of the Poor,* xi.

23. Lutts, "Chemical Fallout."

24. Ibid., 212.

25. Berlant, "Slow Death," 759. Berlant poses the environment as different temporally from the event. I very much appreciate Berlant's analysis, although I continue to use the term *event* not or not only to describe crises but with a more expansive temporality in mind.

26. Nixon, *Slow Violence and the Environmentalism of the Poor,* 9–10.

27. Povinelli, *Ethics of Abandonment,* 120.

28. Murphy, *Sick Building Syndrome and the Problem of Uncertainty,* 10. Murphy brilliantly tracks how both imperceptibility and perceptibility—seeing and

not seeing, knowing and not knowing—is produced in the case of the emergent illnesses of late capitalism: sick building syndrome and multiple chemical sensitivity.

29. One favorable reviewer writes, "Some of the most interesting material in this book is contained in the later chapters which deal with energy transformations and metabolic cycles in the cell. Miss Carson relates pesticide function to cellular physiology and builds a fascinating hypothetical relationship between cancer and pesticides." Thompson, "Review of *Silent Spring* by Rachel Carson," 107.

30. In *The Sea around Us,* Carson discusses ecological evidence, which she describes as both "the testimony of the earth's most ancient rocks" and the "indirect evidence we may infer that life existed in some abundance before its record was written in the rocks" (3). In her work on the sea, Carson posits what she calls a "material immortality," noting, "Nothing is wasted in the sea; every particle of material is used over and over again, first by one creature, then by another" (30).

31. Murphy, *Sick Building Syndrome and the Problem of Uncertainty,* 91.

32. Ibid., 92.

33. As I will discuss in more detail in chapter 6, thorazine, the first antipsychotic drug, was introduced in 1955 and would be one of the key factors in the deinstitutionalization and neoliberalization of mental health care. In the same year that thorazine became available for clinical use, the Cancer Chemotherapy National Service Center was also established. DeVita and Chu, "A History of Cancer Chemotherapy."

34. In a letter to Beverly Knecht, a young artist and would-be writer who corresponded extensively with Carson in the late 1950s and who was blind and diabetic, Carson enthusiastically recommends vitamin therapies, writing: "From sources other than Dr. Biskind, I have recently become aware of the wonderful properties of Vitamin C in combatting infection and aiding in the repair and healing of tissues. In fact, I gave it a trial myself this winter, when I had grown tired of a long persisting sinus infection. My specialist's treatments were only temporarily helpful, and the same could be said of the antibiotics he prescribed. When he began to talk of more drastic procedures, I decided I would listen to the advice of friends who had tried it, and began taking large quantities of Vitamin C. Almost immediately there was improvement. My specialist was able to discharge me and I have had no need to return to him. This was some six weeks ago. I suppose I cheated a little in that I did not tell him what I had done on the side, but just smiled to myself when he commented on the remarkable change in the appearance of the mucous membranes. Probably I should tell him." Rachel Carson to Beverly Knecht, March 8, 1959, box 103, folder 1957, Rachel Carson Papers, Beinecke Library, Yale University.

35. Gammon et al. "The Long Island Breast Cancer Study Project"; "Environmental Toxins and Breast Cancer on Long Island. I."; and "Environmental Toxins and Breast Cancer on Long Island. II." The three articles articulate the "moments"

of emergence very similarly, which is not surprising considering that the same people wrote all three articles, although "The Long Island Breast Cancer Study Project," which introduces the multi-institutional collaborative study, provides more extensive background information than the other two about the political and scientific factors that led to the studies.

36. Thanks go to Emily Boyce for her extensive review of the literature on the enactment of the multiple object "breast cancer on Long Island." For further analysis of this enactment, see Diedrich and Boyce, "'Breast Cancer on Long Island.'"

37. See, for example, Ferraro, "The Anguished Politics of Breast Cancer."

38. Thomas, *The Lives of a Cell*, 3. Thomas's essay "The Lives of a Cell" was first published in the *New England Journal of Medicine* on May 13, 1971. My quotations are from the collection of these essays published in 1974 and hereafter will appear parenthetically in the text.

39. Thomas, *The Youngest Science*, 10. Citations hereafter will appear parenthetically in the text.

40. For work "against health," see, for example, Metzl and Kirkland, eds., *Against Health.*

Snapshot 4

1. For a fascinating discussion of Fanon at Blida, from one of Julien's interviewees, an Algerian who worked with Fanon as an intern at Blida in 1956–57 and is now a psychoanalyst, see Cherki, *Frantz Fanon.* For a comprehensive biography of Fanon, see Macey, *Frantz Fanon.*

2. Foucault, *History of Madness*, 464.

3. Julien and Nash, "Fanon as Film," 15. Many of the themes that Julien and Nash discuss in this essay were first addressed in an interview with Julien by Coco Fusco. See Fusco, "Visualizing Theory."

4. The text was first published in French in 1961 and translated into English in 1963 as part of *The Wretched of the Earth* by Constance Farrington. Recently, Richard Philcox has provided a new translation, with a foreword by Homi K. Bhabha. Citations here are from the 1963 English translation and will be made, heretofore, parenthetically in the text.

5. For an insightful account of Fanon as "clinician and revolutionary," see Keller, "Clinician and Revolutionary."

6. In her book about the Black Panther Party's social health work, Nelson notes that the "ideas of Ernesto 'Che' Guevara, Mao Zedong, and Frantz Fanon provided a conceptual bridge between the Party's political philosophy, its community service ethos, and its health politics. These theorists' influence could be seen in how the Party afforded an integral role to medicine in its imagination of a 'robust' social body: in its valorization of lay expertise, in its critique of 'bourgeois'

healthcare and medical power, and in its aim to foster medicine for and by 'the people.'" *Body and Soul,* 17.

7. In his preface to Fanon's text, Sartre writes, "The status of 'native' is a nervous condition introduced and maintained by the settler among colonized people *with their consent.*" Sartre, preface to Fanon, *The Wretched of the Earth,* 20. Tsitsi Dangarembga uses the first part of Sartre's sentence as an epigraph for her novel *Nervous Conditions* about colonialism in Rhodesia. She doesn't name Sartre as the author of the epigraph but only mentions that the words are from a preface to Fanon's *Wretched of the Earth,* thus willfully obscuring Sartre's role in introducing Fanon to a European readership.

8. Julien and Nash, "Fanon as Film," 14.

9. For a recent film that also works to give substance to Fanon's ideas and words, see Göran Olsson's *Concerning Violence* (2014), which mixes a reading of Fanon's text "Concerning Violence" by American singer Lauryn Hill with images from the Swedish film archive of liberation struggles from colonialism in Africa in the 1960s and 1970s. Hill gives voice to Fanon's words, which are often, at the same time, typed across the screen. The spoken words are materialized as word images, creating a kind of echo between voice and text on screen.

10. Julien and Nash, "Fanon as Film," 16.

11. Ibid., 15.

12. Fusco, "Visualizing Theory," 57.

13. Fuss, *Identification Papers,* 162.

14. Ibid.

15. Ibid., 164.

16. Fusco, "Visualizing Theory," 55.

5. Drawing Epilepsy

1. The term *graphic medicine* was first coined by the general practitioner and graphic artist Ian Williams as the name for a website he created in 2007, and since then many other discourses, genres, and practices of graphic medicine have arisen or been identified as operating *avant la lettre.* Along with Ian Williams, feminist science studies scholar and critical theorist Susan Squier and nurse and comics artist MK Czerwiec have been at the forefront of the project of graphic medicine. They are the authors, along with Michael J. Green, Kimberly R. Myers, and Scott T. Smith, of *Graphic Medicine Manifesto.*

2. David B., *Epileptic.* The text's original French title is *L'ascension du hautmal,* which translates as *The climb of the high sickness.* Translating this richly metaphorical phrase into *Epileptic* risks reducing a complex experience to an illness identity category. Subsequent references are cited parenthetically in the text.

3. Foucault, "Of Other Spaces." "Of Other Spaces" is a translation of "Des es-

paces autres," first published in the journal *Architecture-mouvement-continuité* in October 1984. The text comes from a manuscript of a lecture Foucault gave to a group of architects in Paris in 1967. At the time, Foucault was living and teaching in Tunisia, and his own movement between France and Tunisia seems important in his formulation of the concept. In his lecture he describes colonies as heterotopias of compensation: "Their role is to create a space that is other, another real space, as meticulous, as well arranged as ours is messy, ill constructed, and jumbled" (27).

4. Chute, "Review of *Our Cancer Year, Janet and Me, Cancer Vixen, Mom's Cancer, Blue Pills, Epileptic,* and *Black Hole,*" 414. Chute identifies Justin Green's *Binky Brown Meets the Holy Virgin Mary* from 1972 as "widely identified by cartoonists and scholars as the first autobiographical work in the form of comics"; as a story about masturbation and obsessive-compulsive disorder, Green's *Binky Brown* also brings together the domains of mental illness and sexuality (414).

5. Eisner, *Comics and Sequential Art,* 39.

6. Foucault, *Psychiatric Power,* 305.

7. Ibid., 325n18.

8. Ibid., 310.

9. Deleuze and Guattari, *Kafka,* 53.

10. Massumi, "Notes on the Translation and Acknowledgments," in Deleuze and Guattari, *A Thousand Plateaus,* xvi.

11. Deleuze and Guattari, *A Thousand Plateaus,* 13.

12. The character Pierre-François is based on the author/graphic memoirist David B. As the text depicts, in 1970 Pierre-François decides to change his name from Pierre-François to David after learning that his mother almost named him David but decided against that name because her father thought it "sounded too Jewish" (170). David B. explains the name change as a symbolic act suggesting he has "won the war" and "prevailed over the disease," linking the overcoming of epilepsy with the overcoming of antisemitism (165). For Pierre-François, becoming-David is also a kind of becoming-Jewish and the beginnings, perhaps, of his becoming-writer. His mother tells him that "all the best writers are Jewish . . . or homosexual" and admits she "would've liked to be Jewish." David B. speculates that this actually means she wanted to be a great writer (174). Here, becoming-Jewish or becoming-homosexual are creative routes out of the stigmatization of the categories Jew and homosexual. David B. seems to want to suggest various modes of challenging stigmatization, including becoming-epileptic. The text does not provide an explanation for the author's shortening of his family name, Beauchard, to B., but its anonymizing effect is interesting in relation to the impact of both his drawing and his brother's epilepsy on his family.

13. Engel, "The Need for a New Medical Model."

14. *Biocultural* has recently been taken up as a term for signaling the hybridity

of most medical—and for that matter, human—experience. Although I appreciate the work a term like *biocultural* does (and see my work aligned with many of those affiliated with Lennard Davis's Project Biocultures), I think the discordant effects of speaking the neologism *biopsychosocial* demonstrates something of the force of inclusions and exclusions operating between biological, psychological, and social domains. My point is not that these are, in fact, separate domains but that the boundaries between each are policed and contested. Many people have an interest in either maintaining or breaking down these boundaries. For information about Project Biocultures, see www.biocultures.org.

15. Engel, "The Need for a New Medical Model," 129.

16. Ibid., 131.

17. Ibid., 132.

18. Ibid., 135.

19. In his discussion of Guattari's concept and practice of transversality, Genosko explains that Guattari replaced transference with transversality partly because, in Guattari's estimation, transference was "an effect contributing to guruism in psychoanalysis." "The Life and Work of Félix Guattari," 49.

20. The phrase "path of escape in all its positivity" comes from Deleuze and Guattari's analysis of becoming-animal as a challenge to Oedipalization in Kafka's work. *Kafka,* 13.

21. Chute argues that in *Epileptic* "illness is materialized as a character, a physicality sometimes contiguous with, but *outside,* the body, that must be reckoned with; it is shown, in one instance, as physically taking up residence, sitting at the kitchen table." "Review of *Our Cancer Year, Janet and Me, Cancer Vixen, Mom's Cancer, Blue Pills, Epileptic,* and *Black Hole,*" 423.

22. The terms "logic of choice" and "logic of care" are from Mol, *The Logic of Care.* I discuss the impact of these different logics on clinical practice and make an argument that the counterlogic of care is queer in these neoliberal times in chapter 2.

23. Cooper, *Psychiatry and Anti-psychiatry,* 23.

24. Deleuze, *Two Regimes of Madness,* 25.

25. Ibid., 27.

26. Roger Gentis is a psychiatrist who trained at Saint-Alban with François Tosquelles and, like Guattari, participated in the institutional psychotherapy movement. He is the author of several books, including *Traite de psychiatrie provisoire* (*Manual of provisional psychiatry*), *Leçons du corps* (*Lessons of the body*), and *Guérir la vie* (*Curing life*). For interviews with Gentis and others about institutional psychiatry and the La Borde Clinic, see www.cliniquedelaborde.com.

27. Goffman, *Stigma.* Goffman discusses what he calls "the wise": "namely, persons who are normal but whose special situation has made them intimately privy to the secret life of the stigmatized individual and sympathetic with it" (28). One "type of wise person is the individual who is related through the social structure to

a stigmatized individual—a relationship that leads the wider society to treat both individuals in some respects as one" (30).

28. Berger and Mohr, *A Fortunate Man*, 50.

29. Florence, the youngest of the three, who appears in many of the childhood adventures depicted by David B., seems to have taken a somewhat different path from her brothers'. When David B. says that, for him, drawing is his armor (151), he also explains that Florence "has no armor" (152). Moreover, David B. tells us she is the only member of the family not interested in esoterism, which provides another kind of armor for the family. There are signs in the text of mental illness, and an older Florence discussing her younger self pinpoints "the moment her sadness began" and admits, echoing Jean-Christophe's own developmental stasis, "I never got out of that period" (161). We are told that in writing Florence is able to explore her feelings, and she is the author of the two texts that frame David B.'s graphic narrative—a foreword from 1996 and an afterword from 2003. Although we might read Florence's framing texts as an alternative or supplement to David B.'s representation of Jean-Christophe's epilepsy, her account functions more to give credence to David B.'s story than to challenge or expand it. In the next chapter, I discuss two different texts by daughters of a woman with schizophrenia that, although obviously connected in profound and banal ways, nonetheless reveal divergent investments in the stories we tell of others.

30. It is interesting in this regard to consider the figurative meaning of the verb *doctor*: "to treat so as to alter the appearance, flavour, or character of; to disguise, falsify, tamper with, adulterate, sophisticate, 'cook.'" *Oxford English Dictionary Online*, s.v. "doctor," http://www.oed.com.

Snapshot 5

1. Disability Law Center, "Report on Investigation of Bridgewater State Hospital," 1. A similar investigation by the U.S. Attorney in Manhattan has been conducted recently at Rikers Island correctional facility in New York and finds a "deep-seated culture of violence" there. In particular, the report focuses on the treatment of adolescents and finds that the "New York City Department of Correction systematically has failed to protect adolescent inmates from harm in violation of the Eight Amendment and the Due Process Clause of the Fourteenth Amendment of the United States Constitution. This harm is the result of the repeated use of excessive and unnecessary force by correction officers against adolescent inmates, as well as high levels of inmate-on-inmate violence." Office of Preet Bharara, "Civil Rights of Institutionalized Persons Act (CRIPA) Investigation of the New York City Department of Corrections Jails on Rikers Island."

2. Disability Law Center, "Report on Investigation of Bridgewater State Hospital," 2.

3. Disability Law Center, "Report on Investigation of Bridgewater State Hospital," 3. Bridgewater is administered by the Massachusetts Department of Corrections. Such an arrangement is not typical; only one other state, Iowa, has such an arrangement. According to the Massachusetts State Government's Official Website of the Executive Office of Public Safety and Security, men who have been charged with or convicted of a crime or who have been determined to be "in need of strict security because of the potential for endangering themselves or others" are sent to Bridgewater State Hospital. See Official Website of the Executive Office of Public Safety and Security, "Bridgewater State Hospital," www.mass.gov/eopss/law-enforce-and-cj/prisons/doc-facilities/bridgewater-state-hospital.html. Advocates for people with mental illness note that in many instances men who are held at Bridgewater have not actually been charged with a crime.

4. Disability Law Center, "Report on Investigation of Bridgewater State Hospital," 3.

5. Ibid., 4.

6. Goffman, *Asylums*, 12.

7. Anderson and Benson, *Documentary Dilemmas*, 1.

8. Scott, *The Fantasy of Feminist History*, 54.

9. Ibid.

10. For example, Dr. Ross tells Vladimir that if he is not being truthful, then Vladimir can "spit on my face," to which Vladimir responds, "Why would I do that?"

11. Anderson and Benson's important book on the making of *Titicut Follies* and the legal and ethical fallout regarding the question of whether Wiseman had obtained informed consent to film various patients and staff at Bridgewater documents how Vladimir attempted to use the filmmakers: "This subject realized his reproduction on celluloid was something valuable to a filmmaker; it was a commodity to be negotiated. He did not sign a release; yet his frustrated attempts for a transfer from Bridgewater did become a central part of *Titicut Follies*. Vladimir's story is a capsule version of the complexity of the consent dilemma." *Documentary Dilemmas*, 25.

12. Goffman, *Asylums*, 45.

13. For a full transcript of *Titicut Follies*, see Grant, *Five Films by Frederick Wiseman*.

14. Goffman, *Asylums*, 16.

6. Witnessing Schizophrenia

1. Available from Vine Street Pictures, P.O. Box 662120, Los Angeles, CA 90066; for information about purchasing, go to www.outoftheshadow.com.

2. Kotulski, *Saving Millie*. Subsequent references to this text appear in the text.

3. Foucault, *The History of Madness* and *Mental Illness and Psychology*. This

text has been reissued in an English edition entitled *Madness: The Invention of an Idea.*

4. Foucault, *The Government of the Self and Others,* 20–21; and "What Is Enlightenment?" in *Ethics,* 315.

5. Foucault, *Psychiatric Power.*

6. Ibid., 161.

7. Ibid., 54.

8. At the end of *Out of Shadow,* describing her job at a fast food sandwich chain, Mildred tells Susan, "I love work. It's normal people. The bus [she takes to get to work] is normal people. You're normal people."

9. When the film was shown on PBS in October 2006, it was reviewed in the *New York Times* utilizing the clichés of an "overcoming adversity" narrative. Mildred is described as a "true heroine," who "undergoes a transformation, metamorphosing from a minimally functioning mental patient into a loving grandmother. For all their tribulations, the Smileys have something to smile about." Stewart, "A Mother in Shades of Gray, Love, Schizophrenia and All."

10. Guattari, *Chaosophy,* 189.

11. Shadows are also a prominent feature in David B.'s *Epileptic,* where the figures on the page are often drawn emerging out of a flat black background. In her foreword David B.'s sister Florence speaks directly to her brother to say, "You've laid down, in the panels of this book, the shadows of our childhood" (1).

12. Swartz, foreword to Kotulski, *Saving Millie,* xi.

13. For an account of the shift from the dominance of psychoanalytic to biological thought styles in psychiatry, see Metzl, *Prozac on the Couch* and *The Protest Psychosis.* For a compelling critique of the new biological psychiatry, see Lewis, *Moving beyond Prozac, "DSM," and the New Psychiatry.*

14. Foucault, *History of Madness,* 464.

15. For historical accounts and critiques of the practice of deinstitutionalization, see Torrey, *Nowhere to Go* and *Out of the Shadows*; Grob, *From Asylum to Community* and "Deinstitutionalization." In *Out of the Shadows,* Torrey argues that "deinstitutionalization began in 1955 with the widespread introduction of chlorpromazine, commonly known as Thorazine, the first antipsychotic medication, and received a major impetus 10 years later with the enactment of federal Medicaid and Medicare" (8). Torrey calls deinstitutionalization "one of the largest social experiments in American history" (8).

16. There is some confusion between Smiley's film and Kotulski's memoir as to when exactly Mildred Smiley was finally diagnosed with paranoid schizophrenia. In *Out of the Shadow,* Susan's voice-over notes that Mildred was diagnosed after Tina was placed under the care of a psychiatrist after her suicide attempt in 1979. In *Saving Millie,* Kotulski gives a much more detailed account of the relief she felt when Mildred's condition was finally named paranoid schizophrenia in 1985.

17. Recall my discussion in chapter 3 of the changing definition of the term *clinical*. The most recent meaning, in use from the mid-twentieth century, is "coldly detached and dispassionate, like a medical report or examination; diagnostic or therapeutic, like medical investigation or treatment; treating a subject-matter as if it were a case of disease, especially with close attention to detail; serving as part of a case-study." *Oxford English Dictionary Online*, s.v. "clinical," http://dictionary.oed.com.

18. Smiley's work exemplifies the three levels of witnessing that Dori Laub has identified in relation to the Holocaust experience: "the level of being a witness to oneself within the experience; the level of being a witness to the testimonies of others; and the level of being a witness to the process of witnessing itself." "An Event without a Witness," 75.

19. This relates to the discussion in chapter 5 about the difficulty of discerning true from false convulsions. Elsewhere, I have described the constitutive link between lying and the social position of the patient and the many reasons a patient might lie: "They lie to themselves out of fear and as a form of hope; they lie to their loved ones in order to make them (their loved ones) feel better; they lie to others to avoid the stigma and shame attached to many illnesses; they lie to doctors, nurses, and other health care practitioners because they want to be seen as good (read: compliant) patients, or because they want to be eligible to receive certain treatments." Diedrich, "Lying and the Performance of Patienthood," 133. It is also the case that patients are frequently lied to, for many of the same reasons.

20. In her review Stewart critiques the film for its ineffective challenge to the public health system: "The villain of 'Shadow' is the vast and anonymous system that shuttles this woman from one psychiatrist to another without continuity of care or consistency in medication. Health care is an easy target, and 'Shadow' is stronger when it's not tilting at institutional windmills." If health care is such an easy target, then why is taking it on likened to "tilting at institutional windmills"? And what a fascinating choice of idiom to describe what the film is doing.

21. Thanks go to Victoria Hesford for pointing this out to me.

22. Foucault, *Psychiatric Power*, 236.

23. Ibid.

24. Ibid., 237.

25. The first page of the record of Mildred Smiley's stay at Hinsdale Sanitarium and Hospital in 1983 is shown at the beginning of *Out of the Shadow*, but unless one stops the film and reads the text of the medical record, its specific contents remain difficult to discern. Other medical records are also shown in the film, which are scanned and have phrases and partial sentences highlighted for the viewer's perusal, including, for example, "The patient was in total rage" and "homeless, was very paranoid."

26. One of the curious things about Kotulski's memoir is that in most of the

instances in which Mildred is quoted, the quotes come from Smiley's film. In a way this is another kind of witnessing—Kotulski extends Smiley's witnessing in the film by incorporating elements of the film into her own text.

27. Except perhaps in one scene where Smiley and camera follow along as Millie goes to refill her many prescriptions at the pharmacy. In this scene she seems uncomfortable, though it is hard to say whether the discomfort is with being filmed or with having to refill her prescriptions or a combination of the two: being captured on film refilling prescriptions. The one person we see who does not want to be filmed and, indeed, seems a little paranoid about the prospects of being filmed is one of the doctors reviewing Mildred's application for the group home. When Susan tries to film a conversation she has with him, he tells her to turn off the camera. Obviously, there are issues of patient confidentiality at stake, but one of the effects of the more stringent health care confidentiality laws is that they prevent certain kinds of qualitative study of the impact of particular health policies and practices on people who are ill.

28. It is possible that Smiley has edited out footage in which Millie makes it apparent that she doesn't want to be filmed, but even if this were the case, I'm not sure it would call into question the impression that Mildred likes being in front of the camera. In a later addition to the website for the film, Smiley has added a note about the making of the film, which addresses directly the question of Mildred Smiley's consent: "I would not, or could not have made the film without my mother's unequivocal consent and support." Susan Smiley, *Out of the Shadow* website, accessed June 17, 2009, http://www.outoftheshadow.com/about_susan_family.html.

Afterimage

1. From the *New Sydenham Society Lexicon* from 1879 as cited in *Oxford English Dictionary Online*, s.v. "afterimage," www.oed.com.

2. As I was working on this conclusion, I presented some of this material at the Society for Science, Literature, and Arts Conference in October 2014. Karen Barad delivered one of the keynotes at that conference, "Shifting Sands of Time," and her presentation resonated with what I am doing in this chapter in particular and the book more generally. To attempt to get around a binary that would argue things are either continuous or discontinuous, she argued for a concept and method that emphasized dis/continuity, which suggests both cut and link, a both/and concept and method that runs throughout *Indirect Action*. In response to a question about scale, she also said we need to unthink what we have learned about the distinctions between micro and macro. In her view scale itself is performative, meaning that scale is not already there, prior to our determinations of its workings. According to Barad, measurements are intra-actions, and they make worlds, across multiple spaces and times.

3. Here, I gesture to the work of Elizabeth Povinelli, especially *Events of Abandonment*.

4. See also Smith and Siplon, *Drugs into Bodies*.

5. Lyotard's concept of the differend is useful for thinking about a certain incommensurability between different "mode[s] of presenting a universe" that are not translatable from one "phrase regimen" to the next. Lyotard, *The Differend*, 128.

6. Guattari, *Chaosophy*, 189.

7. Brier, *Infectious Ideas*, 168.

8. I formulate this as an equation to echo that other AIDS activist equation, Silence = Death.

9. Kane Race's *Pleasure Consuming Medicine* informs my analysis here. Race discusses multiple practices of drug use, offering a savvy biocultural analysis of what drugs do and why people do them. He describes the emergence of neoliberal discourses of drug use and misuse and the possibility of counterpublics queering these dominant discourses.

10. Like Brier and also citing Gould's important work on ACT UP, Duberman discusses the growing "rift over priorities" in ACT UP. According to Duberman, "Some members insisted that ACT UP's prime goal of speeding up medical research and getting more 'drugs into bodies' should remain its singular focus. Others remained committed to the more expansive social agenda of combatting sexism, racism, and classism within ACT UP itself and in the culture at large." *Hold Tight Gently*, 188. See also Gould, *Moving Politics*, 285–86. Duberman notes the contrasting priorities generally pitted the Treatment and Data Committee against the Majority Action Committee, the Women's Caucus, and the Housing Committee (which would eventually break from ACT UP to form Housing Works) (191–92).

11. Duberman, *Hold Tight Gently*, 228.

12. Ibid.; emphasis in original.

13. For a discussion of the controversies surrounding AIDS causation, including Sonnabend's ecological immune-overload theory, see Epstein, *Impure Science*. Epstein also includes a chapter titled "Drugs into Bodies," focusing on the first two years of ACT UP's existence, 1987 and 1988. After HIV was identified as the virus that caused AIDS, Sonnabend and Callen would be associated with what would come to be called dissident theories of AIDS causation. Duberman is emphatic that neither Sonnabend nor Callen denied that HIV caused AIDS; nonetheless, they argued that other factors were crucial in the spread of AIDS. In his brilliant analysis of Thabo Mbeki's alliance with HIV dissident scientists, Didier Fassin doesn't simply reject Mbeki's stance out of hand but tries "to grasp the particular rationality of Mbeki's thinking, suggesting a sociological interpretation of the epidemic," by seeking "a kind of third way, a means of making biological and social

theories compatible, as was done more than a century ago for tuberculosis." *When Bodies Remember*, 15. This also relates to Paul Farmer's delineation of structural violence as a key factor in the cause of AIDS in *Infections and Inequalities*.

14. Wojnarowicz quoted in Guattari, "David Wojnarowicz."

15. The full list of the cast for the film on IMDb names everyone identified in the film in both archival and present-day footage, beginning, in order of appearance, with Ed Koch, former Mayor of New York. See IMDb's for the cast and crew of *How to Survive a Plague* at http://www.imdb.com/title/tt2124803/fullcredits. Only a few women are named, and even fewer people of color are named. Yet the impression from some of the archival footage of meetings and protests is of a diverse mix of activists, and it isn't that there are no women or people of color in the film—ACT UP member Ann Northrop is shown in archival footage and interviewed in the near present; scientist and ACT UP member Iris Long figures prominently in interviews with Treatment and Data Committee (T&D) members; Garance Franke-Ruta, one of the few women in T&D, also appears in footage from the past and present; and Ray Navarro appears as Jesus Christ at ACT UP's Stop the Church demonstration and with his loving mother as he is dying. Nonetheless, the white guys in the T&D dominate the interviews and archival screen time. It really is their story.

16. Description found at the official *How to Survive a Plague* website at http://surviveaplague.com.

17. Barad, "Shifting Sands of Time."

18. For an example of an artist whose film work attempts to make visible and provide a meditation on the evidence of experience, see Sharon Hayes's work, including her exhibition at the Whitney Museum entitled *There's So Much More I Want to Say to You*, especially the film project *Gay Power (2007–2012)*.

19. I say "at the time of the making of the film" because, as I discussed at the end of the snapshot of Bordowitz's work, Spencer Cox, one of the people interviewed for *How to Survive a Plague*, would die not long after the release of the film from complications of AIDS after he stopped putting into his body the drugs he had worked so hard to get approved.

20. In a review of the film in the *Huffington Post*, tellingly entitled "Please, Oscars: Don't Give 'Dallas Buyers Club' Any Awards," Jack Mirkinson dismisses the whole premise of the film, questioning its canonization of Woodroof and its forgetting of LGBT AIDS activists. Mirkinson summarizes the film as about "a homophobic womanizer who, after contracting AIDS thanks to a variety of drug-and-sex-related behavior, is stunned to find that the medicine the US government is pushing is no good for him and goes about setting up a 'buyers club' for drugs from other countries." Mirkinson's point is that the film oversimplifies Woodroof's story, including the fact that many people who knew him said he was bisexual and not homophobic.

21. Rayon is played by Jared Leto, who won an Academy Award for Best Supporting Actor, alongside McConaughey's award for Best Actor. Despite the Academy Award, Leto's performance has been criticized by some LGBT activists. In an article in *Time* magazine, Steven Friess compares Rayon to Mammy in *Gone With the Wind*. "Don't Applaud Jared Leto's Transgender 'Mammy.'" Although Leto claimed he was determined to play Rayon not as a drag queen but as transgender, in one interview clip on the film's official website of Leto discussing Rayon, he uses the male pronoun for Rayon.

22. "AIDS Activism in the Time of Dallas Buyers Club," official website of *Dallas Buyers Club,* http://www.focusfeatures.com/article/aids_activism_in_the_time_of_dallas_buyers_club?film=dallas_buyers_club.

23. Ibid.

Bibliography

Agamben, Giorgio. *Homo Sacer: Sovereign Power and Bare Life.* Translated by Daniel Heller-Roazen. Stanford, Calif.: Stanford University Press, 1998.

———. *Means without Ends: Notes on Politics.* Translated by Vincenzo Binetti and Cesare Casarino. Minneapolis: University of Minnesota Press, 2000.

Ahmed, Sara. *The Cultural Politics of Emotion.* New York: Routledge, 2004.

Alonso, Ana Maria, and Maria Teresa Koreck, "Silences: 'Hispanics,' AIDS, and Sexual Practices." *Differences: A Journal of Feminist Cultural Studies* 1 (Winter 1989): 101–24.

Althusser, Louis. "Ideology and Ideological State Apparatuses." In *Lenin and Philosophy and Other Essays.* Translated by Ben Brewster. New York: Monthly Review Press, 1972.

Altman, Lawrence K. "Rare Cancer Seen in 41 Homosexuals." *New York Times,* July 3, 1981.

Anderson, Carolyn, and Thomas W. Benson. *Documentary Dilemmas: Frederick Wiseman's "Titicut Follies."* Carbondale: Southern Illinois University Press, 1991.

Armstrong, David. "The Emancipation of Biographical Medicine." *Social Science and Medicine* 13A (1979): 1–8.

———. "Space and Time in British General Practice." In *Biomedicine Examined,* edited by Margaret Lock and Deborah Gordon. Dordrecht: Kluwer, 1985.

———. "The Rise of Surveillance Medicine." *Sociology of Health and Illness* 17, no. 3 (1995): 393–404.

B., David. *Epileptic.* Translated by Kim Thompson. New York: Pantheon, 2005.

Balint, Michael. *The Doctor, His Patient and the Illness.* London: Churchill Livingston, 1957.

Barad, Karen. "Shifting Sands of Time: Liquid Time, Solid Memories, and Diffracted Histories." Paper presented at the Society for Science, Literature, and the Arts Conference, Dallas, Tex., October 11, 2014.

Barlow, Tani. *The Question of Women in Chinese Feminism.* Durham, N.C.: Duke University Press, 2004.

Barnes, Mary, and Joseph H. Berke, *Two Accounts of a Journey through Madness.* New York: Other Press, 2002.

Baxandall, Rosalyn, and Linda Gordon, *Dear Sisters: Dispatches from the Women's Liberation Movement.* New York: Basic Books, 2000.

Berger, John. *Ways of Seeing*. 1972. London: Penguin Book, 1990.

Berger, John, and Jean Mohr. *A Fortunate Man: The Story of a Country Doctor*. New York: Pantheon Books, 1967.

———. *A Seventh Man: Migrant Workers in Europe*. New York: Viking, 1975.

———. *Another Way of Telling*. New York: Vintage, 1982.

Berlant, Lauren. "Slow Death (Sovereignty, Obesity, Lateral Agency)." *Critical Inquiry* 33 (Summer 2007): 754–80.

———. *Cruel Optimism*. Durham, N.C.: Duke University Press, 2011.

Bernstein, Jacob. "Surviving AIDS, but Not the Life That Followed." *New York Times*, February 24, 2013.

Bindé, Jérôme. "Toward an Ethics of the Future." *Public Culture* 12, no. 1 (2000).

Bordowitz, Gregg. *The AIDS Crisis Is Ridiculous and Other Writings, 1986–2003*. Cambridge, Mass.: MIT Press, 2004.

Boston Women's Health Book Collective. *Our Bodies, Ourselves*. New York: Simon and Schuster, 1973.

Bourg, Julian. *From Revolution to Ethics: May 1968 and Contemporary French Thought*. Montreal: McGill-Queen's University Press, 2007.

Brennan, Teresa. *Transmission of Affect*. Ithaca, N.Y.: Cornell University Press, 2004.

Brier, Jennifer. "Locating Lesbian and Feminist Responses to AIDS, 1982–1984." *Women's Studies Quarterly* 35, nos. 1–2 (Spring 2007): 234–48.

———. *Infectious Ideas: Political Responses to the AIDS Crisis*. Chapel Hill: University of North Carolina Press, 2009.

Campbell, Carole A. "Male Gender Roles and Sexuality: Implications for Women's AIDS Risk and Prevention." *Social Science and Medicine* 41 (1995): 197–210.

Canguilhem, Georges. *A Vital Rationalist: Selected Writings of Georges Canguilhem*. Edited by Francois Delaporte. Translated by Arthur Goldhammer. New York: Zone Books, 2000.

Carson, Rachel. *The Sea around Us*. 1950. New York: Oxford University Press, 1989.

———. *Silent Spring*. 1962. Boston: Houghton Mifflin, 2002.

Castiglia, Christopher. "Sex Panics, Sex Publics, Sex Memories." *boundary 2* 27, no. 2 (2000): 149–75.

Castiglia, Christopher, and Christopher Reed, *If Memory Serves: Gay Men, AIDS, and the Promise of the Queer Past*. Minneapolis: University of Minnesota Press, 2012.

Chen, Mel. "Racialized Toxins and Sovereign Fantasies." *Discourse* 29, nos. 2–3 (Spring and Fall 2007): 367–83.

———. *Animacies: Biopolitics, Racial Mattering, and Queer Affect*. Durham, N.C.: Duke University Press, 2012.

Cherki, Alice. *Frantz Fanon: A Portrait*. Translated by Nadia Benabid. Ithaca, N.Y.: Cornell University Press, 2006.

Chow, Rey. *The Age of the World Target: Self-Referentiality in War, Theory, and Comparative Work*. Durham, N.C.: Duke University Press, 2006.

Chute, Hillary. "Review of *Our Cancer Year, Janet and Me, Cancer Vixen, Mom's Cancer, Blue Pills, Epileptic,* and *Black Hole.*" *Literature and Medicine* 26, no. 2 (Fall 2007): 413–29.

Cixous, Hélène, and Catherine Clément. *The Newly Born Woman*. Translated by Betsy Wing. Minneapolis: University of Minnesota Press, 1986.

Coburn, Judith. "Off the Pill." In *Dear Sisters: Dispatches from the Women's Liberation Movement,* edited by Rosalyn Baxandall and Linda Gordon. New York: Basic Books, 2000.

Code, Lorraine. *Ecological Thinking: The Politics of Epistemic Location*. New York: Oxford University Press, 2006.

Cohen, Cathy J. "Punks, Bulldaggers, and Welfare Queens: The Radical Potential of Queer Politics." In *Black Queer Studies: A Critical Anthology,* edited by Patrick Johnson and Mae G. Henderson, 21–51. Durham, N.C.: Duke University Press, 2005.

Cohen, Peter F. *Love and Anger: Essays on AIDS, Activism, and Politics*. New York: Haworth Press, 1998.

Collings, Joseph S. "General Practice in England Today: A Reconnaissance." *Lancet* 255, no. 6604 (March 1950): 555–85.

Concerning Violence: Nine Scenes from the Anti-imperialistic Self-Defense. DVD. Directed by Göran Hugo Olsson. Sweden: Kino Lorber, 2014.

Conley, Verena Andermatt. *Ecopolitics: The Environment in Poststructuralist Thought*. New York: Routledge, 1997.

Cooper, David. *Psychiatry and Anti-psychiatry*. London: Tavistock, 1967.

Crimp, Douglas, ed. *AIDS: Cultural Analysis/Cultural Activism*. Cambridge, Mass.: MIT Press, 1988.

Crimp, Douglas, and Adam Rolston. *AIDS Demo Graphics*. Seattle: Bay Press, 1990.

Cvetkovich, Ann. *An Archive of Feelings: Trauma, Sexuality, and Lesbian Public Cultures*. Durham, N.C.: Duke University Press, 2003.

———. *Depression: A Public Feeling*. Durham, N.C.: Duke University Press, 2012.

Czerwiec, MK, et al. *Graphic Medicine Manifesto*. University Park: Pennsylvania State University Press, 2015.

Dallas Buyers Club. DVD. Directed by Jean-Marc Vallée. Universal City, Calif.: Focus Features, 2013.

Dangarembga, Tsitsi. *Nervous Conditions*. Seattle: Seal Press, 1988.

Davis, Flora. *Moving the Mountain: The Women's Movement in America Since 1960*. Urbana: University of Illinois Press, 1999.

Davis, Kathy. *The Making of "Our Bodies, Ourselves": How Feminism Travels across Borders*. Durham, N.C.: Duke University Press, 2007.

Delany, Samuel R. *The Motion of Light in Water: Sex and Science Fiction Writing in the East Village*. Minneapolis: University of Minnesota Press, 2004.

Deleuze, Gilles. "Coldness and Cruelty." In *Masochism*. Translated by Jean McNeil. New York: Zone Books, 1989.

———. *The Fold: Leibniz and the Baroque*. Translated by Tom Conley. Minneapolis: University of Minneapolis Press, 1993.

———. *Negotiations: 1972–1990*. Translated by Martin Joughin. New York: Columbia University Press, 1995.

———. *Essays Critical and Clinical*. Translated by Daniel W. Smith and Michael A. Greco. Minneapolis: University of Minnesota Press, 1997.

———. *Spinoza: Practical Philosophy*. Translated by Robert Hurley. San Francisco: City Lights, 2001.

———. *Desert Islands and Other Texts, 1953–1974*. Edited by David Lapoujade. Translated by Michael Taormina. New York: Semiotext(e), 2004.

———. *Two Regimes of Madness: Texts and Interviews, 1975–1995*. Edited by David Lapoujade. Translated by Ames Hodges and Mike Taormina. New York: Semiotext(e), 2007.

Deleuze, Gilles, and Fèlix Guattari. *Anti-Oedipus: Capitalism and Schizophrenia*. Translated by Robert Hurley, Mark Seem, and Helen R. Lane. Minneapolis: University of Minnesota Press, 1983.

———. *Kafka: Toward a Minor Literature*. Translated by Dana Polan. Minneapolis: University of Minnesota Press, 1986.

———. *A Thousand Plateaus: Capitalism and Schizophrenia*. Translated by Brian Massumi. Minneapolis: University of Minnesota Press, 1987.

———. *What Is Philosophy?* Translated by Hugh Tomlinson and Graham Burchell. New York: Columbia University Press, 1994.

DeVita, Vincent T., Jr., and Edward Chu. "A History of Cancer Chemotherapy." *Cancer Research* 68, no. 21 (November 1, 2008): 8643–53.

Diedrich, Lisa. *Treatments: Language, Politics, and the Culture of Illness*. Minneapolis: University of Minnesota Press, 2007.

———. "Gathering Evidence of Ghosts: W. G. Sebald's Practices of Witnessing." In *Searching for Sebald*, edited by Lise Patt, 256–79. Los Angeles: ICI Press, 2007.

———. "Complexity and Cancer: The Multiple Temporalities and Spaces in Richard Powers' *Gain*." In *Global Science/Women's Health*, edited by Cindy Patton and Helen Loshny, 87–116. Youngtown, N.Y.: Teneo Press, 2008.

———. "Lying and the Performance of Patienthood." In *The Patient*, edited by Harold Schweizer, 131–52. Lewisburg, Penn.: Bucknell University Press, 2010.

———. "Speeding Up Slow Deaths: Medical Sovereignty Circa 2005." *Media Tropes eJournal* 3, no. 1 (2011).

———. "Graphic Analysis: Transitional Phenomena in Alison Bechdel's *Are You My Mother?*" *Configurations* 22 (Fall 2014): 183–203.

Diedrich, Lisa, and Emily Boyce. "'Breast Cancer on Long Island': The Emergence of a New Object through Mapping Practices." *BioSocieties* 2, no. 2 (2007): 193–218.

Disability Law Center. "Report on Investigation of Bridgewater State Hospital." July 11, 2014. http://www.dlc-ma.org/BSHReport.pdf.

Dosse, François. *Gilles Deleuze and Félix Guattari: Intersecting Lives*. Translated by Deborah Glassman. New York: Columbia University Press, 2010.

Dreifus, Claudia. *Seizing Our Bodies: The Politics of Women's Health*. New York: Vintage, 1977.

Dresser, Rebecca. "What Bioethics Can Learn from the Women's Health Movement." In *Feminism and Bioethics: Beyond Reproduction*, edited by Susan M. Wolf, 144–59. New York: Oxford University Press, 1996.

Dreyfus, Hubert, and Paul Rabinow, eds. *Michel Foucault: Beyond Structuralism and Hermeneutics*. Chicago: University of Chicago Press, 1983.

Duberman, Martin. *Hold Tight Gently: Michael Callen, Essex Hemphill, and the Battlefield of AIDS*. New York: New Press, 2014.

DuPlessis, Rachel, and Ann Snitow, eds. *The Feminist Memoir Project: Voices from Women's Liberation*. New York: Three Rivers Press, 1998.

During, Simon. *Foucault and Literature: Towards a Genealogy of Writing*. New York: Routledge, 1992.

Echols, Alice. *Daring to Be Bad: Radical Feminism in America, 1967–1975*. Minneapolis: University of Minnesota Press, 1989.

Egler, Frank E. "Pesticides—In Our Ecosystem." *American Scientist* 52, no. 1 (March 1964): 110–36.

Ehrenreich, Barbara, and Deirdre English. *For Her Own Good: 150 Years of the Experts' Advice to Women*. New York: Anchor, 1978.

Eisner, Will. *Comics and Sequential Art: Principles and Practices from the Legendary Cartoonist*. New York: W. W. Norton, 2008.

Engel, George L. "The Need for a New Medical Model: A Challenge for Biomedicine." *Science* 196 (1977): 129–36.

Epstein, Steven. *Impure Science: AIDS, Activism, and the Politics of Knowledge*. Berkeley: University of California Press, 1996.

Evans, Sara. *Personal Politics: The Roots of Women's Liberation in the Civil Rights Movement and the New Left*. New York: Vintage, 1980.

Faderman, Lillian. *Surpassing the Love of Men: Romantic Friendship and Love between Women from the Renaissance to the Present*. New York: William Morrow, 1981.

Fanon, Frantz. *The Wretched of the Earth*. Translated by Constance Farrington. New York: Grove, 1963.

Farmer, Paul. *Infections and Inequalities: The Modern Plagues*. Berkeley: University of California Press, 1999.

Fassin, Didier. *When Bodies Remember: Experiences and Politics of AIDS in South*

Africa. Translated by Amy Jacobs and Gabrielle Varro. Berkeley: University of California Press, 2007.

Fast Trip, Long Drop. Directed by Gregg Bordowitz. Chicago: Video Data Bank, 1993.

Ferguson, Denzel E. "Review of *Silent Spring* by Rachel Carson." *Copeia* 1963, no. 1 (March 30, 1963): 207–8.

Ferguson, Roderick A. *The Reorder of Things: The University and Its Pedagogies of Minority Difference.* Minnesota: University of Minnesota Press, 2012.

Ferraro, Susan. "The Anguished Politics of Breast Cancer." *New York Times Magazine,* August 15, 1993.

Fortun, Kim. *Advocacy after Bhopal: Environmentalism, Disaster, New Global Orders.* Chicago: University of Chicago Press, 2001.

Foucault, Michel. *Mental Illness and Psychology.* Translated by Alan Sheridan. 1954. Berkeley: University of California Press, 1987.

———. *The History of Madness.* Translated by Jonathan Murphy and Jean Khalfa. 1961. New York: Routledge, 2006.

———. *The Birth of the Clinic: An Archeology of Medical Perception.* Translated by A. M. Sheridan Smith. 1963. New York: Vintage, 1973.

———. *Death and the Labyrinth.* Translated by Charles Ruas. 1963. London: Continuum, 2004.

———. *The Order of Things: An Archaeology of the Human Sciences.* 1966. New York: Vintage, 1970.

———. *The Archaeology of Knowledge and the Discourse on Language.* Translated by A. M. Sheridan Smith. 1969. New York: Pantheon, 1972.

———. *The History of Sexuality.* Vol. 1, *An Introduction.* Translated by Robert Hurley. 1976. New York: Vintage, 1978.

———. *Discipline and Punish: The Birth of the Prison.* Translated by Alan Sheridan. New York: Vintage, 1977.

———. *Language, Counter-memory, Practice: Selected Essays and Interviews.* Edited and translated by Donald F. Bouchard. Ithaca, N.Y.: Cornell University Press, 1977.

———. *Power/Knowledge: Selected Interviews and Other Writings, 1972–1977.* Edited and translated by Colin Gordon. New York: Pantheon Books, 1980.

———. "Of Other Spaces." Translated by Jay Miskowiec. *Diacritics* 16, no. 1 (Spring 1986): 22–27.

———. *Ethics: Subjectivity and Truth.* Vol. 1 of *The Essential Works of Foucault, 1954–1984.* Translated by Robert Hurley and others. New York: New Press, 1997.

———. *Power.* Vol. 3 of *The Essential Works of Foucault, 1954–1984.* Translated by Robert Hurley and others. New York: New Press, 2000.

———. *Psychiatric Power: Lectures at the Collège de France, 1973–1974.* Edited by

Jacques Lagrange. Translated by Graham Burchell. Houndmills, U.K.: Palgrave Macmillan, 2006.

———. *The Government of the Self and Others: Lectures at the Collège de France, 1982–1983.* Edited by Frédéric Gros. Translated by Graham Burchell. Houndmills, U.K.: Palgrave Macmillan, 2010.

———. *Madness: The Invention of an Idea.* Translated by Alan Sheridan. New York: Harper Perennial, 2011.

France, David. "Pictures From a Battlefield." *New York Magazine,* March 25, 2012. http://nymag.com/news/features/act-up-2012-4.

Frankfort, Ellen. *Vaginal Politics.* New York: Bantam Book, 1973.

Frantz Fanon: Black Skin, White Mask. DVD. Directed by Isaac Julien. United Kingdom: Arts Council of England, 1996.

Freccero, Carla. *Queer/Early/Modern.* Durham, N.C.: Duke University Press, 2007.

Freeman, Elizabeth. *Time Binds: Queer Temporalities, Queer Histories.* Durham, N.C.: Duke University Press, 2010.

Friedan, Betty. *The Feminine Mystique.* New York: W. W. Norton, 1963.

Friess, Steven. "Don't Applaud Jared Leto's Transgender 'Mammy.'" *Time,* February 28, 2014. http://time.com/10650/dont-applaud-jared-letos-transgender-mammy/.

Fusco, Coco. "Visualizing Theory: An Interview with Isaac Julien." *Nka: Journal of Contemporary African Art,* nos. 6–7 (Summer/Fall 1997): 54–57.

Fuss, Diana. *Identification Papers.* New York: Routledge, 1995.

Gallop, Jane. *Around 1981: Academic Feminist Literary Theory.* New York: Routledge, 1991.

Gammon, M. D., et al. "The Long Island Breast Cancer Study Project: Description of a Multi-institutional Collaboration to Identify Environmental Risk Factors for Breast Cancer." *Breast Cancer Research and Treatment* 74 (2002): 235–54.

———. "Environmental Toxins and Breast Cancer on Long Island. I. Polycylic Aromatic Hydrocarbon DNA Adducts." *Cancer Epidemiology, Biomarkers, and Prevention* 11 (August 2002): 677–85.

———. "Environmental Toxins and Breast Cancer on Long Island. II. Organochlorine Compound Levels in Blood." *Cancer Epidemiology, Biomarkers, and Prevention* 11 (August 2002): 686–97.

Genosko, Gary. "The Life and Work of Félix Guattari: From Transversality to Ecosophy." In *The Three Ecologies,* by Félix Guattari, 46–78. Translated by Ian Pindar and Paul Sutton. London: Continuum, 2008.

Gentis, Roger. *Traite de psychiatrie provisoire.* Paris: F. Maspero, 1977.

———. *Leçons du corps.* Paris: Flammarion, 1980.

———. *Guérir la vie.* Paris: F. Maspero, 1978.

Gever, Martha, John Greyson, and Pratibha Parmar, eds. *Queer Looks: Perspectives on Lesbian and Gay Film and Video.* New York: Routledge, 1993.

Goffman, Erving. *Asylums: Essays on the Social Situation of Mental Patients and Other Inmates.* New York: Anchor, 1961.

———. *Stigma: Notes on the Management of Spoiled Identity.* New York: Simon and Schuster, 1963.

Gould, Deborah. *Moving Politics: Emotion and ACT UP's Fight against AIDS.* Chicago: University of Chicago Press, 2009.

Grant, Barry Keith. *Five Films by Frederick Wiseman: "Titicut Follies," "High School," "Welfare," "High School II," "Public Housing."* Berkeley: University of California Press, 2006.

Griffin, Fred L. "The Fortunate Physician: Learning from Our Patients." *Literature and Medicine* 23, no. 2 (Fall 2004): 280–303.

Grob, Gerald N. *From Asylum to Community: Mental Health Policy in Modern America.* Princeton, N.J.: Princeton University Press, 1991.

———. "Deinstitutionalization: The Illusion of Policy." *Journal of Policy History* 9 (1997): 48–73.

Guattari, Félix. "David Wojnarowicz." *Rethinking Marxism* 3, no. 1 (Spring 1990).

———. *The Three Ecologies.* Translated by Ian Pindar and Paul Sutton. London and New York: Continuum, 2008.

———. *Chaosophy: Texts and Interviews, 1972–1977.* Edited by Sylvère Lotringer. Translated by David L. Sweet et al. Los Angeles: Semiotext(e), 2009.

———. *The Machinic Unconscious: Essays in Schizoanalysis.* Translated by Taylor Adkins. Los Angeles: Semiotext(e), 2011.

Habit. DVD. Directed by Gregg Bordowitz. Chicago: Video Data Bank, 2001.

Hammonds, Evelyn. "Missing Persons: African American Women, AIDS, and the History of Disease." *Radical America* 24 (1992): 7–23.

Hartsock, Nancy. "The Feminist Standpoint: Developing the Ground for a Specifically Feminist Historical Materialism." In *The Second Wave: A Reader in Feminist Theory,* edited by Linda Nicholson, 216–40. New York: Routledge, 1997.

Healy, Patrick. "A Lion Still Roars, with Gratitude: Larry Kramer Lives to See His 'Normal Heart' Filmed for TV." *New York Times,* May 21, 2014.

Hesford, Victoria. *Feeling Women's Liberation.* Durham, N.C.: Duke University Press, 2013.

Hesford, Victoria, and Lisa Diedrich. "Experience, Echo, Event: Theorizing Feminist Histories, Historicising Feminist Theory." *Feminist Theory* 15, no. 2 (August 2014): 103–17.

———. "On 'The Evidence of Experience' and Its Reverberations: An Interview with Joan W. Scott." *Feminist Theory* 15, no. 2 (August 2014): 197–207.

Hollibaugh, Amber. *My Dangerous Desires: A Queer Girl Dreaming Her Way Home.* Durham, N.C.: Duke University Press, 2000.

Howard, John. *Men Like That: A Southern Queer History.* Chicago: University of Chicago Press, 1999.

Howell, Mary C. "What Medical Schools Teach about Women." *New England Journal of Medicine* 291, no. 6 (August 8, 1974): 304–7.

How to Survive a Plague. DVD. Directed by David France. New York: Public Square Films, 2012.

Hudson, Martyn. "The Clerk of the Foresters Records: John Berger, the Dead, and the Writing of History." *Rethinking History* 4 no. 3 (2000): 261–79.

Huffer, Lynne. *Mad for Foucault: Rethinking the Foundations of Queer Theory.* New York: Columbia University Press, 2010.

Huntley, J. S. "In Search of *A Fortunate Man.*" *Lancet* 357 (2001): 547.

Ingelfinger, Franz J. "Doctor Women." *New England Journal of Medicine* 291, no. 6 (August 8, 1974): 303–4.

Jewson, Nicholas. "The Disappearance of the Sick Man from Medical Cosmology, 1770–1870." *Sociology* 10, no. 2 (1976): 225–44.

Joseph, Miranda. *Against the Romance of Community.* Minneapolis: University of Minnesota Press, 2002.

Julien, Isaac, and Mark Nash. "Fanon as Film." *Nka: Journal of Contemporary African Art,* nos. 11–12 (Fall/Winter, 2000): 12–17.

Kamau, Pius. "Feminists Asleep in AIDS Fight." *Denver Post,* July 21, 2004.

Keller, Richard C. "Clinician and Revolutionary: Frantz Fanon, Biography, and the History of Colonial Medicine." *Bulletin of the History of Medicine* 81, no. 4 (Winter 2007): 823–41.

Kingsland, Sharon. *Modeling Nature: Episodes in the History of Population Ecology.* Chicago: University of Chicago Press, 1995.

Kotulski, Tina. *Saving Millie: A Daughter's Story of Surviving Her Mother's Schizophrenia.* Madelia, Minn.: Extraordinary Voices Press, 2006.

Kramer, Larry. "1,112 and Counting." *New York Native,* March 14–27, 1983.

———. *The American People.* Vol. 1, *Search for My Heart.* New York: Farrar, Straus and Giroux, 2015.

Kuhn, Thomas. *The Structure of Scientific Revolutions.* 50th anniversary ed. Chicago: University of Chicago Press, 2012.

Kushner, Rose. *Why Me? What Every Woman Should Know about Breast Cancer to Save Her Life* (originally titled, *Breast Cancer: A Personal History and Investigative Report*). New York: New American Library, 1975.

Lalonde, Beth. "I Hate *The Normal Heart.*" *StyleCon,* May 29, 2014. http://www.thestylecon.com/2014/05/29/hate-normal-heart/.

Laub, Dori. "An Event without a Witness: Truth, Testimony, and Survival." In *Testimony: Crises of Witnessing in Literature, Psychoanalysis, and History,* edited by Shoshana Felman and Dori Laub, 75–92. New York: Routledge, 1992.

Lear, Linda. *Rachel Carson: Witness for Nature.* New York: Henry Holt, 1997.

Lewis, Bradley. *Moving beyond Prozac, "DSM," and the New Psychiatry: The Birth of Postpsychiatry.* Ann Arbor: University of Michigan Press, 2006.

Lippincott, Robin. "One Big Canvas: The Work of John Berger." *Literary Review* 35, no. 1 (Fall 1991).

Lorde, Audre. *The Cancer Journals*. San Francisco: Aunt Lute, 1980.

Lotringer, Sylvère, and Giancarlo Ambrosino, eds. *David Wojnarowicz: A Definitive History of Five or Six Years on the Lower East Side*. New York: Semiotext(e), 2006.

Love, Heather. "Truth and Consequences: On Paranoid Reading and Reparative Reading." *Criticism* 52, no. 2 (Spring 2010): 235–41.

———. "Diary of a Conference on Sexuality, 1982." Special issue, *GLQ* 17, no. 1 (2011): 49–78.

———. "Queer." *TSQ: Transgender Studies Quarterly* 1–2, no. 1 (2014): 172–76.

Loyd, Jenna. "Where Is Community Health? Racism, the Clinic, and the Biopolitical State." In *Rebirth of the Clinic: Places and Agents in Contemporary Health Care*, edited by Cindy Patton, 39–67. Minneapolis: University of Minnesota Press, 2010.

———. *Health Rights Are Civil Rights: Peace and Justice Activism in Los Angeles, 1963–1978*. Minneapolis: University of Minnesota Press, 2014.

Lutts, Ralph H. "Chemical Fallout: Rachel Carson's *Silent Spring*, Radioactive Fallout, and the Environmental Movement." *Environmental Review: ER* 9, no. 3 (Autumn 1985): 210–25.

Lyotard, Jean-François. *The Differend: Phrases in Dispute*. Translated by Georges Van Den Abbeele. Minneapolis: University of Minneapolis Press, 1988.

Macey, David. *The Lives of Michel Foucault*. New York: Pantheon Books, 1993.

———. *Frantz Fanon: A Biography*. New York: Verso, 2012.

Macherey, Pierre. *The Object of Literature*. Translated by David Macey. Cambridge: Cambridge University Press, 1995.

Mass, Lawrence D. "Interview with a Writer." In *We Must Love One Another or Die: The Life and Legacies of Larry Kramer*. New York: St. Martin's Press, 1997.

Massumi, Brian. "Notes on the Translation and Acknowledgments." In *A Thousand Plateaus: Capitalism and Schizophrenia*, by Gilles Deleuze and Félix Guattari, ix–xv. Minneapolis: University of Minnesota Press, 1987.

McPhee, John. "Heirs of General Practice." *Table of Contents*. New York: Farrar Straus Giroux, 1985.

Metzl, Jonathan. *Prozac on the Couch: Prescribing Gender in the Era of Wonder Drugs*. Durham, N.C.: Duke University Press, 2003.

———. *The Protest Psychosis: How Schizophrenia Became a Black Disease*. Boston: Beacon Press, 2009.

Metzl, Jonathan, and Anna Kirkland, eds. *Against Health: How Health Became the New Morality*. New York: NYU Press, 2010.

Mirkinson, Jack. "Please, Oscars: Don't Give 'Dallas Buyers Club' Any Awards." *Huffington Post*, February 28, 2014. http://www.huffingtonpost.com/jack-mirkinson/dallas-buyers-club-oscars_b_4871217.html.

Mol, Annemarie. *The Body Multiple: Ontology in Medical Practice*. Durham, N.C.: Duke University Press, 2002.

——. *The Logic of Care: Health and the Problem of Patient Choice*. New York: Routledge, 2008.

Morgen, Sandra. *Into Our Own Hands: The Women's Health Movement in the United States, 1969–1990*. New Brunswick, N.J.: Rutgers University Press, 2002.

Morton, Timothy. *The Ecological Thought*. Cambridge, Mass.: Harvard University Press, 2010.

Muñoz, José Esteban. *Cruising Utopia: The Then and There of Queer Futurity*. New York: NYU Press, 2009.

Murphy, Michelle. "Immodest Witnessing: The Epistemology of Vaginal Self-Examination in the U.S. Feminist Self-Help Movement." *Feminist Studies* 30 (2004): 115–47.

——. *Sick Building Syndrome and the Problem of Certainty: Environmental Politics, Technoscience, and Women Workers*. Durham, N.C.: Duke University Press, 2006.

——. *Seizing the Means of Reproduction: Entanglements of Feminism, Health, and Technoscience*. Durham, N.C.: Duke University Press, 2012.

Nelson, Alondra. *Body and Soul: The Black Panther Party and the Fight against Medical Discrimination*. Minneapolis: University of Minnesota Press, 2011.

Nettleton, Sarah. "The Emergence of E-Scaped Medicine?" *Sociology* 38, no. 4 (2004): 661–79.

Nixon, Rob. *Slow Violence and the Environmentalism of the Poor*. Cambridge, Mass.: Harvard University Press, 2011.

——. "Rachel Carson's Prescience." *Chronicle of Higher Education* 59, no. 2 (September 3, 2012). http://find.galegroup.com.

Normal Heart, The. DVD. Directed by Ryan Murphy. New York: Home Box Office, 2014.

Office of Preet Bharara, U.S. Attorney, "Civil Rights of Institutionalized Persons Act (CRIPA) Investigation of the New York City Department of Corrections Jails on Rikers Island." http://www.nytimes.com/interactive/2014/08/05/nyregion/05rikers-report.html.

Omi, Michael, and Howard Winant, *Racial Formations in the United States, from the 1960s to the 1990s*. New York: Routledge, 1994.

Osmond, Marie Withers, K. G. Wambach, Diane Harrison et al. "The Multiple Jeopardy of Race, Class, and Gender for AIDS Risk among Women." *Gender and Society* 7, no. 1 (March 1993): 99–120.

Out of the Shadow. DVD. Directed by Susan Smiley. Los Angeles: Vine Street Pictures, 2004.

Patton, Cindy. *Sex and Germs: The Politic of AIDS*. Boston: South End Press, 1985.

——. "AIDS Industry: Construction of 'Victims,' 'Volunteers' and 'Experts.'" In

Taking Liberties: AIDS and Cultural Politics, edited by Erica Carter and Simon Watney, 113–25. London: Serpent's Tail, 1989.

———. *Inventing AIDS.* New York: 1990.

———. *Last Served? Gendering the AIDS Pandemic.* London: Taylor and Francis, 1994.

———. *Globalizing AIDS.* Minneapolis: University of Minnesota Press, 2002.

Patton, Cindy, ed. *Rebirth of the Clinic: Places and Agents in Contemporary Health Care.* Minneapolis: University of Minnesota Press, 2010.

Petchey, Roland. "Collings Report on General Practice in England in 1950: Unrecognised, Pioneering Piece of British Social Research?" *BMJ* 311 (July 1995): 40–42.

Petryna, Adriana. *Life Exposed: Biological Citizenship after Chernobyl.* Princeton, N.J.: Princeton University Press, 2002.

Pisacano, Nicholas J. "History of the Specialty." American Board of Family Practice website. www.theabfm.org/about/history.aspx.

Povinelli, Elizabeth A. *Events of Abandonment: Social Belonging and Endurance in Late Liberalism.* Durham, N.C.: Duke University Press, 2011.

Preston, John, and Glenn Swann. *Safe Sex: The Ultimate Erotic Guide.* New York: New American Library, 1986.

Race, Kane. *Pleasure Consuming Medicine: The Queer Politics of Drugs.* Durham, N.C.: Duke University Press, 2009.

Rees, Geoffrey. "The Clinic and the Tearoom." *Journal of Medical Humanities* 34, no. 2 (June 2013): 109–21.

Riley, Denise. *Am I That Name? Feminism and the Category of Women in History.* Minneapolis: University of Minnesota Press, 1988.

Rizk, Mysoon. "Looking at 'Animals in Pants': The Case of David Wojnarowicz." *Topia: Canadian Journal of Cultural Studies* 21 (Spring 2009): 137–59.

Rodenbeck, Judith. "Madness and Method: Before Theatricality." *Gray Room* 13 (Fall 2003): 54–79.

Román, David. *Acts of Intervention: Performance, Gay Culture, and AIDS.* Bloomington: Indiana University Press, 1998.

———. "Not-about-AIDS." *GLQ: A Journal of Lesbian and Gay Studies* 6, no. 1 (2000): 1–28.

Rose, Nikolas. *The Politics of Life Itself: Biomedicine, Power, and Subjectivity in the Twenty-First Century.* Princeton, N.J.: Princeton University Press, 2006.

Rosen, Ruth. *The World Split Open: How the Modern Women's Movement Changed America.* New York: Penguin, 2000.

Rosman, N. Paul. "Review of *Epilepsy: A Clinical Textbook.*" *New England Journal of Medicine* 280, no. 17 (April 24, 1969): 966–67.

Ross, Kristin. *May '68 and Its Afterlives.* Chicago: University of Chicago Press, 2002.

Rotello, Gabriel. *Sexual Ecology: AIDS and the Destiny of Gay Men*. New York: Dutton, 1997.

Ruzek, Sheryl Burt. *The Women's Health Movement: Feminist Alternatives to Medical Control*. New York: Praeger, 1978.

Ryan, Hugh. "How to Whitewash a Plague." *New York Times*, August 3, 2013.

Schneider, Beth E., and Nancy E. Stoller, eds., *Women Resisting AIDS: Feminist Strategies of Empowerment*. Philadelphia: Temple University Press, 1995.

Schulman, Sarah. *People in Trouble*. New York: Dutton, 1990.

———. *My American History: Lesbian and Gay Life during the Reagan/Bush Years*. New York: Routledge, 1994.

———. *The Gentrification of the Mind: Witness to a Lost Imagination*. Berkeley: University of California Press, 2012.

Scott, Joan W. "The Evidence of Experience." *Critical Inquiry* 17, no. 4 (Summer 1991): 773–97.

———. "Fantasy Echo: History and the Construction of Identity." *Critical Inquiry* 27, no. 2 (Winter 2001): 284–304.

———. "Feminist Reverberations." *differences: A Journal of Feminist Cultural Studies* 13, no. 3 (2002): 1–23.

———. *The Fantasy of Feminist History*. Durham, N.C.: Duke University Press, 2011.

Seaman, Barbara. *The Doctors' Case against the Pill*. New York: Peter H. Wyden, 1969.

Sedgwick, Eve Kosofsky. *Tendencies*. Durham, N.C.: Duke University Press, 1993.

———. *Touching Feeling: Affect, Pedagogy, Performativity*. Durham, N.C.: Duke University Press, 2003.

Signorile, Michelangelo. "641,086 and Counting." *Out*, September 1998.

Slater, Lauren. *Lying: A Metaphorical Memoir*. New York: Random House, 2000.

Smith, Michael. "'Silence, Miss Carson!' Science, Gender, and the Reception of *Silent Spring*." In *Rachel Carson: Legacy and Challenge*, edited by Lisa H. Sideris and Kathleen Dean Moore, 136–48. Albany: State University of New York Press, 2008.

Smith, Raymond A., and Patricia D. Siplon's *Drugs into Bodies: Global AIDS Treatment Activism*. Westport, Conn.: Praeger, 2006.

Sontag, Susan. *Illness as Metaphor*. New York: Farrar, Straus and Giroux, 1978.

———. *AIDS and Its Metaphors*. New York: Farrar, Straus and Giroux, 1989.

Spiro, Howard M. "Myths and Mirths: Women in Medicine." *New England Journal of Medicine* 292, no. 7 (February 13, 1975): 354–56.

Spivak, Gayatri Chakravorty. *Outside in the Teaching Machine*. New York: Routledge, 1993.

———. "Can the Subaltern Speak?" In *Colonial Discourse and Post-colonial Theory: A Reader*, edited by Patrick Williams and Laura Chrisman, 66–111. New York: Columbia University Press, 1994.

Staiger, Janet, Ann Cvetkovich, and Ann Reynolds, eds. *Political Emotions.* New York: Routledge, 2010.

Steedman, Carolyn Kay. *Landscape for a Good Woman: A Story of Two Lives.* New Brunswick, N.J.: Rutgers University Press, 1986.

Steingraber, Sandra. "The Fracking of Rachel Carson." *Orion,* September/October 2012. http://www.orionmagazine.org/index.php/articles/article/7005.

Stewart, Kathleen. *Ordinary Affects.* Durham, N.C.: Duke University Press, 2007.

Stewart, Susan. "A Mother in Shades of Gray, Love, Schizophrenia and All." *New York Times,* October 7, 2006.

Stoler, Ann Laura. *Race and the Education of Desire: Foucault's "History of Sexuality" and the Colonial Order of Things.* Durham, N.C.: Duke University Press, 1995.

Stoll, Mark. "Rachel Carson's *Silent Spring,* a Book That Changed the World." Environment and Society Portal. 2012. http://www.environmentandsociety.org/exhibitions/silent-spring/personal-attacks-rachel-carson.

Swartz, Marvin. Foreword to *Saving Millie: A Daughter's Story of Surviving Her Mother's Schizophrenia,* by Tina Kotulski. Madelia, Minn.: Extraordinary Voices Press, 2006.

Tadiar, Neferti. *Things Fall Away: Philippine Historical Experience and the Making of Globalization.* Durham, N.C.: Duke University Press, 2009.

Thomas, Lewis. *The Lives of a Cell: Notes of a Biology Watcher.* New York: Penguin, 1974.

———. *The Medusa and the Snail: More Notes of a Biology Watcher.* New York: Penguin Books, 1979.

———. *The Youngest Science: Notes of a Medicine Watcher.* New York: Viking, 1983.

Thompson, Daniel Q. "Review of *Silent Spring* by Rachel Carson." *Wilson Bulletin* 75, no. 1 (March 1963): 106–7.

Tierney, John. "Fateful Voice of a Generation Still Drowns Out Real Science." *New York Times,* June 5, 2007.

Titicut Follies. DVD. Directed by Frederick Wiseman. United States: Zipporah Films, 1967.

Torrey, E. Fuller. *Nowhere to Go: The Tragic Odyssey of the Homeless Mentally Ill.* New York: Harper and Row, 1988.

———. *Out of the Shadows: Confronting America's Mental Illness Crisis.* New York: John Wiley and Sons, 1997.

Trouillot, Michel-Rolph. *Silencing the Past: Power and the Production of History.* Boston: Beacon Press, 1995.

United in Anger: A History of ACT UP. DVD. Directed by Jim Hubbard. Los Angeles: Film Collaborative, 2012.

Vance, Carole, ed. *Pleasure and Danger: Exploring Female Sexuality.* New York: Routledge/Kegan Paul, 1984.

Viego, Antonio. *Dead Subjects: Towards a Politics of Loss in Latino Studies.* Durham, N.C.: Duke University Press, 2007.

Voelcker, John. "The Death of Activist Spencer Cox: Wounded AIDS Warriors Suffering, Dying on Their Own." *Huffington Post,* January 7, 2013.

Wachter, Robert M. "AIDS, Activism, and the Politics of Health." *New England Journal of Medicine* 326, no. 2 (January 9, 1992): 128–33.

Wells, Susan. *"Our Bodies, Ourselves" and the Work of Writing.* Stanford, Calif.: Stanford University Press, 2010.

Went, Frits. "Review of *Silent Spring.*" *American Institute of Biological Science Bulletin* 13 (February 1963): 42.

Wiegman, Robyn. "The Times We're In: Queer Feminist Criticism and the 'Reparative Turn.'" *Feminist Theory* 15, no. 4 (2014): 4–25.

Williams, Raymond. *Culture and Society, 1780–1950.* New York: Columbia University Press, 1958.

———. *Keywords: A Vocabulary of Culture and Nature.* New York: Oxford University Press, 1983.

———. *Marxism and Literature.* London: Oxford University Press, 1977.

Wojnarowicz, David. *In the Shadow of the American Dream: The Diaries of David Wojnarowicz.* Edited by Amy Scholder. New York: Grove Press, 1999.

Wolfe, Maxine. "The Mother of Us All." In *We Must Love One Another or Die: The Life and Legacies of Larry Kramer,* edited by Lawrence D. Mass, 282–86. New York: St. Martin's Press, 1997.

Woolf, Virginia. *Three Guineas.* 1938. San Diego: Harcourt Brace Jovanovich, 1966.

Index

ACT UP (AIDS Coalition to Unleash Power), 1, 6, 7, 8, 29–30, 49–51, 201, 204–11, 222–23n17, 223n20, 256n10, 257n15; "Drugs into Bodies," 16, 34, 188, 200–215, 256n10, 257n19; mission statements, 221n2; Oral History Project, 26, 33, 36–39, 41; origin story of AIDS activism, 7, 9, 12, 20, 25–28, 53, 202, 204; "Seize Control of the FDA" demonstration, 33, 34–35; sexual relationships in, 38–39, 40; Silence = Death, 256n8; Treatment and Data Committee, 202, 206, 209, 257n15; video collectives, 205, 231n16. See also DIVA TV; Testing the Limits

affect, 7, 22, 27, 28, 31, 33, 38, 39, 40, 49, 50, 55, 63, 150, 154, 180, 184; negative, 135; transmission of, 63, 69, 234n38, 251n29

affective/effective: communities, 32, 36, 37, 39; histories, 28, 37, 38, 40, 80, 232n1; responses, 80; strategies, 41

afterimage, 199–201

Agamben, Giorgio, 4, 77, 233n33

agency, 20, 120, 159, 174, 241n58

Ahmed, Sara, 223n21, 234n38

AIDS, 1–2, 4–6, 16, 17–43, 49, 50–51, 53–57, 66, 71, 77, 87, 110–11, 115, 129, 131, 141, 159, 164, 175, 199–215, 223n21; in Africa, 17–18, 19, 41–43, 71; Buddy program, 26, 202; de-

mentia, 168; discrimination and, 215; false stories of, 36, 39; global conference, in Montreal, 209; global conference, in Thailand, 17, 19; origin story of activism, 7, 9, 12, 20, 25–28, 53, 200–201, 202; rumors about virus's origins, 71; science of, 206, 209–10; theories of causation, 203, 224–25n32, 256–57n13. See also ACT UP; prehistory: of AIDS

Algerian war of liberation, 9–10, 11, 14–15, 66, 133–39, 179

alternative medicine, 148–49, 155, 187, 202, 246n34

Althusser, Louis, 240n39

Altman, Lawrence K., 227n27

Andrews, Bob, 26

antinuclear movement, 225n32

antipsychiatry movement, 13, 70, 149, 150–51, 180; as heteronormative, 70; as paranoid critique, 72

anxiety, 99, 115, 135, 137, 138, 150; of identification, 13

archeological method, 5, 79, 83, 93, 98, 174

archive, 80, 139; activism, 2; of feelings, 41; undoing the colonial, 136

Armstrong, David, 86–87, 95, 239n35

art, 1, 9, 14, 28, 41, 45, 46, 47, 67, 76, 77, 78, 107, 111, 112, 154, 204, 257n18; practices, 16, 39; therapy, 151–52

articulation, 75–76

103, 213–14, 233n30, 234n44; clinics, 58, 61–64, 65, 69; criticism of, 64–65; and transmission of affect, 63, 64

Self Help Clinic (Price), 63–64

Self-Help Manual for Women (Marshall, Vogel, and Bogas), 61–62

sexism, 59–60, 244n8, 256n10. *See also* heterosexism

Sex Series (Wojnarowicz), 74, 76–77, 78

sexual abuse, 167

sexuality, 4, 19, 20, 23, 24, 29, 39, 47, 48, 50, 54, 64, 76–77, 78, 108, 110, 111, 148, 186, 207, 214–15, 225n32, 226n10, 228n50, 234n39, 238n21, 242n4, 249n4, 257n20; illness and, 5, 14, 22–23, 25, 108, 112, 201

sexual politics, 5, 19, 54, 55, 110–11

sex wars, 25, 29

shadow, 51, 77, 163, 179, 186, 189–90, 191, 192, 193, 253n11; being the, 194; concept of, 176–77

shame, 23, 30–31, 135, 176, 193, 223n21, 228n60, 254n19

sick building syndrome, 122, 245–46n28

Signorile, Michelangelo, 226n2

slow death, 120, 221n5

slow violence, 118, 120–21, 221n5

Smith, Daniel W., 222n16

Smith, Michael, 244n8

snapshot, 12, 13, 14, 15, 45, 78, 108, 136, 139, 156, 169, 177, 194, 195; concept of, 12; function like gestures, 77; of a snapshot, 134, 179; term in Bordowitz, 45, 46

social movements, 5, 6, 10, 11, 13, 14, 25, 27, 30, 39, 48, 53, 55, 77, 78, 110, 114, 119, 149, 151, 222–23n17, 225n32, 225n38, 226n11

Sonnabend, Joseph, 202–3, 256n13

Sontag, Susan, 7, 232n12

spatiality, 11, 12, 89, 95, 109, 111, 115, 119, 123, 141, 142, 151, 156, 168, 169, 204, 207, 242n60; of witnessing, 177

specialization, 11, 14, 61, 80, 84, 85, 86, 95, 98, 113, 119, 126, 145, 239n33. *See also* generalism

Spinoza, Baruch, 127, 243n4

Spiro, Howard M., 58, 60

Spivak, Gayatri Chakravorty, 8, 17, 18, 223n26, 226n7

split dioptre, 136

Squier, Susan, 248n1

Staley, Peter, 49, 205–6, 209, 211, 214; on *Crossfire,* 207–8

Steedman, Carolyn Kay, 240n38

Stein, Gertrude, 46–47

Steingraber, Sandra, 243n3

Stewart, Kathleen, 222n9

stigma, 23, 53, 146, 152–53, 154, 155, 176, 193, 215, 231n4, 249n12, 250–51n27, 254n19

Stoler, Ann Laura, 241n44

Stoll, Mark, 244n9

Stonewall Riots, 27, 54

structural: analysis, 19, 55, 64, 175–76, 185, 193, 201; complexity, 46; inequality, 42, 59, 201; response, 61, 86, 187

structural violence, 104, 188–89, 193, 241n58, 257n13

structures of feeling, 47, 48, 49, 50, 230–31n11, 240n38. *See also* "queer structures of feeling"

subjectivity, 11, 16, 23–24, 69–70, 81, 84, 89, 99, 108, 111, 112, 119, 177, 190, 205, 233n30, 240n39. *See also* desubjectification

superorganism, 129

surveillance, 153, 238n24

survivor's guilt, 159, 211, 222n8

LISA DIEDRICH is associate professor of women's, gender, and sexuality studies at Stony Brook University. She is the author of *Treatments: Language, Politics, and the Culture of Illness* (Minnesota, 2007) and coeditor with Victoria Hesford of *Feminist Time against Nation Time: Gender, Politics, and the Nation-State in an Age of Permanent War.*